Dedication

This is dedicated to my precious mother,
Alma Christine Buck
for her unconditional love and support.
I will paint her beautiful face and sweet smile
when we meet again in heaven.

To Marilyn,
never, never give up
and follow your dreams!
God Bless you,
Linda Weatherspoon

Can I Paint in Heaven?

Linda Baumann Weatherspoon's Story of Survival and Victory

by the
Weatherspoon Family

Pp
PROSEPRESS
www.prosepress.biz

Can I Paint in Heaven ?
Copyright © 2014
by The Weatherspoon Family

Comments: jwxspoon@gmail.com

Find Linda Baumann Weatherspoon at
www.lindaweatherspoon

ISBN: 978-1-941069-13-4

Prose Press
Pawleys Island, SC   29585
proseNcons@live.com

Preface

This is a true story about my near-death experience due to a brain aneurysm and stroke that damaged or destroyed thirty percent of the left hemisphere of my brain. After weeks in a coma, the grim prognosis was that death was expected and survival meant living in a chronic vegetative state. By God's Grace, I survived and recovered.

The purpose of writing my story is to share my experience and hope with others who are facing similar situations. A stroke is a life-changing event. It has a traumatic effect on the survivor that lasts a lifetime. Victims live with the knowledge that death by stroke is a ticking time bomb. We learn to live with it one day at a time.

Sharing my strength and the details of my road to recovery may help others keep hope alive that significant restoration of brain function is possible. Hopefully, my strenuous efforts to learn, store, and retrieve information will inspire other survivors to seek daily progress. Starting at ground zero, I dedicated eight hours of my daily routine to improve my brain and continue my recovery to this day.

A catastrophic illness has major consequences for the family and closest friends of the victim. My family suffered tremendous emotional, physical, and financial pain. Their lives have been forever altered. Sharing their stories may help other families to realize they are not alone in their struggles. Their survival strategies, feelings, and fears may be a source of strength and comfort to others.

My ultimate purpose is to encourage individuals to be proactive in their health care and relentless in their pursuit of answers to their health concerns. The health care system failed in my case. In all likelihood, my stroke could have been prevented with a referral to the proper specialists after diagnostics identified the underlying causes. That failure placed me on a collision course.

The final chapter, my personal life story, was written first. My remote memory is more intact. Revisiting my personal history allowed me to gain perspective on the values and lessons learned about myself. Putting my life's lessons in order has been tremendously therapeutic and gave me new confidence.

The events in our lives happen in
a sequence in time,
but in their significance to our selves,
they find their own order...
the continuous thread of revelation."
– Eudora Welty

"Painting is another way of keeping a diary."
–Pablo Picasso

Acknowledgements

I survived a traumatic brain injury in 2007. Despite significant recovery of cognition and speech, writing my story in a cogent manner would have been impossible without the help of others. First, I want to thank my editor, Peggy Weatherspoon, for her support and commitment to this undertaking. Due to my aphasia, this was a time-consuming labor of love for her. I also want to thank author Carrie Penner of Southern California for her thoughtful guidance and outlining the table of contents. I especially want to thank her for suggesting the title Can I Paint in Heaven? after reading my very first draft.

Special acknowledgments go to my family members who shared their devastation and coping strategies. Thank you to my son, Larry; my daughter, Elena; my sister, Gail; and my husband, Jeff, for their willingness to relive and write about the worst experience of their lives.

I am grateful to my dearest friends, former colleagues, and extended family for their encouragement, suggestions, and support throughout this project, notably among them my lifelong friend Linda Roney. Finally, I thank my dear and wonderful husband who is always there for me. Thank you, Jeff, for your patience, tolerance, and love.

Linda Weatherspoon

Table of Contents

The Event
Jeff Weatherspoon

The week of spring break 2007 was a busy one. The girls were out of school and underfoot all the time. Linda was visiting her dad in Ripley, Tennessee, a trip she had both dreaded and anticipated for quite a while. She dreaded the trip because she feared flying worse than anyone I have ever met, but was looking forward to the time with her dad in his new Tennessee home.

Linda had lost her mom to a five- year battle with cancer the previous October and the loss was still fresh in her mind. With her dad fighting cancer as well, Linda felt she couldn't afford to wait on the visit. Linda was in her second year as a high school art teacher for Horry County Schools. Teaching was something she loved but the schedule was difficult; spring break would be her first real chance to get out to Tennessee.

Linda had been seeing a doctor for recurring high blood pressure problems. Her doctor would prescribe medicine to treat her and the blood pressure numbers would come down, but it wouldn't be long before they began creeping up again. It became a cycle over a year or so with the doctor constantly increasing, changing, or adding medication. It was something we were aware of but weren't terribly concerned about. We felt that Linda's doctor would eventually hit upon the correct combination of meds that would take care of the problem.

Linda had also been having headaches for two to three weeks prior to spring break '07. Headaches were rare for Linda and it was odd to see her reaching for the ibuprofen from time to time. I've had migraines for twenty years or so, ever since a minor skull fracture in a restaurant parking lot fight while in the Army, but in 17 years of marriage I could only recall Linda having had a serious headache once or twice.

I attributed the headaches to Linda dealing with our oldest daughter, Christina. At 15, Christina was a real handful. She seemed to thrive on confrontation and pushed us up to the edge of control. We had seen behavior and grade problems with Christina since middle school. Lying and sneaky behavior had evolved over a couple of years into blatant verbal disrespect and petty theft around the house. After a neighbor advised me that he had seen Christina locked in an embrace with a boy on the school bus, Linda and I made the decision to pull her out of the local high school and have her attend school at North Myrtle Beach High School where Linda taught.

At first that seemed to work, but soon Christina began to be disrespectful with Linda and, on occasion, me. I decided to allow Christina to get a job at the local McDonald's, hoping that the hard work in a minimum wage job would motivate her more to focus on school. Unfortunately, she quickly found a new boyfriend who worked there and her behavior didn't improve. As her relationship deteriorated with Linda she became more disrespectful and had confrontations with other teachers at Linda's school. Christina even ran away overnight. This was disappointing to us because we didn't want Christina's misbehavior to affect Linda's job and we felt the behavior was approaching this point. It was so frustrating because Christina was beautiful, smart, and had a great personality. She could influence and manipulate people easily and never thought to use her gifts to do well in school or help out around the house. It was very frustrating, and certainly more than a good cause for a headache.

Luckily, our two younger daughters were the other end of the spectrum. Carmelita and Elena were great students, helpful, respectful, and a real joy to have around the home. Carmelita was just turning 11 and Elena was 9.

As for me, my mortgage business was chugging along and paying all the bills. I was busy going to college full time to finish the prerequisites for school at the Medical University of South Carolina, where I would be taking course in their master's program to become a physician assistant. The PA program at MUSC didn't require a four-year degree, just a specific recipe of roughly 115 semester hours of courses, which I was finally close to completing.

Linda's return from Tennessee was a relief for all of us. Wearing the dad hat, the cook hat; handling basic housekeeping, and also going to school full time and working full time was a real drain, even if Linda was only gone for a few days. When she came back from her flight, Linda looked terrible. She had a headache and seemed exhausted. One of the things I have always loved about Linda is that she is always the same person, very predictable. Steady and solid as a rock, with an unbelievable work ethic and an inner drive that would rival even the most dedicated in any profession. Now she seemed absent-minded, irritable, and sick of dealing with a headache.

Linda told me her dad was living way out in the country, over an hour's drive from the nearest metropolitan area through difficult mountain roads. She couldn't understand why, with her dad's medical problems, he would subject himself to the long drive necessary to reach his medical appointments. Even worse, if something happened to him while he was at home it could take hours to get him proper medical care.

Linda told me that driving the rental car down the unfamiliar roads back to the airport was really a challenge for her. Even at the best of times Linda can be directionally challenged while driving, but when describing this drive she shook her head and said, "I really don't know how I found the airport. I don't even remember the drive."

She followed up by telling me she had a headache and that the flights had been difficult. She felt she might be getting sick. I told her that a good meal, being at home and around the kids, and a good night's sleep would help her a lot. This was April 4th, 2007. Linda's blood pressure was very elevated and I was concerned enough to call her doctor's office and ask for a change in her medicine. I spoke to the nurse and received a call back to double Linda's dose of Clonidine, one of her BP medications. I was told to watch her carefully because that increase could have some minor side effects; not to let her drive, etc.

Thursday was a busy day. Linda slept in uncharacteristically long and I was up and in the office working. I tried to get my mortgage stuff done in the mornings so that I could be prepared for any school classes in the afternoon. That day my only class was an Anatomy & Physiology lab, basically two to three hours in a science classroom doing whatever related experiments were required. Usually the labs went quickly because after some initial instruction one could work at his own pace. I'd need to leave the house at 3:30 pm or so to get into the lab.

The morning work was mostly some phone calls, emailing, and light paperwork. Periodically I went upstairs to see what the family was doing. I noticed Linda sort of absently moving around the house. She looked pale and stressed out. When I asked her how she was feeling I had to repeat myself a couple of times. She told me she felt light-headed and still had the nagging headache from the day before. An hour or so later I came up and she was standing in the kitchen area. I said something funny to her I had seen on the Internet and she watched me intently and sort of shook her head. I repeated the story and finally she said, "I'm sorry I'm just not getting it, probably because I'm not feeling well. I'm having a hard time concentrating today."

I told Linda she should probably go take a nap and as usual she shook her head. Getting Linda to rest and relax is like getting a kid to the dentist. She said she had a lot to do to prepare for what she would be teaching when spring break ended and classes began the following week, but she just didn't feel up to it. She told me she would probably work on her sculpture for a few minutes.

Linda was often doing different types of art around the house. Since the school had purchased a kiln and pottery wheel Linda was able to do some clay sculpture, which she absolutely loved. She was actually working on a 12-inch tall version of the Geico Insurance gecko. A few minutes later she moved downstairs to where she had her sculpture area set up on a table.

Just before lunchtime I talked with Rick, a good friend of mine who periodically fed me loans through his investment and annuity business. Rick wanted to bring me by some paperwork for one of his clients. He mentioned he and his girlfriend might drop by soon. I told him he was welcome any time before I went to my class at 3:30. I also mentioned that Linda might seem a little distracted or dazed and that it was because we had doubled one of her medications and she was feeling some side effects.

Around lunchtime Rick and his girlfriend Marilyn did come by. They came through the area where Linda was doing her gecko sculpture. Rick teased Linda about the sculpture and she smiled but didn't say much. Rick was only there a few minutes and then he and Marilyn

4

headed off to grab some lunch.

At one point around lunchtime I came out of my office and Linda was just sitting there at the table, holding her head in her hand.

"Headache still there?" I asked. She nodded and said, "Worst I have ever had."

I suggested that she go lay down for a bit and she nodded, "I think you're right. But don't let me sleep too long."

I didn't know how long too long was but I intended to let her sleep as long as she could. She went upstairs slowly to our bedroom to lie down.

The girls were busy enjoying their last days of spring break. Carmelita had a friend over, Ashlyn, who was planning to spend the night. Elena was in and out of the house playing with some of the neighborhood kids. Christina, as usual, was in her room with the door closed and locked.

As time went by I got my anatomy book and my lab book and other school materials together. I felt uncomfortable leaving Linda when she was feeling so bad. What if her reaction to the Clonidine intensified and I wasn't here? I delayed leaving for the lab until it was almost certain that I would be late. Then I waited some more until I KNEW I was already late ... but still I couldn't leave the house.

I heard Linda's voice upstairs and went to the base of the stairs. Linda was standing on the stairs about two steps down from the top, one hand on the stair rail and the other on her forehead. She seemed to be in tremendous pain. I asked her if she was okay and she looked up at me and said, "Honey, I need the appointment."

I said, "Appointment? We don't have an appointment today."

"I need the appointment," she repeated, "I need ____." She began to say it over and over, substituting different words that made no sense. I realized weeks later she was asking for ibuprofen.

Linda began to get angry that I didn't understand what she was saying. After trying to talk with her for a minute or so I realized the smart thing would be to take her to the doctor's office. I asked her to go get her shoes on and her purse, but she didn't seem to understand me, still mumbling nonsensically. I took her by the hand and she roughly pulled away, cursing, upset that I wouldn't help her. I was speaking sternly to her, telling her "Linda, get your shoes on, let's go please."

I was dimly aware of the kids coming in and out, hearing our conversation. Linda switched and asked one of the girls the same questions, I think it was Carmelita. Unable to understand her mom, Carmelita looked puzzled and a little scared. Linda was obviously very agitated and upset.

"Screw it," I said, "I'm not going to keep fighting you." I went and got the house phone. I dialed 911 and asked for an ambulance. In the background Linda very upset, "GODAMMIT I need ____!" over and over. I tried to talk to her in a calm voice, letting her know she was scaring the girls, to just sit down and calm down, the ambulance was coming and they would help, etc. Tears were streaming down Linda's face, and probably a few on mine as well.

The ambulance came in 10 minutes or so, speeding past the house. I was pretty stressed and was out on the front porch watching for them; I cursed until they saw me waving and came over. The first paramedic was a tall white guy in his twenties; he bounded up the stairs and I quickly explained what was going on with Linda. I told him I thought she was having a severe reaction to her blood pressure medication. He went in and spoke with Linda and then said, "She needs to go, help me get her down the stairs."

We walked beside Linda as she went down the stairs. She had one or both of her hands on her head at all times; at this point she was reduced to saying "Oh God … oh" repeatedly. I knew that we were closer to Waccamaw Regional Hospital but I also knew that Grand Strand Regional was bigger and had more facilities. Also, Linda's doctor's office was near Grand Strand. I told the paramedics to take her to Grand Strand and that I would be right there as soon as I could.

As they put Linda into the ambulance and strapped her down and prepared to leave, I went inside. All the girls were in the living room sitting on the couch, looking scared. Carmelita's friend Ashlyn was there with them as well.

"Your mom is going to be fine," I told them, "I think she's having a reaction to some new medicine. I just want to be safe so I'm going to go meet the ambulance at the hospital." I told the girls that unfortunately Ashlyn could not sleep over tonight due to what was going on, and that her mom needed to come and get her. All the girls nodded somberly. Christina was as concerned as the younger girls. I told Christina to keep an eye on them and that I would call her as soon as I knew something.

I got into our Toyota Corolla as soon as possible and headed up toward the hospital. I called her doctor's office while I was driving and spoke to the receptionist, asking her to have the doctor give me a call and that I was following an ambulance to the hospital. The doctor quickly called me and I explained the symptoms. He was very calming and said "Jeff I am sure this is a reaction to the Clonidine. You're doing the right thing by having her taken to the emergency room, but I really feel like the increase in dosage of the Clonidine is causing her problems."

I thanked him for calling back and hung up. At this point I really wasn't too concerned. I felt concern for Linda but never in my wildest dreams did I suspect she had ruptured an aneurysm and was currently having a stroke. When I got to the hospital I identified myself and filled out some basic information, insurance, etc. An ER doctor came out and told me they were having a quick CT scan done on Linda's brain to determine if there was any bleeding.

I sat for a few minutes. I can't remember if I called Gail or Carol, two of Linda's sisters; I think it was Gail that I called. I told her that Linda was in the emergency room and that we weren't sure what had happened. I asked Gail to let the other sisters know what was going on. Gail told me they would be on their way down to Myrtle Beach as soon as possible from their homes in Fayetteville, N.C. I told her that I would call her with any updates.

Soon there was an update; a doctor came out and told me that Linda's CT scan indicated there was bleeding in the brain. He told me that Grand Strand was not equipped to deal with brain injuries and that they would be transporting Linda to either McLeod Hospital in Florence, S.C., or MUSC in Charleston as soon as they had confirmation of available space. I asked how they would transport her; the doctor told me it would be by helicopter.

I was absolutely stunned. I had never considered the possibility of a stroke, a ruptured aneurysm, or any major brain injury. How could I? Linda was healthy; she exercised regularly, controlled her diet, didn't smoke or do drugs, drank only occasionally. How was this possible?

A nurse led me into the secured patient area and I was brought into a dark room where Linda was lying on a bed. The nurse told me they could not give her any additional medication because of the brain injury. Linda was in tremendous pain. I tried to console her and hold her hand but it was unbearable for me to see her so uncomfortable. I stood at the door of the room, watching the bustling emergency room and trying to control my increasing frustration. I knew it wasn't true, but it seemed as if Linda had been put into a dark room and forgotten about.

In a few minutes a nurse came in and told me that they had gotten confirmation that space was available at MUSC. The medical helicopter would be taking off from Charleston soon and heading to Myrtle Beach to pick Linda up. There was one other patient who was also going to be transported with Linda. The nurse told me that Linda had to be intubated for the flight. She asked me if I wanted to remain in the room while they inserted the tubes. I absolutely did NOT want to be in the room as I have seen people intubated and knew the amount of discomfort Linda might go through in addition to what she was going through already. I told Linda I loved her and that I would see her soon. I couldn't tell if she could hear me or not, the pain and pressure in her head was so great that she was semi-conscious at this point.

I went back out into the lobby and called Gail and told her that her sister was being flown to MUSC. Gail and Carol were en route to Myrtle Beach and Roxanne was preparing to head down as well with her husband Arthur. We agreed that I would meet Gail and Carol at our home in Surfside Beach.

I waited at Grand Strand Hospital until the helicopter had arrived and I knew Linda was headed to MUSC. Then I got into the Corolla and drove home. My mind was a blur. Somewhere along the line I called my stepson Larry and told him what I knew. Larry was a regional manager for a restaurant chain in Florida. Ever practical and efficient, Larry said simply that he would be there as fast as possible, and that he would meet me in Charleston at MUSC. I knew that he would do whatever it took to get there.

When I arrived at home it was dark and Gail and Carol were there. I really don't remember too much of what happened there, if we waited long enough for Roxanne to arrive or not. I packed a backpack quickly with my laptop computer and a couple of extra T-shirts and hugged the girls, telling them their mom was on the way to another hospital that could take better care of her. Gail and Carol drove in Gail's Chevy Avalanche and followed me down to Charleston.

It was the worst drive of my life. I had no idea what to expect when I arrived in Charleston. It took 2 to 2.5 hours to get there and I was alone in the car with my thoughts and my fears. I called my parents along the way and told them what was going on. I also got a call from my stepson Nathan and Eddie (Carol's husband) that they were on the way to Charleston from Fayetteville. I had a terrible feeling of foreboding the closer I got to Charleston. I was scared to death I would arrive and be told Linda had died already. I was also angry with myself for even thinking of that possibility.

As we got into Mount Pleasant, which is a northern suburb of Charleston, I had to focus on exactly how to get to MUSC. It was very late, between 11 p.m. and midnight. I followed the signs to MUSC and both Gail and I parked near each other on a side street near the hospital. Amazingly, we drove right to the hospital area with no issues.

MUSC is a medical complex as well as a medical university and there are buildings everywhere. We walked through a parking garage and followed the signs to an emergency room. There I asked where a brain injury transport patient would be and was told to go to the neurology wing on one of the upper hospital floors.

We rode the elevator up and the doors opened onto a completely dark waiting room. Everything was locked up tight and closed. There was nobody to ask and nobody on duty. What kind of facility was this?

I found a phone and dialed the operator. When she came on I explained that my wife had been brought to the hospital several hours ago by helicopter and I was just arriving. The operator told me there was no person registered in the hospital by the name Linda Weatherspoon.

My heart absolutely stopped beating. Thoughts flashed through my mind that if Linda had been DOA she might not ever have been registered as a patient. Somehow I managed to convey my confusion and the operator asked, "Are you sure you have the right hospital?"

"Right hospital?" I replied, "They flew her down to MUSC. Here we are. Where else is there to go?"

The operator answered by telling me I was in the Roper Hospital. MUSC was literally right next door. Two completely separate hospitals right next door to each other in downtown Charleston! Who knew? She gave me directions and Gail, Carol, and I trouped back downstairs and through the emergency room entrance. We crossed the street and sure enough soon found another emergency room entrance. When I identified myself there we were told to go up to the after hours waiting room, several floors up. Linda was in the Cardio-Thoracic Intensive Care Unit, I was told.

That obviously didn't make a whole lot of sense. Her injuries, as far as I knew, were brain focused. Why the C-T Intensive Care? Eventually things sorted out. When Linda had arrived, the only intensive care space available was in the C-T ICU. She was put there temporarily until space opened up in the neurological ICU.

The after hours waiting room in MUSC was an awful place. Basically it was a large room with lots of chairs and some partial room dividers. During the day it would be a busy place as people came and went for various cardio- or thoracic-related appointments. In the evening, the hospital was pretty much shut down and it became the only waiting room in the hospital that was officially open. As such all the lights were on and multiple TV's were going in different corners of the room. People came and went, many obviously exhausted or extremely stressed out with whatever situation had brought them there, and kids ran unsupervised throughout the room. Babies cried and noise came from everywhere. The elevators constantly dinged and the doors opened and closed.

I imagine we looked the same as everyone else in there, wide-eyed, scared, and wondering what was to come for the night. I identified myself to a hospital employee who sat at a desk in the room and she disappeared for a few minutes. When she returned she said that in a few minutes we could see Linda! I was excited at the prospect. This all seemed to be a bad dream; now I was ready to collect my wife and go back home. I half expected a doctor to tell me that they had overreacted and that Linda really had suffered a reaction to her blood pressure medicine. I would be gracious at accepting their apologies and we would be done with this place.

Gail, Carol, and I were led to the entrance of the C-T Intensive Care Unit. MUSC builds the ICUs that I have seen as very secure areas with only one main entrance, which is secured electronically and guarded by the staff on duty inside. One cannot just walk in. The Cardio-Thoracic Intensive Care Unit had a set of white metal doors at the entry. A young doctor introduced himself to us as a resident neurosurgeon from MUSC. He was kind of short, had a slight Hispanic accent, and came across as quiet and competent. Carol and Gail thought he was extremely good-looking.

The doctor told me that Linda had been sedated just prior to the helicopter flight and was still heavily sedated. They had a battery of tests scheduled over the next few hours, mostly MRIs and CT scans of the brain. He said Linda had a significant bleeding blood vessel in her brain and was in very serious condition. Gail asked what the prognosis was and the doctor shook his head, replying that it was way too soon, and that in all probability Linda was still experiencing additional bleeding. All the hospital could do at this point was provide support until all test results were in. Any kind of surgery was out of the question until they had more information.

The doctor explained that Linda was only going to be in the C-T ICU for a short time, and that a bed should be open in the Neurological ICU shortly. Linda would be leaving soon for her battery of tests and then would be sent up to Neuro ICU on the eighth floor. We asked the doctor if the Neuro ICU had a waiting room, and if he would tell us the results of the tests. He agreed to meet us there but told us it would be very late. It was already almost 1 am on Friday morning.

Gail, Carol, and I were allowed into the C-T ICU to see Linda. She was, of course, unconscious and hooked up to all sorts of machinery, but it was good to see her and reassure ourselves that she was still there. She looked peaceful and asleep if one could discount the ventilation tubes and all the machinery. I looked at her head and just couldn't imagine the bleeding that was going on in there. How could this have happened? There was no outward bruising or other indication of the devastation being wrought within her skull.

We weren't there long, perhaps five minutes. Then we made our way back into the big common waiting room. More people had come in since we had left and the din was terrific. We kept to our thoughts for a few minutes and all made our own phone calls.

Linda's sister Roxanne and her husband Arthur had driven straight to our home. Roxanne had offered to take care of the kids. It was a great idea; the kids loved her and I knew Roxy would not only do her best to help them keep a normal routine, but also add her own flair and fun to their lives with neat recipes and activities. It was a huge help to me and a load off of my mind at a critical time.

I knew Larry was on the way, somehow and somewhere. North of Florida and south of Myrtle Beach there are some desolate stretches of road. I said a little prayer that he would be safe on the way. How terrible would it be for someone to get in an accident rushing to Charleston! Carol's husband Eddie and my stepson Nathan were still on their way as well. It's about a four- to five-hour drive from Fayetteville to Charleston. I wondered when they had left. It would be good to see Nathan, even under these circumstances.

Nathan was married in his early 20's and, like me, had married a lady a few years older than he was. His wife Angie had a son from a previous relationship named Vincent. Vince was a good kid, around 10 years old at the time, and he and Nathan adored each other. I didn't know Angie very well, I knew that she and Nathan had a stormy relationship sometimes but they seemed to get along well when I was around them, and Nathan seemed happy.

After a few minutes and by mutual agreement we decided to go ahead and move on up to the Neuro Intensive Care waiting room. This after-hours waiting room was a miserable place to wait because of the excessive noise and the number of kids running around. We took the elevator from the fourth floor on up to the eighth floor, where the Neuro IC was supposed to be.

When the doors opened it was like we were in a different world. Most overhead lighting was off and there was no sound but the quiet hum of generators and air conditioning. Following the signs, we discovered a small waiting area with an L-shaped desk near the entrance. The desk was unmanned and the lights were off. The waiting room had perhaps six small couches and a few chairs, arranged in such a way that there were two separate areas inside the waiting room. Two groups of people could be in the waiting room and still remain apart in the relatively small room. At the far end of the waiting room was a large window. I could see the lights of Charleston on the other side of the window, and somehow it made me feel better. Out there people were going about their lives normally and it was somehow reassuring amid all the uncertainty and fear that I felt. There was an old style desktop phone sitting in the room, which we would come to know well. The phone number to the phone was written on it.

Our home away from home

One of Linda's sisters wandered down the hall a little bit and found the entrance to the Neuro ICU. It looked like a bank vault door, a large windowless steel door. A camera was set above the door and there were various warning signs around it. To the left and a little before the door was a wall panel with an intercom and a button with a visiting hours list. Visiting hours were very restricted. Immediate family visitors could see a patient for a short time, a few minutes really, every few hours. Our lives would come to revolve around these times. We would make sure we had breakfast prior to the first visiting hours at 930 am; we would be prepared to see Linda again at 2 pm or so when the second set of hours were available, and would again be ready around dinner time. After that we would have to wait all night, dreading a phone call and hoping for a status update. It would become an odd reality over the next month that I would spend all day waiting for my time to see Linda, prioritizing and anticipating it to the exclusion of all else, but when I was in the room with her I could not bear to be there for more than a few minutes at a time.

Now that we had found the waiting room and the door to the Neuro ICU we were set. Of course I hadn't packed anything significant before coming to Charleston. I was acutely aware that it was after 1 am on Friday morning and I had been up since 6 am the previous morning. Brushing teeth or washing up was not really an option in the short term. Around this time Nathan and Eddie arrived from Fayetteville. There was a real feeling of comfort in having Gail, Carol, Eddie, and Nathan there with me, knowing Larry was also on the way. This was my first inkling of the power of a family united in a time of crisis. We drew strength from one another even at this early point when everything was unknown.

About 2:30 am the elevators dinged and there was some activity. We peeked around the corner of the waiting room and saw people wheeling a patient – Linda! They quickly moved her with all her accompanying equipment into the "vault" of Neuro ICU and the door shut. A few minutes later the short doctor came into the ICU holding some information. He looked at our hopeful expressions, thought for a moment, and said "I will be right back."

The doctor returned a few minutes later wheeling a small cart. On top of the cart was a laptop computer. He wheeled the computer over to one of the couches at the entrance to the waiting room and told us it would be easier for him to show us visually what was happening to Linda. Of course, he meant it would be easier for us to understand, but we very much appreciated the gesture on his part as he fired up the computer and pulled up an MRI viewer.

"Mrs. Weatherspoon has suffered a break, or rupture, in a blood vessel in her brain. This is what we would call a ruptured aneurysm. This may have been sudden or the bleeding may have been occurring for a period of days or even weeks. There is no way to know. However, it is evident that yesterday this became a large bleed. This is very dangerous and her situation is critical. The blood vessel is still bleeding, and as it bleeds a large clot forms on the left side of her brain. This causes her problems in two main areas. First, the large clot that forms will destroy any brain tissue that it comes into contact with. Second, inside the skull is a very compact space. There is very little extra room, so that when a bleed like this occurs the brain matter is pushed to the side and a great deal of pressure builds up inside the skull. The brain does not handle this kind of pressure well and is damaged or destroyed easily."

He brought up Linda's MRI tests and flipped through a series of pictures, showing us the blood clot inside her brain. I was shocked because it looked huge. I asked him how big it was. He deliberated for a moment and then replied that it was the size of a small plum.

My brain reeled at this picture. Since I was about to start at MUSC as a physician assistant student, I had enough general anatomy and physiology knowledge to know that the brain really isn't that large, basically my two fists put together. Inserting a growing, deadly, clot of blood the size of a small plum … that was a large percentage of brain mass! How could Linda possibly recover from something like this? How could she live if this continued bleeding? Why weren't they doing surgery to try and fix it? I had so many questions at that point.

One of Linda's sisters asked if this was like having a stroke. The doctor nodded. "It is exactly a stroke. One can have a stroke from a blood clot or from a bleed. In this case the bleed IS the stroke." I digested this, thinking about the stroke victims I had seen while doing rounds in a rehab clinic at Waccamaw Hospital with a PA friend of mine, Brian Forbus. Those stroke victims seemed old, frail, and almost non-functioning. I could vividly remember the feeling of sadness going into a room with Brian and meeting a man who had had a stroke. He was in his 70s and was obviously a solid, successful man. His dignity and confidence were palpable, and yet he could no longer talk. I remember tears in his eyes as he tried to communicate. It was hard for me to reconcile that vision with the picture in my mind of Linda.

We asked about surgery and the doctor shook his head. "We will discuss all treatment options with all of our surgeons in a meeting today. Dr. Chalela, the head of our neurosciences division, will be returning from a conference later this afternoon." I made a mental note to look up Dr. Chalela's credentials as the doctor continued. "Treating this injury. ... It is difficult." He seemed uncomfortable and chose his words carefully, "this injury is ... unusual. Not exceptional but very rare. Mrs. Weatherspoon has suffered a ruptured aneurysm in a vein and not in an artery. That in itself is unusual. Now from a treatment perspective we have two options that seem to be contraindicating. If it were a simple blood clot, we would introduce medication to dissolve the clot and restore blood flow. If it were a continuing slow bleed, we would attempt to stop the bleeding by introducing medication to force the bleed to slow or stop via clotting.

"In this situation, we have both an extremely large blood clot AND a continuing bleed. Treating one does not help the other. It is a difficult situation and does not call for surgery at this point. The best we can do at the moment is to watch Linda closely and attempt to respond to any changes that occur."

As we digested this information the doctor packed everything up. He asked us if there was anything he could get for us to make us more comfortable. We just answered that if he took care of Linda we would be okay.

Larry arrived a few hours later. As soon as I had called him the previous day he had gotten a ride to the airport, only to find that he had missed the last flight to South Carolina. Larry had immediately rented a car and drove through the night to get to MUSC in Charleston, arriving at first light. As the sun came through the window of the waiting room the hospital began to come alive, lights came on, and people came around. Two older women came into the waiting room and sat down, obviously waiting for visiting hours.

Soon Gail's daughter Chasity arrived, as did Carol's daughter Taylor. We had quite a little group there in the waiting room as the first visiting hours for the neurological ICU opened.

When visiting hours rolled around I was standing in front of the door to the ICU along with Larry and the two women we had seen in the waiting room. Only two visitors were allowed per patient at a time. When we were allowed in we saw a central desk area ahead and to our left. It was set up as the hub of a wheel. The rooms began to our right and the corridor curved around ahead of us and to the left. As we hesitantly walked down the corridor I saw an elderly man in the first room, swathed in bandages. He didn't look good and appeared to be just lying there, staring off into space. I wondered what kind of accident he had been in.

Linda was in the second room on the right. I was to find out later they had nine rooms in the Neuroscience ICU. There was quite a bit of turnover. (I don't know the exact numbers but from my own observation over the course of a month, I would say at least half of the people we saw in the ICU didn't make it.) The entrance to Linda's room was sort of a sliding glass door that faced the central hub of the nurse's station. There was a blond female nurse working around Linda's bed and a male working on a large set of equipment. Hoses led from the equipment to Linda and I realized the man must be a respiratory therapist and the machinery was breathing for Linda, some sort of ventilator machine. Linda's eyes were closed and she still had mascara around her eyes. The nurse saw me notice this and said, sort of defensively, "I don't know what kind of mascara she uses but it doesn't come off. We have tried everything."

There were no visitor's chairs. Linda's bed was slightly elevated. She had feeding tubes, breathing tubes, multiple IVs, ECG leads, you name it. I felt a rush of emotion seeing her as my fear was pushed back just a little. I felt like I was in a dream world. This was the most important human being in the world to me lying there in that bed, totally helpless. I put my right hand into her left hand but there was no response from her. Her hand felt cold.

The nurse had a clipboard and told me that she was going to conduct Linda's neurological function tests. She explained that these tests would be conducted several times a day and would provide detailed feedback of Linda's sensory recovery over time; whether or not her pupils dilated, whether she responded to verbal and physical stimuli, etc. As the nurse went through her checks it was disconcerting to see her reach out and place her palm on Linda's breastbone, pushing vigorously and shaking Linda's entire body, calling out "Linda!" loudly. I felt like grabbing her hand and asking her if she didn't realize how fragile Linda was? Larry's eyes met mine and I knew he felt the same way.

The tests got worse. After telling us "You may not want to be in here for this, we have to pinch her in various places to test her reaction to pain," the nurse waited a moment to see if we would stay and then reached out and grabbed about an inch of flesh on Linda's chest, just inside of her armpit, between her thumb and bent forefinger. She twisted viciously and I winced, gritting my teeth. No response from Linda; the nurse made a mark on her clipboard and then proceeded to grab the other side, repeating the pinch.

This was horrible! I mumbled something to Larry about letting someone else in and slowly moved out of the ICU. Gail went in next as I came out. I went into the waiting room and didn't have many words to describe what I had seen. I told the family members waiting that Linda looked okay under the circumstances, just that there was a lot of equipment hooked up to her and that she was non-responsive.

The gravity of the situation was fully upon me. Less than 24 hours before my wife had suffered from bleeding in the brain and was being kept alive on life support in the ICU two hours from home. Our children were waiting at home to find out how their mom was doing, probably fearing the worst. I had to call them and reassure them somehow, but I didn't know what to say. I knew Roxanne would be taking good care of the girls and giving them lots of love, but I knew they must be in great fear for their mom. I hadn't slept in more than 24 hours and couldn't remember when my last meal had been, maybe lunch the previous day before Linda woke up from her nap.

As some of the family visited Linda's room I made some phone calls, updating Linda's fellow art teacher at North Myrtle Beach High School, Toby. Toby was shocked and saddened and agreed to help out by interfacing immediately with the school administration. Spring break didn't end until the next Monday, and it was only Friday, so hopefully the school could get a substitute in there.

I called Linda's best friend for life, Linda Roney. Linda Roney had been a next-door neighbor as a young Army lieutenant at Fort Bragg when Linda was divorced from her first husband, Larry. When I had originally met my Linda, I had to "pass muster" with her best friend, Linda Farley. Over the years a strong friendship had developed and Linda Farley was now Linda Roney. She had also been promoted and was a U.S. Army Reserve lieutenant colonel and lived in Ohio with her husband Rich. When I called, Linda Roney was visiting her parents down in Florida. She was absolutely devastated and told me she would find an immediate flight to South Carolina.

Then I called my friend Rick. Rick thought the world of Linda and sounded so sad over the phone. He offered to do anything I asked; unfortunately at this point I didn't know what to ask. I told him to say prayers and he replied that soon his entire church and everyone he had ever met would be praying for Linda.

In a daze I went down to the main floor of the hospital where the cafeteria was located. There was a tiny Subway restaurant there, and then they had regular cafeteria fare. All things considered, it was pretty good food, at least during the day. By walking around just a bit on the main floor of the hospital I discovered a small gift shop and bought some candy, also noticing that they sold MUSC T-shirts. I made a mental note of this as I would need extra clothing soon.

The day passed with no new news as far as Linda's condition, just the beginning of a month-long routine for us of waiting for visiting hours. As it got dark, some of the family left and others stayed sprawled out in the tiny waiting room.

In the beginning Larry and I decided to sleep each night in the small NICU waiting room. I had slept in many worse places in the Army. On the second day, Larry, Nathan, and I went to a nearby Wal-Mart. We bought clothes, underwear, and toiletries. Near the sporting goods section, we found small roll-up pallets similar to thin sleeping bags. Excited about our good fortune, we took these back to the NICU waiting room and when it got late we shut the waiting room lights off and unrolled them near the back of the waiting room. This worked great for a couple of days, and then one night we were awakened by a security guard.

The guard ordered us to move out of the waiting room and told us that we would have to go to the loud, busy waiting room on the fourth floor. That waiting room, the guard explained, was the only one open at night. We dutifully moved to the fourth floor room but it was terrible, just as on the first night we had arrived there was blasting noise from multiple TV's, crying babies, and people constantly coming in and out.

Larry, Nathan, and I had done enough exploring inside the MUSC buildings to know that there were a bunch of hidden waiting and recreation rooms throughout the nine floors of the main hospital. If the security was going to force us out of the NICU waiting room, we would simply move to another. There soon began a cat and mouse game in which Larry or I tried to periodically convince the hospital administration to allow us to spend the night in the NICU waiting room, while simultaneously dodging the roving security patrols.

There was some sympathy for us on the part of the hospital administration. Early on we were staying in one of the alternate waiting rooms we had found while exploring the hospital, and a guy came into the room and introduced himself to us. He told us his uncle was there in the hospital and he had been spending the nights there as well. He had no money and wanted cigarettes from us; neither Larry or I smoked. It became evident to us after a while that this guy was homeless and hanging out in the hospital. Unfortunately for the legitimate family of patients, the hospital would try to restrict their movements after regular business hours due to the constant problem they had of homeless people roving through the hospital.

I felt homeless, though. Linda's sister Roxanne and her husband Arthur were back in Myrtle Beach, watching the three girls. Linda's other two sisters were at the hospital during the day and then stayed each night in a hotel room. Various family members came around and then left. Larry and I had this repeating cycle of finding new places to sleep each night. We were determined not to leave the hospital until Linda was out of danger.

My stepson Nathan stayed as long as he could, but his wife gave him a very hard time about staying in Charleston. We couldn't understand why Nathan was so upset each time he talked to his wife Angie on the phone, but after overhearing part of a conversation we realized that Angie was threatening Nathan, telling him (among other things) that for every day he stayed by his mom's side at the hospital, she would refuse to go in to work. Therefore, the bills would be piling up, and if she lost her job (a call center operator at Verizon – good job with good benefits) it would be all Nathan's fault.

Poor Nathan was miserable. He felt in his heart that he needed to be near his mom, but his relationship with his wife was deteriorating rapidly. While we always had felt that Nathan's wife was a bit too domineering in their relationship, we had all stayed out of their business out of respect for Nathan. However, now we were all stressed and upset and worried, and Angie became the target of a lot of our anger. Her relationship with the rest of the family was irreparably damaged during the weeks we spent in Charleston. After a few days Nathan had to head back to North Carolina to try and patch things up with his wife. Nathan would keep things together, but five miserable years later he split from Angie.

Gail and Carol stayed in Charleston for the early portion of Linda's hospital stay. Both of them were teachers in Fayetteville and were utilizing the 'family medical leave act' to spend their time down in Charleston waiting to see how Linda's condition progressed. They spent two weeks each off of work with their husbands and children coming periodically to visit and provide support. I have to say that my respect for Gail and Carol increased immensely during the time they spent in Charleston with me and Linda. While Linda and I had been married for 16 years at the time of her brain injury, I had always felt like an outsider with the rest of her family. Thus in Charleston I really got to know Gail and Carol for the first time. It was an enforced stay and we all had to make the best of it, and during that time I developed a tremendous respect for them and for their love of their sister.

Family is so powerful. I never understood it growing up. I had always been a loner, a bookworm, very self-reliant. My parents had divorced when I was a baby and I had lived in many different cities and states growing up: Maui, Hawaii; Tucson, Arizona; Dallas, Texas; Great Falls, Montana; and Anaheim, California. I went to four high schools before I graduated a year early and joined the Army. When young I didn't make friends easily and was very self-conscious about being tall and skinny. In the Army I chose the hardest routes I could – Airborne, Rangers, Special Forces … I drove myself to excellence in the military because it was the only family I felt I had.

When I met Linda and subsequently got out of the military, I felt adrift in a sea of civilian mediocrity. Over the years I came to admire the success qualities I saw in Linda that I aspired to in myself: honesty, loyalty, perseverance, work ethic, compassion. Linda embodied them all. Linda was the kind of person who inspired you to live up to her own ideals. Of course, along with that came strong opinions and a stubborn streak a mile wide! Thinking back now I realize all of these qualities were needed by Linda as she recovered from this injury.

About halfway through Linda's stay in ICU (perhaps 10-12 days in) she developed a significant pneumonia infection in her lungs and began to display the symptoms of swelling in her brain. From time to time during the first week in ICU she would respond in a limited fashion to the external stimulus testing, but at this point she stopped responding altogether. The neurosurgeons showed me copies of tests in which they referenced a midline shift in her brain. In such tests there is a line dividing the center of the brain; when the line shows up in the test as curved it is reflecting pressure within the brain that is distorting the brain's shape. This was perhaps the most dangerous point of her stay at MUSC and I felt constantly panicked and helpless. I know that I sounded such when I called my parents or my sister Kelly daily to update them on Linda's status. Her status never seemed to get better and it seemed each day I was providing incrementally worse news.

Larry and I found a bar and grill near the hospital and a couple of times swapped shifts with Gail or Carol and went out to eat and have a beer. It is amazing how oppressive the hospital can become. Looking back now, I believe it is critical for a caregiver/loved one to escape his or her duties from time to time. Although we always made sure one of our party was at the hospital, the brief hour respite was often enough to recharge our mental batteries and keep us going. During this time I also began to feel the guilt that would end up plaguing me throughout Linda's recovery. Here I was in a bar, drinking a beer and eating chicken wings, having "fun" while my wife barely clung to life a couple of blocks away. What kind of a husband was I?

Larry and I must have looked pretty shabby, because one of the volunteer workers at the hospital told us about the Ronald McDonald room in the children's hospital area of the MUSC complex. It was a room for the parents of child patients in the hospital. It had a TV, refrigerator, etc. Best of all, it had a shower! We incorporated the use of this room for showering daily and felt much more comfortable as a result.

There came a time during Linda's second week in NICU that I was questioning one of the neurosurgeons with all of the typical family member questions. This doctor, the short (short to me is relative, I stand 6' 1" tall) one who had helped inform us about Linda on the first night at the hospital stopped me during my questioning about how Linda might recover from these injuries.

"Mr. Weatherspoon, please. You must understand, there are varying degrees of brain injury. This is a major injury ... catastrophic. There is catastrophic damage inside Linda's brain. You must not expect too much in terms of recovery." I chewed on this for a long time. The picture this doctor was painting did not reconcile with the image I had in my mind of my wife.

"Mr. Weatherspoon, a patient with Linda's injuries will present significant impairment, but it is unclear which direction this will go. Assuming she recovers, she might lose her memory, all or years of it. She might be unable to perform even the most basic and simple functions. She may be immobile; whatever the damage, there WILL be significant damage."

I spoke with Larry about this conversation. He was pragmatic and said that we would do whatever it took. I was filled with pride at what kind of a man he had become. He was fully willing to do anything necessary to help his mother in her time of need. I knew that with Larry's help I could handle whatever came.

In the third week of her stay the powerful IV antibiotics began to help. The pneumonia began to subside and Linda's brain showed signs of decreasing pressure in her tests. By this time, Gail and Carol had returned to their teaching jobs in Fayetteville, N.C. My mom, Peggy Weatherspoon, flew out from California to see us and her charm and warm, loving comfort helped us all. While my mom was still in South Carolina, Linda began to show signs of improvement. She began to respond better to the stimulus testing. However, we soon found out there was another problem rearing its head.

There is only so long a period of time a person can be intubated. I had never thought of it before, but breathing and feeding tubes certainly count as foreign bodies. Their extended presence in Linda's airway and esophagus could lead to a dangerous buildup of bacteria and additional infection. The doctors in the ICU told me that soon they would have to remove the breathing and feeding tubes that were keeping Linda alive. If she were unable to breathe on her own, they would be forced to perform a tracheotomy for breathing and also put in a "peg" in her stomach for feeding access.

Linda began to improve a bit every day. Her eyes would open sometimes when I went in to visit. Looking in them they seemed full of pain and confusion. It was almost as if I was looking in a wounded animal's eyes. I couldn't tell if Linda knew that I was there or not. I told myself she knew it was me, and I made sure the little girls' get well cards and drawings were conspicuously posted.

For a period of three days the doctors tried removing the breathing apparatus, but Linda was unable to begin breathing on her own. Finally, the doctors brought me the permission forms for my signature to perform the two procedures. In a daze, I signed them.

There was a nurse who worked in the ICU who was our favorite; her name was Leah. We came to find that the quality of nursing care varied greatly in the hospitals. Some were better and some were worse; one we even had banned from Linda's room. Leah in particular was our favorite; gentle, knowledgeable, and very patient. She convinced the doctors to postpone the procedure and give Linda one more day and one more try at removing the breathing equipment. On this fourth try, Linda was able to breathe on her own! I will always be grateful to Leah for her insight and for caring enough to persuade the doctors to give Linda another day. This saved Linda a surgical procedure and there was no telling what kind of complications could have ensued.

Finally, on Linda's 19th day in neurological ICU, she was deemed well enough to move out of the ICU and into a regular room. However, there were a few complications.

First, the MUSC staff advised us that patients recovering from a brain injury are confused, in pain, and often combative. We were warned that even if Linda's language abilities had been damaged, she might still be able to remember words that would shock us.

This seemed funny when they first told us but it became prophetic. Even without the breathing tubes and ventilator, Linda had feeding, elimination and IV tubes still in place, in addition to a PICC line that was inserted into an artery near her collar bone, providing instant medication access. It was critical that Linda not pull out these tubes and lines. For this reason, the MUSC staff told us that initially they might have to restrain Linda with physical straps.

Larry and I moved our backpacks out of the waiting room and over to Linda's new room. We were excited about this change. First, it would end our nomadic existence inside the hospital as we would be allowed to sleep in this room without a guard trying to kick us out. Also, the room had its own bathroom and small shower, which meant we no longer needed the Ronald McDonald room in the children's hospital. The room had a TV and, best of all, a door that could be closed from time to time for a small amount of privacy. Larry and I would not have to adhere to any set visiting hours, which meant that one of us could be with Linda at all times.

We anxiously awaited Linda's transfer into the room. When she finally came, it was a bit of a letdown. Linda's arms and legs, even on her paralyzed right side, were firmly strapped down to the sides of the bed with leather straps and belt buckles. Linda was awake and looked frightened and angry. It was obvious she was confused and didn't know what was going on. The next order of business would be getting the feeding tube out and seeing if Linda still had the reflex to swallow. If she didn't, eating would be a dangerous exercise of choking and risking food material going down her airways. If she couldn't eat, the surgery to place a "peg" into her stomach and feed her by this method was the only option.

In her confusion and anger, the risk of Linda ripping out her tubes and trying to escape her situation was very real. I could only imagine her falling off of the bed and striking her head again, reopening a barely closed blood vessel. It might be fatal. The MUSC medical staff, Larry, and I all took it very seriously.

The non-nurse staff members who came in didn't get it and it was very frustrating to me and Larry. Sure, Linda was injured and had spent the last 18 to 19 days in NICU; however, she had been going to the gym for more than 30 years every single week. She was shockingly strong, even with only one usable hand. There were incidents in which Larry or I had to pin her left arm to prevent her from trying to escape. Linda cursed at us during these times and it was evident she thought she was being held against her will in some kind of facility. Sometimes she felt we were the enemy and sometimes she seemed to know who we were. Linda didn't understand anything we tried to tell her so communication was a difficult process. Sometimes we would think we had gotten the message across and Linda would appear to have calmed down and understand she was injured, and then as soon as our guard was down she would grab for her feeding tube or PICC line and try to rip them out quickly. Then would come a wrestling match until she gave up and her arms would be buckled back down.

It was horrible.

There came a day in which I wasn't in the room and Larry was. A staff member came in and wanted to take Linda to the bathroom to clean up. Mindful of how deceptive Linda could be until she made her move, Larry insisted that a second person be called in to help. The two ladies were irritated by Larry's request and assured him that they knew how to handle patients; that they did this for a living. Still, Larry felt better when Linda went into the bathroom with both nurses.

It didn't matter. By the time they all came out of the bathroom Linda had broken free of the nurses and ripped the remaining feeding tubes out. Luckily, the startled nurses were able to prevent Linda from removing her PICC line. So now that Linda couldn't be fed via the feeding tube, we were at our next quandary.

Linda still couldn't eat. Even assuming she were conscious and cognizant enough to understand what she needed to do, her right side was still paralyzed and there was concern that she might not remember how to swallow. If that happened she could choke, or food could be aspirated into her airways and cause infection, etc.

There is a set procedure to teach a patient how to eat. The MUSC staff explained to us that Linda would have a horrible sore throat from the weeks of intubation. They would start her on liquids only, chicken broth, etc, then graduate to jello, then more substantive food. The MUSC staff also told us that Linda would be ravenously hungry for real food. They cautioned us about having food in the room and eating in front of her.

One thing about Linda that didn't change after the injury was that she loved to eat. A dedicated workout fanatic, Linda had always been able to eat what she wanted for the most part, as she always knew she could work it off in the gym. Linda enjoyed eating as much as any human being I have ever met.

At mealtime in the hospital the meals are brought on large carts around to the various rooms. The smell of the meals would permeate the halls. Larry and I were sitting in Linda's room, Linda sitting angrily in the bed, strapped down. A worker brought in a tray and Linda immediately perked up, looking hungrily at the covered tray, obviously imagining what might be on it. A staff member came in and fed Linda a bowl of clear soup broth with a spoon. It obviously was not enough for Linda and she was visibly irritated when it was gone and there was nothing else to eat. She gave me a look of pure frustration as they took away the tray. Then, a few minutes later, another worker came in and set a tray down on the table. This tray had roasted chicken, mashed potatoes and gravy, bread rolls, jello, and a cup of coffee. Linda had just long enough to get excited about the meal and crack the first smile I had seen in weeks when the worker came back in the room.

"Whoops, wrong menu, sorry!" The worker snatched up the tray and left the room. Linda was dumbfounded and outraged and it was all I could do to maintain a straight face as I tried to explain to her that she wasn't ready yet to eat that food.

Communicating with Linda was an interesting endeavor. She didn't understand any words. There was some kind of disconnect in her brain between the things she wanted to say to us and the things she heard. She was completely aphasic, meaning when she tried to talk only mixed up words came out, none of them meaning what she intended to say. The only time that she made sense was when she was cursing at us. In 16 years of marriage I rarely had heard Linda curse, but during her stay at MUSC I heard curse words from Linda I never realized she even knew. Larry and I repeatedly tried to tell her that she had suffered an aneurysm and a stroke and that she was recovering in the hospital. Sometimes she appeared to understand us, but without effective communication it was very difficult to tell.

Peggy was still in South Carolina, spending some time with our three daughters. While our oldest daughter, Christina, had come and stayed for a day when Linda was still in the intensive care, the two smaller girls hadn't seen their mom since she was taken away in an ambulance almost three weeks ago. Peggy was planning to come back to Charleston and visit Linda one more time before flying to California. We agreed that Peggy would bring the two little girls down to Charleston. We would play it by ear depending upon Linda's mental status as to whether or not the girls would see her.

Peggy brought the girls down and they stayed in a hotel. We brought them to the hospital and they got to see Larry and the places in the hospital that we had been staying for the last few weeks. Although the girls wanted to see their mom, at the last minute Larry and I both agreed that Linda was too combative to see the girls. We were unsure how she would react or even if she would know the girls.

To get out of the hospital and into the parking garage we had to walk the girls past the entrance to a corridor. About 50 feet down that corridor was Linda's room. Larry was in the room with Linda and I was walking with the girls past the corridor entrance. Sure enough, as we walked past the corridor entrance the nurses had Linda out of her room and in a wheelchair while they did something in the room. Larry shrugged helplessly at my glare but it was too late. Carmelita said "Mommy!" and Linda looked over and saw the girls.

Linda gave a shocked and excited look when she saw them – she obviously knew them! They ran down the corridor to her and gingerly hugged their mom. Many tears were flowing on all our parts. It was a little awkward because Linda couldn't communicate with the children, but it was so good for them to see their mom after the longest absence of their lives from her.

As Linda slowly regained the ability to eat normal food, her communication ability was still almost nonexistent. She was often frightened and confused. One day Peggy was in the room with her, brushing her hair and putting lotion on her skin. Peggy spoke to her in a soft, calm voice, telling Linda how loved she was, how special she was. Peggy told her that as soon as she was recovered enough that they would go on a trip together to anywhere in the world. Linda, of course, didn't understand a word, but Peggy's tone was soothing and reassuring.

Now that Linda was able to eat her next step was to transition to a rehabilitation facility. It so happened that a good friend of mine named Brian was a physician's assistant in a rehabilitation facility at Waccamaw Hospital, in Murrells Inlet, SC, just a few miles south of our home. I called Brian and explained the situation. Once he was over the initial shock of Linda's injury, he agreed to pull whatever strings were necessary to see that Linda was transferred to his facility. I will always be grateful to Brian for his unhesitating willingness to do anything in his power for Linda.

The trip from MUSC in Charleston to Murrells Inlet was about an hour and a half by transport ambulance. Larry and I discussed it and decided that Larry would ride with Linda in the ambulance and I would settle accounts with the hospital and meet him at the new hospital. Now that we knew Linda would survive, it was time to help her with her recovery.

1

THE STROKE

Linda Weatherspoon

"If you return the Almighty, you will be restored" – John 22:23

"Jeff, the ibuprofen is not helping! I have so much to do and my head is hurting so bad!"

I am in here with a headache, not accomplishing anything. I need to get downstairs to my studio and work in the clay. My students will be so excited when I show them a clay gecko and teach them how to work in this medium. They will love sculpture and the gecko will make them laugh.

No wonder I have a headache! There is so much stress in our lives right now. I lost my mom to lung cancer just six months ago and I miss her sweet face every single day. I returned from visiting with my dad yesterday in Tennessee. We have not been close much of my life, but we try to communicate and I know we love each other. I visited him this week because he is terminally ill with adrenal gland cancer and not doing well. It is so sad losing both parents within six months of each other. My husband, Jeff, is also under a lot of pressure. The downturn in the economy has practically destroyed his mortgage business and he is just starting coursework to establish a new career as a physician's assistant. He's also trying to find another house for us closer to my job so I can cut down on the long commute. I leave home at 6 A.M. and return twelve hours later in time for dinner. I have a new job teaching art at North Myrtle Beach High School. I love it, but I am new and it is challenging when you first begin teaching.

I need to find the ibuprofen bottle again.

My head is pounding so hard it is impossible to think and focus on what I am doing. I was trying to figure out why my headache was so severe. I remembered I had a headache and high blood pressure before I left school. I just didn't feel right—light headed, vertigo, fuzzy thinking. I stopped in to see our high school nurse and asked her to check my blood pressure. She told me it was dangerously high. I cannot recall the number. How high was it? I went directly to my doctor's office and he adjusted my medication. I was worried. I had already gained excessive weight and knew something was medically wrong with me. I felt like no one was listening. I was seeing my doctors regularly for checkups. I was being treated for high blood pressure. I was working out at the gym, following a diet plan of 1500 calories, exercising and still continuing to gain weight. I was getting depressed about my awful appearance.

I know something else is causing this problem—but I don't know what. In July of 2006, I was diagnosed with a small tumor on my adrenal gland. The doctor decided it was too small to be concerned about, and told me to return for another test in six months. Since my dad had already been diagnosed with adrenal gland cancer—I was really scared and still am. I didn't want to wait for the damn thing to grow. Why won't he just take it out—now?

Thinking about that—I'm feeling more irritated and remind myself that we are starting spring break and there will be time to rest. Still, I feel overwhelmed with all there is to do today—and this awful headache won't go away. I cannot expect Jeff to do anything else to help me. He already runs his own business, cooks most of our meals, pays the bills and takes the girls to and from school. Where are the little girls right now? Christina has been asleep almost all day. Typical teenager! At least she could have helped with the laundry. "Jeff, this medicine is not working and I'm dizzy. I have been working on my clay and I haven't accomplished anything." Jeff is sweet and says, "Why don't you lie down and take a nap?" I hurt so badly I don't protest.

It is about one o'clock when I lay down, and I sleep for two hours. When I wake up, my head is exploding—I feel the worst pain I have ever known. I sit up and suddenly become so dizzy I am stumbling out of bed to look for Jeff. I have difficulty walking and am losing my balance. I cry out, "Jeff, my head is hurting so bad, I need some medicine." The words are twisted coming out of my mouth. I make it to the living room and see Jeff. He looks alarmed and says, "Linda, what are you saying? I can't understand you? What is wrong?" This time, I scream the words at him and he firmly commands, "Linda, I am not going to argue with you. Put your shoes on. I am taking you to a hospital right now!" I remember nothing after those words.

Medical University of South Carolina Gilligan's Island

Linda Weatherspoon

When I wake up, I feel stiff. The bed I am sitting on is a hammock. There is a door open in front of me and it looks like the ocean— just like Myrtle Beach. Then I recognize my doctor....*what was his name? No, he's not my doctor, he is The Professor. Where am I? What has happened to me?*

I try to focus my eyes—everything looks distorted—as if I am seeing things through someone else's thick glasses. Nothing in the room looks familiar. My eyes scan the room in slow motion...just an inch at a time. I see a table and then a computer. It is such an odd computer, I know it must be old—it looks ancient. *Why are they using that strange old-fashioned computer?*

I am trying to focus my eyes and my brain—to make sense of what I see. My thoughts seem rational to me. I am somewhere...the past... the present...the fog in between. I cannot comprehend anything. *I am so lost. Help me.*

I have no point of reference. I am on the edge of a strange scene... an observer to my present life. I feel disconnected and scattered. *What are they doing here? What are they doing in my room? Why am I here?* This room does not make any sense to me. Nothing in here is making sense to me. *What are they doing hovering around my bed? What are they looking at on those ancient machines? What happened to me? I am searching my mind for answers to bring some order to the chaos in my head. I edge toward panic. Then a tiny resemblance of something comforting seeps in...just a fleeting thought I cannot hang on to. What was it? It was so vague—like trying to capture a puff of smoke in your hand. I am so lost in my own mind. I sleep.*

When I wake up, I manage to find my voice—finally! Now I have the key—the ability to speak, to assert myself, and get the answers. Communication will illuminate the awful darkness in my head. I ask them, *"Why am I here? What are you doing? Why are you staring at me? Why are you looking right at me—but ignoring all my questions? Why won't you answer me?"* There are so many questions rumbling through my mind like a freight train—still, they give me no answers. My frustration grows and I get more agitated with their lack of basic courtesy. They all ignore me and act like I am invisible. I see them— *why can't they see me and give me the courtesy of responding to my basic logical questions? What the hell is going on here?*

Reaching the pinnacle of fury—I am talking louder and louder— then finally I am screaming at them. *Why in the hell won't you bastards answer me?* Just as quickly, my feelings plummet to despair because I realize my lips are not moving. I am not speaking out loud. They cannot hear my silent thoughts. I have lost myself. Hot tears spill over my cheeks. It is almost comforting to at least feel the wetness of the tears. *Have I lost my mind?* Silenced by despair, I slip into blessed sleep.

Every time I open my eyes again, my questions are the same. No matter how many times I formulate these very simple questions in my mind, I realize no one can hear me. My lips are not moving and my vocal chords are not working—so no one will answer until I can make myself heard. *How can they hear me if I cannot communicate? Oh, my God, what is happening?* I have only three emotions now— anger, fear, and despair. I am overwhelmed and lost. I am searching for a way home. I close my eyes and drift away from this madness.

When I open my eyes, I notice that Jeff is right beside me standing up. I know he is my husband. It is so comforting to see his familiar face—finally something makes sense. This is Jeff, he is my husband, I am safe, he will explain everything—he always knows the answers. I implore him to tell me what happened. He explains, "Linda, I know you are scared. If you can hear me, you need to know that you had a brain aneurysm. One of the veins that remove blood to your brain ruptured." I have no idea what he is saying to me. I stare at him and he starts speaking in the same calm voice, "When your vein ruptured you experienced a major bleed in the brain which caused a stroke. You immediately lost all of your brain function. Do you understand? You

31

had an aneurysm and a stroke." I am getting more confused. Is my husband looking directly at me and mocking me with gibberish? He is talking calmly, looking me in the eyes, I hear his familiar voice— but his words are jumbled. *Is this a cruel joke? Doesn't he know how scared I am?* He is talking to me but not responding to the questions! I am so confused. I am searching for answers and struggling to comprehend. I ask him the same questions again. He is very close to my face—eye to eye. He has his hand on me. "You have been in a coma—unconscious for a long time. Do you understand?" *Am I dreaming this? What is he saying? What is going on in here? Why are these people hovering over me? What happened to me? Where am I? How long has this been? I have to go....go where? Where is it I was going to go?* I close my eyes and lose myself.

Searching inside my head is depleting my resolve. I am always ignored by them for some reason. It is important that they answer my questions. My mouth is so dry. My tongue is swollen and thick and I am so thirsty. I want to ask for water, but I can't remember that word "to drink!" I can't even remember "drink!" *I want to scream..... why won't you answer me? What is wrong with my voice?* They are they not cooperating. I want to get up and leave...now! Broken by the unbearable fatigue, I fall from the scaffold I was climbing and rest my head on something. I am falling through the hammock. I fall asleep on the sand.

I awaken to the stillness of the beach and the rhythmic sounds of the ocean. I can see the sand on my floor. Jeff is looking right at me now and talking—stroking my cheek—but still not answering my questions. He is calm and soothing. He is talking in his kindest voice...he is so intelligent and he can explain anything. He is...like Gilligan on Gilligan's Island...but he is saying nothing that helps me. I cannot comprehend his language. *Oh, God, why is my own husband ignoring the answers to my specific questions? Why can't he see that I desperately need to know what is going on?* He talks to me again—and he says what he wants to say and uses word salad! I do not care about the things he is saying to me. I just want *my* questions answered. I am confused, afraid, and angry all at the same time. It is exhausting just to be awake. I close my eyes again to escape from the madness. I feel the sting of hot tears on my cheeks. I wonder if I am insane. The weight of this insanity is too much. Exhausted, I drift away.

I open my eyes sometime later and Jeff is still there. I know the men with him—are they my sons? I do not know their names but they are familiar. I am beginning to despise them. Again, I beg Jeff to answer me. I walk the plank—moving from hysteria to bewilderment and back again. Sometimes I see other men I know. I am not sure who they are. They are kind—but they do not answer me. I realize that either they do not hear me or they do not care. Everyone is hovering, busy, and using a language I do not recognize. *Why are they keeping me in this bed against my will? Who tied me down?* I am getting more and more furious with my husband. *Jeff, do something about it! Help me! How can you let this happen?* I know I can get up and walk just fine—but they have me in ropes. Am I being tortured? What did I do? If they would untie me—I could get up. I could take care of myself if they would let me. I probably look awful. *Is someone combing my hair? Have I had a bath? Am I clean?*

What happened to my head? How long have I been here? *No, I don't want to smile! I might smile if you get me out of here and let me have some water!* I just want to tear everything out of my body. I try to calm down and ask the questions again. They smile but I do not agree to smile back at them and act as if nothing is wrong. If I smile, then that means I agree with my situation whatever it is. *No, hell no! I am not going to smile or let you keep me here unless you answer some of my questions. Get away and don't try to kiss me. This is hell—this is not the way to treat any human being.*

I see things they don't think I can see. Visions—hallucinations— but I do not follow the police I see in my room. Time is a mystery. I have no idea how long I've been here. Perhaps it is irrelevant. I just need to get out of here so I can figure everything out. I vaguely remember something—my horrible headache. I remember that I had an excruciating headache. It was so unbearable I could not breathe. It was so overwhelming it blinded me. I could not see. *Then what happened?* I can recall nothing. My memory is blank—everything after the headache until this moment is erased. *How long ago did that happen? How much time did I lose? Is this real or am I dreaming?* I must figure this out or I will choke on my fear.

I am trying to get up. I am trying so hard —but I cannot find the key. I cannot find the way out of my own mind. I realize something else—I am not in a real doctor's office! That professor is smiling, too. I know I am in a hammock, rocking gently over the sand. I can see the beautiful serene ocean. It is a place made of palm trees and bamboo. Those trees are not in Myrtle Beach. *I am in Gilligan's Island! This is insane. I am lost in a world I do not understand.*

I remember my mother, Christine, was here. *What happened to her? Why did she leave?* I remember how much she comforted me when she came to me. I feel safer—knowing she is here with me. She is here…oh, something finally makes sense. She is here because she did not want me to feel alone. She knows I do not like the darkness— and her presence is so calming. I am not agitated now. When we are together again, everything will be okay. Her smile and laugh will make everything work. My mother is here—right on my shoulder. I feel safer and more serene. She told me not to worry. I must be safe. I drifted in and out of awareness for many days and nights. I do not know how long. Intuitively, I know my mother will not return.

Warm feelings flow over me. I feel lighter. I remember she always provided her unconditional love for me. She was the very best mother she could possibly be. Oh, n*ow I remember*… she had lung cancer… *and died.* I could not save her. I could not help her. I cried endlessly. Then I remembered those damn cigarettes she smoked all those years. No matter how mad I got at her…. but *no, no, no I can't think about that now.* She could have lived to be 100 years old. She had more courage than anyone I know. Even Jeff said, "Your mother has more guts than any Ranger in my troops." *No, no, no, I can't think about that right now. She was here. You are safe.*

Jeff or Larry stay with me at night. I see things. I remember visions—hallucinations—but I do not follow the police I see in my room. I am not crazy so it must be a result of the medications and damage but I am not sure. *I am glad that one of them is here because we did not leave my mother alone and that was a good thing. The nurses are overwhelmed sometimes. My mother was so contented and never complained. I never stop complaining. The nurses probably cannot wait to get off their shifts and hope that I am gone when they get back! I don't care. I want out of here.* Sleep is a blessing and a curse. I can escape the insane chaos around me when asleep. But if I'm asleep, I cannot figure a way out of this hell hole.

When I come back to the moment—all I think about is to just get up and get out of this place. *Why am I strapped to a bed in a room that I have never seen before except on television? I do not have time to watch television! How can I be on television? I am so busy. I am a mother, a teacher, a wife, a woman with a million things to take care of. I have to make sense of this. My life is upside down. My mind is inside out. Am I insane?*

Doctors, nurses, Jeff, and young men I know but cannot remember their names come and go. I cannot just smile and act pleasant when so much has happened. I do not understand what is happening to me and why I feel so strange at this very moment. *What on earth did I do to deserve this?* I am so lost and so confused. *I drift in space comforted only by the gift of sleep and the silence of my mind.*

I remember that I enjoyed watching Gilligan's Island. I remember the conversation I had with Debbie at Kelly Springfield where I used to work. She asked me what my new boyfriend looked like. When I tried to describe him I said, "Well, he is handsome and yet he reminds me of the guy with the hat on Gilligan's Island." Another pleasant flashback comes to me. When I met Jeff, my husband, I told Debbie I was attracted him to because he had American Indian features. She laughed, "Jeff was an Indian but looked like Gilligan with his hat?" She did not make the connection. I thought that was a good description in an artist's mind. *That is why all of this sand is on my floor?*

I am slipping in and out of awareness. I struggle to stay in the present. My thoughts are slow and muddled—then piercingly sharp and clear as they emerge again. I am lucid—but no one else has any idea what I am saying and I am furious with them. Is this a cruel hoax? I know with absolute certainty I have only one purpose now— to get out of this hammock at any cost. Determined to get loose, I visually scan the room for help. Searching for a way out of this prison, my eyes focus on my sons. *What are their names? Thank God there is finally someone familiar who will help me escape!* Aware they are here and watching over me, I feel hopeful. I ask them to help me sit up; they do not move a muscle. I ask them to untie me; they just stare at me with blank expressions. I ask them why they are staring at me; and they refuse to respond. I begin to feel my blood boiling. I am choking on the rage and I am furious at them for disrespecting their own mother. Heaven help me—even my sons will not help me get free. I am bitterly spitting out the words....*I am your mother and you need to answer me! What are their names? I am cursing now—something I have rarely done with my children. I am cursing with fury and still they defy me. You bastards!*

Now, all three of them are here beside me—but I cannot remember their names—no, I only have two sons—the other one is my husband. My confusion and frustration are pushing me harder to find answers. My anger is growing into rage with them. These are my sons and they will not help me. I ask them all the same questions I've been asking since I woke up—and none of them will explain anything! Their words do not match my questions. Then, they are getting up and moving toward me. I am so relieved. They will finally untie me and save me. Then they say they are leaving! *Where are you going? Oh! Don't you dare try to kiss me after abusing me this way! How dare you ignore your own mother's plea for help? Just get out and don't come back if you cannot respect me! You dirty bastards! I will show you bastards!*

No one treats me this way. Now I was determined to show them I don't need their help—I can do it myself. I fight against the restraints with all my strength and might, and use every fiber of my being to force myself free. Feeling defeated is foreign to me. Never do I give up. I begin to panic and the fear is getting away from me. I am screaming obscenities, fighting for my life, to gain my freedom. I see them going to the ocean and they will not take me! *What did I do? Tell me the reason I cannot go?* Then the ladies are coming at me—they will try to stop me. I fight harder but i*t is not working...the nurse is shooting me. I am so heavy and losing my body, my eyes are going out, I am falling. My breath is so heavy. I am losing the fight. I sink into a black hole.*

I wake up calmer. *How long has it been? What happened to me?* I am confused, but not frightened. I am not in the hospital—but this is not my home, either. I find myself relaxed in thoughts about the past. I am thinking about my life when I first met Jeff. He was the tall, dark, and handsome man that most girls dream of meeting. He was wearing his Army Ranger uniform. When we talked, I was in complete awe of his intellect and commanding presence. For now, I am more peaceful. Only the remote past makes any sense to me. My recent memory is gone. I will think about the past for a while. I sleep—not knowing that I had been in a coma for weeks.

My Best Friend
Lt. Col. Linda Roney

Linda is my best friend. We met as next-door neighbors in Fayetteville, N.C. in 1984. When I moved in 1988 we kept in touch by email, phone, and once or twice a year visits. She is like a sister to me. I love her dearly.

I'm now a school teacher in Ohio and my parents live in Florida. Whenever I drive to visit them, I always stop on my way down or my way back to visit Linda and her family in Myrtle Beach. However, during my spring break of 2007, I had purchased a round trip plane ticket to fly to Florida, so I wasn't planning to visit the Weatherspoons on that trip.

It was Thursday evening, the day before I was to fly to Florida, that I got a call from Linda's husband, Jeff. He told me that Linda had had a stroke and was in critical condition at a hospital in Charleston. I felt like he had punched me in the gut. I couldn't breathe. I sat down – my mind was reeling. I felt numb. I asked questions – when? How? But I don't really remember much of the conversation. I was sick. I had to think about what I would do and then I'd call him back. I called Jeff back quickly and said I'd be there on Saturday.

I decided to keep my reservations to fly to Florida. I called my parents and told them about Linda. They graciously allowed me to borrow their car to drive to Charleston the day after I arrived in Ocala to visit them. So on Saturday morning I drove seven hours to the hospital in Charleston. It was an awful, lonely, scary drive. I was filled with fear and anxiety. How could this have happened to my beautiful, sweet, healthy, *young* friend?

I was in touch with Jeff via phone and he gave me directions to the hospital and the ICU where Linda was. I was overwhelmed when I got there. The waiting room was filled with her family. I remember her sisters Gail and Carol were there, as well as both of her sons, Larry and Nathan. They had been there since Thursday. I was warmly welcomed; we hugged and cried. Her sister, Roxie, wasn't there

37

because she had dropped what she was doing and went to their home in Myrtle Beach to care for the three girls, Christina, Carmelita, and Elena.

Linda was in a coma. The prognosis was not good. There was a tangerine-size clot in her brain where she was bleeding. It was terrible. Only two could visit Linda at her bed at one time, and only for a few minutes every few hours. Everyone let me and Jeff go in when we were next allowed.

Lying there on the bed with tubes and wires connected to her was my friend. I felt so helpless. I'm not an overly religious person, but God is a big part of my life. I pray to Him frequently, but usually in private. I felt an overwhelming need to pray to God – fervently – and out loud to save my friend and heal her. I asked Jeff if it would be okay with him and of course he said yes. I put my hands on Linda and I begged God to heal her. I don't remember exactly what I said, but that was one of the most intense moments of my life. It was in His hands.

Our visiting time was up and we went back into the waiting room and visited with Linda's family for a while. It was late Saturday night and Jeff hadn't been home yet (since Thursday). So I left my car there at the hospital and drove back to Myrtle Beach with. He needed to sleep, take a shower, get clean clothes, and most of all, hug his girls.

Carmelita and Elena were making their mom get well cards. They are both quite artistic – just like their mom! Roxie and her husband visited with us for a while. Linda and Jeff's oldest daughter, Christina, had recently been giving Jeff and Linda a hard time, acting kind of rebellious. She and I spoke briefly and she agreed that it was time for her to step up to the plate and act responsibly. She said she'd try to be a good role model for her younger sisters. That made me feel good and I knew Linda would appreciate it when she regained consciousness.

I don't remember much of the rest of the visit. I slept in one of the girls' beds and Jeff and I got up early the next morning and drove back to the hospital. I visited with everyone a little while that morning, got to see Linda once again, and then headed back to Ocala.

Jeff kept me posted on the rest of Linda's miraculous recovery via phone. The doctors thought she might not recover at all – that she'd die in the ICU. They warned Jeff and her family that if she did recover, she might not be able to walk or talk. Her brain damage was quite severe. Linda's family was especially concerned that if she did survive the stroke that she wouldn't still be able to paint and draw. The doctors weren't hopeful.

They were wrong!

Just a few weeks later, she awoke and a few weeks after that she was in a rehab center. But not for long. She was back home within a month of awaking from her coma.

About two months after I visited Linda in the hospital, I visited her at her home. She was walking and talking! She was struggling with her speech, but improving daily. She was seeing a speech therapist and I went to one visit with her). She could speak clearly, but couldn't remember the words for most things. She knew what they were she just couldn't say them. She had post-it notes all over her house for ordinary items such as "plate – chair – table – cup." Over the next several months, her improvements were obvious. She could clearly communicate verbally and was getting better every day! When talking if she couldn't come up with the word she wanted, she would describe it. Such as "it's round and you bounce it" for a "ball." Her daughters Carmelita and Elena were extremely helpful, too. They were (and are!) so cute! Linda called them her Brain One and Brain Two.

My friend is a living, breathing miracle. I am so grateful to God and the awesome medical staff at the hospital in Charleston for saving her. She is still beautiful and sweet and still an awesome artist! I still see her once or twice a year and we talk and send emails.

Linda will be coming up for about a week to paint an ocean/beach mural on two of the walls of a new addition my husband built onto our home. I can't wait! I'll not only benefit from her awesome artistic ability, but I'll get to spend some quality time with her. Lucky me!

A Son's Devotion
Larry Bond

"To one he gave five talents, to another two, to
another one, to each according to his ability"
Matthew 25:15

*The only reason I am writing this is because I love my mother so
very much. She has asked me to put my memories on paper and I
cannot tell her no. It is very hard to revisit the suppressed memories
of the worst experience of my entire life. Even today, the sequence of
events is somewhat jumbled in my mind. But the feelings of fear and
anguish are still there – still fresh. I will do my best to recall as much
as I can and as accurately as I can.*

I have not allowed myself to relive that day ... that life-changing
moment when I received a phone call that my mother had suffered
a massive stroke. I still do not remember who made that call to me.
In the present day, I only think of her tragedy when someone asks if
I am willing to consider relocating from Myrtle Beach. Then I am
reminded why I vowed never to move away from my family again.
Hearing the grim and devastating news about my mom by telephone,
I have never felt so helpless and powerless. My family needed me
right then in South Carolina. As the oldest of five children in a close-
knit family, I knew that my brother and three sisters were suffering
terribly. I knew that Jeff loved my mother beyond measure and that
it would take everything we had to face this tragedy head-on, as a
family should. I don't think I will ever be comfortable living so
far apart from the people I love most. When tragedy strikes, family
matters more than anything else.

I don't remember who called that day. It was someone from my
family, someone I trusted so I knew it was a real emergency. Someone
called and informed me that my mom had a brain aneurysm and was
being transported by helicopter to the Medical University of South
Carolina, a prestigious teaching hospital in Charleston. I stopped
breathing. They also prepared me that she might not make it through

the night. I went numb, then went into action.

I hung up the phone and immediately called my cousin who lived close by. He just recently moved to Florida and I had loaned him my truck for the day. I told him of the urgency at hand, and he picked me up within five minutes. I instructed him to drop me off at the front of the airport. I had one objective: to get to my mom and my family as quickly as possible.

I had just missed the last flight heading anywhere close to where I needed to be. I remember airport security officers looking at me suspiciously as I desperately looked for a flight out, probably because I looked scared and frantic. I didn't want to take the time to call my cousin back, so I rented a car from the rental counter, jumping into the shortest line. With speed and laser-like focus, I headed north on Interstate 95 to Charleston, South Carolina. For the average driver, it is a nine-hour trip. I was not the average driver that night.

I don't remember stopping for anything. I know I had to stop for gas but I have no recollection of it. I drove straight through without breathing or blinking. I was on a mission. I burst through the doors of MUSC and immediately found my family waiting there. Jeff broke the news. "They don't expect her to make it through the night." It was surreal … a moment I had never considered. *She is so young … she is so healthy … this cannot be real.* My heart stopped. *Oh God. What will I do without her?*

The initial panic and denial gave way to the seconds, minutes, and hours of that black night. It was all about waiting for news at this point. I was sick and terrified inside, but I knew I had to be strong for my family. Pretending confidence was the best I could muster. I had to keep a clear head. She lived through the night but the prognosis was so grim. We wanted her to live at any price, in any condition. We were a devoted family. If she lived, we would take care of her no matter what. Sometimes we didn't know what to pray for. After that, my days and nights (for what seemed like years) would be spent in the neurology ICU waiting room. My stepfather, Jeff, and I sat helplessly. We planned, plotted and strategized with each other, knowing all the while that we had no power over the situation. The fate of my loving mother was in the hands of others – not in ours.

We waited in suspense for any and every report from a nurse or surgeon. The waiting was agonizing but we were buoyed with the thought that every hour she survived was in her favor. We never left the hospital without one of us being in the waiting room "on watch." We were in it for the long haul and we knew instinctively what had to be done.

We were lifted by whoever stopped by and visited us throughout the day. It was a constant emotional rollercoaster with such drastic extremes of hope and desperation. Family members came and went. Doctors and nurses kept us informed, but we were not permitted to see her for what seemed like forever.

We had not planned on the security guards who had a nightly ritual of demanding that Jeff and I leave the hospital after visiting hours. Security always lost that battle. We managed to circumvent them. But I felt certain that no one in their right mind would have forced us to leave, especially after getting the sense of what repercussions would have been like if my mother had not made it through the night. Leaving her alone was impossible. We were staying and that fact was not negotiable.

The following days seemed like eternities. Days and nights were spent waiting for the opportunity to visit her and for updates on her condition. Finally, we were elated when the doctor told my family that my mom was doing a better! At last, we had concrete hope … until later that night. We were asleep in the waiting room. Awakened by the nurse, Jeff and I were informed that the pressure around Mom's brain was building dangerously. They were unable to reduce the swelling and with that pressure, "It doesn't look like she will make it." Again, we fought the plummeting depths of despair.

Having spent hours in the family waiting room, we developed an extended family with the parents of a young woman who suffered traumatic brain injury in a car accident. They were warm and wonderful people. They, too, had a large circle of family support coming and going. People in harm's way often pull together in hospitals. It was a good feeling to have others in the boat with us, all of us supporting each other and praying for each other. We shared every new bit of news and reports with each other, and we shared snacks and pizza. The ICU was our home and we were all family. We reveled in the good reports and we ached with the bad reports. Sometime later, we heard the doctor tell their family that their daughter had pressure building around her brain. Their daughter died a few hours later. We were grief-stricken for them. Again, we fought against the panic that this could happen to my mother.

The waiting room at the Neurological Unit at MUSC is a tough place to be. You meet families in the ICU, and they leave, most of the time losing their loved ones. It threatened our resolve that Mom will pull through. But waiting rooms are also places of hope we had to keep hope alive. There was little room in my psyche for anything except my mom's life, which was hanging in the balance. My focus was on the medical staff – the neurologists, neurosurgeons, specialists, my mom's nurses, the medical technicians – anyone who was helping her stay alive. For that first 48 hours, the emergency medical staff worked around the clock to keep her alive. They were the best of the best in neurological medicine. The other matter that had my nightly attention was all the ways to avoid the security guards so we could stay in the unit after hours. The prospect of her dying was too much to bear, for all of us. The prospect of seeing her in a persistent vegetative state was equally difficult to bear.

Despite the grim prognosis, we were grateful that we could at least be with her for brief minutes of time. But even that was agonizing. Watching your mother being poked, prodded, and pinched where she already had enormous bruises was tough to watch. Knowing that this was a necessity to be able to assess her neurological status did not alleviate the emotional toll that it takes to see someone physically hurting your loved ones.

Days turned into weeks. There were few improvements, then immense downturns in the likelihood of recovery. It was surreal when the doctors recommended the family permit removal of the breathing tube. This was a heart-stopping decision, but it was essential. There was no way of knowing where she would be able to breathe on her own. The brain damage was exacerbating and she would surely die if they did not take immediate, aggressive steps. The life-threatening complications outweighed the risks of continued intubation.

By some miracle, Mom pulled through the day and the night. Slowly, we saw a few hopeful signs. She progressed from a comatose state to opened but vacant eyes. She could not move nor speak. We had been prepared by the medical staff that the damage to her brain was massive and affected almost every system; the brain is the command center for the entire body and her brain was swelling by the second and the brain bleed was out of control. If she lived, what would her quality of life be like? That was a haunting and daunting concern.

After weeks of soaring happiness to the depths of despair, my mom squeezed a hand. Later, she uttered a few jumbled words. She was vocalizing but the words were incoherent. She spoke in a word salad. Her modulation was a quiet monotone and hoarse. But I was so damn happy to hear her precious voice, even if it was guttural.

Although there were modest improvements, she was still in grave condition. We had a very small window of time to be permitted at her bedside and visitors were limited to most immediate family. On one visit, my mom looked at me very confused and asked me what sounded like, "Who are you?" I was so excited that she was alive I don't think that it mattered right then whether she knew who I was or not. I had already made up my mind that I would be there for every step of her recovery whether she knew who I was, wanted me there, or didn't. I would take it one hour at a time and that would continue as long as necessary.

She was paralyzed on her entire right side. After weeks in ICU, the doctors kept Mom in restraints. That was a painful sight but I knew it was necessary. Approaching one full month at the hospital, her condition was eventually stable enough to move her to the Critical Care Unit on the same floor. We had a little more access to her and that was good. They inserted a PICC line, a feeding tube, a catheter, oxygen mask, and she had an assortment of other devices connected to her. It was a crushing vision. She was puffy and swollen like a balloon on her face, torso, and all extremities. Her body was covered in large black, blue, and purple bruises. We were permitted to stay with her the entire time that she was in this room. And we did. We never left her alone for 34 days.

My mom had limited mobility in her left hand and arm. She had been in bed for weeks, unconscious or semi-conscious, and appeared totally helpless. She had little motor control, yet she fought continuously to remove the straps that held her inside the bed. She would constantly work the straps to get free until the nurses or doctors came. When she thought a doctor was coming, she immediately removed her hand from the strap. As soon as the doctor would leave or walk past, she was back working at the strap. I was certain that she was now in survival mode. This was encouraging to me but I hated to see her struggle against those restraints and feared she would hurt herself or have another stroke trying to get herself free.

Jeff and I were constantly researching and studying everything we could find on her condition and the procedures the doctors performed. Keeping the PICC line in my mom's chest was one of my primary goals now. I knew she would do everything possible to break her bondage. Doing my research I learned that a PICC line was by definition and per its acronym, a peripherally inserted central catheter. It is inserted into a peripheral vein, usually in the upper arm, and it terminates into a large vessel near the heart. To me that translated to: if she rips the PICC out, it could be fatal. I also had a huge fear of her pulling her feeding tubes out.

The restraint on her wrist was hooked by a plastic buckle that is similar to one that you would find on a life jacket. I watched her hand and the latch closely but tried not to interfere too much with her efforts to release the buckle. I wanted my mom to know that I was there to help her and I didn't want her to associate me with keeping her captive. When she finally managed to release the buckle, she went straight for those tubes. My hand grabbed hers at the exact moment her hand reached the tubes. She was so strong at that second and I thought to myself, "She thinks that we are harming her and she is fighting me because she is scared for her own life." I am strong and physically fit male, yet I had to use both hands and all my strength to pull her arm down toward the bed. I pray that no one reading this ever has to do this to anyone. Her look pierced my soul and I was overtaken with an unimaginable range of feelings. I was wracked with anguish by the physical and emotional pain that I witnessed. I could only imagine what she was thinking in her head as I took every ounce of physical and mental strength I had and forced her arm down to click that buckle back into place.

Mom was always healthy and fit. She took pride in her appearance and she was a beautiful woman with jet black hair. She worked out at the gym four or five days a week for as long as I could remember. She lifted weights and exercized for hours. She was physically very strong, surpassed only by her tenacity and determination. I respected her for both of those assets, and fully understood the meaning of her defiant nature in light of the current circumstances in CCU. The nurses may have been professionals but I knew they were no match for her self-will run riot. Her resolve is intractable.

Shortly after my arm-wrestling to get her back into the restraints, a nurse walked in and asked me to leave the room so she could take my mom into the bathroom for a sponge bath. I told her that was fine if she brought two more nurses to help her. I explained the situation with my mom's feeding tubes and the strength in her arm. The nurse told me she does this every day with other patients and she is fully capable. I then explained to the nurse that there was no way in hell that I would leave the nurse by herself with my mom. She returned later with a second nurse that assured me that they would pay very close attention to the PICC line and would make sure that they kept her hand far away from her feeding tube. I agreed on the condition they would leave the door cracked so I could hear. Within 30 seconds my mom had ripped the feeding tubes out.

Four nurses strapped my mom back into the bed and I resumed my buckle duty. It wasn't long until Mom released the strap again and went straight for the PICC line. I grabbed her hand just in time and relived the trauma of forcing her arm back into the buckle. When I clicked the buckle, she looked me in the eyes and harshly spit her words at me, "I won't forget this. I will get you, mother fucker." She then laid her head back on her pillow with a sigh of frustration and closed her eyes. The nurses had warned me earlier that it is common for coma patients to awaken in a barrage of swear words and to not take it personally. I was so stunned that I didn't know whether to cry or laugh.

I moved the straps around and tied them in a knot so that she was unable to get them off anymore. I realized that my hopes of having her feel comforted and protected by me were not to be. The hope of her realizing that I was there to help her was shattered the first time I clicked that buckle into place. We would both have to just get over it. Right now it was about keeping her alive and safe from herself, whether she wanted me there or not.

After a month, we were able to get Mom into rehab at Waccamaw Rehabilitation Center in Surfside, South Carolina. One of the conditions of her admission as a patient was that she had to go 24 hours without restraints. The doctors came into her room and removed the straps from her wrists, ankles and body. I held my mom's hand

and slept with my head on her arm … she did not resist.

The next day, an Emergency Medical Team crew came in to transfer her by ambulance to the Waccamaw Rehabilitation Center. Again, I insisted on riding in the back of the ambulance with my mom. They refused at first to let me ride with her. Then I gave them a rundown of her behavior and physical strength and they knew that I would not take no for an answer so they relented. Jeff drove his car ahead of us. He had to go home first to check on my little sisters. He was amazing and did everything humanly possible to keep their little lives as normal as possible while dealing with any husband's worst nightmare. He was already at the rehab center by the time we arrived. Unbelievably, we were a little closer to home base. I began to really believe that she would make it home.

Heartcry for Mommy

Elena Weatherspoon

We lived in Myrtle Beach, South Carolina—my mom and dad and my two older sisters. I was the baby of the family. I had two older brothers who would do anything for us but they were also strict with us. Sometimes it felt like I had three dads.

It was Thursday, April 5, 2007. I was ten years old and thinking below the past and above the future. To many this was just another regular day, breakfast at 9, lunch at noon, dinner at 6. But to me it was the eve of the worst day of my life. The next day was different. It was the day that shattered my childhood. It became a *black Friday*—a day of distortion, modification, and refinement. It was the end of the innocence of my childhood and the day I began to learn that adjustment and reconstruction were to become my best friends.

On Thursday evening, we were giddy with excitement because spring break was coming! No school, no homework, and no alarm clocks! It was 5:00 P.M. when my friend, Kelly, and I had just finished eating my mom's golden crispy French fries, our favorite. Mom made the best French fries, and she made them all the time. Kelly was my best friend; she was always with me or I was always with her. About two hours later, I asked my mom if I could spend the night at Kelly's. She lived three doors down from us in Bermuda Bay. She said I could as I watched her emptying the grease off of the fryer. I excitedly ran upstairs and packed an overnight bag.

I liked Kelly's house, it felt like my house. I felt welcomed and safe and had fun. She had a pool in her backyard and I remember swimming, jumping off her diving board, and playing marco polo. When we were finished at the pool, we took turns in the shower, then we went to sleep. I remember waking up with a wide grin on my face because the feathers from the comforter were poking through my tank top. Kelly woke up five minutes earlier.

We slept in and at one o'clock in the afternoon we decided to go over to Kelly's friend Stephanie's house. She was a little bit younger than we were. Kelly told me that Stephanie had a new puppy and that we should go see it. Still a little bit tired, Kelly and I made our way five houses down to Stephanie's. I remember seeing the little Maltese puppy, he was fluffy, white, and had cute ears. Stephanie invited us inside because the puppy needed to eat. We heard a doorbell ring as soon as the puppy started eating.

Kelly ran to open the door. It was Carmelita, my sister. I noticed a tear stuck in her eye, and she was trying to hold it back. She grabbed my hand and led me out of the house. She was with her friend, Ashlynn. She told me that Dad said to come and get me. Curious and uneasy about what was going on, I looked at our house with trepidation. I looked in front of the driveway and I saw an ambulance. *Why is an ambulance parked in front of MY house?* I started questioning Carmelita, "What happened? Do they have the wrong house?" Carmelita tried to be calm and reassure me, saying, "It's nothing big, don't worry." But I could tell by the expression on her face she was afraid and wondering the same thing. Thoughts ran through my mind so fast that I could not think without panic. I even started questioning myself as well. Fear took over and I started sprinting to the side door of the house, still wondering what was going on.

I opened the door carefully then I rushed inside. I was at the foot of the stairs about to go up, but then I saw my mom. I paused. I was shocked. She had this weird look on her face, as if she'd seen a ghost, almost like she didn't even know who I was. That's when I knew that there was something horribly wrong. Something was horribly wrong with my mom.

She was screaming words that didn't make sense. She was physically fighting and yelling at Daddy. She did not look like my mommy, she did not act like my mommy; her eyes were wild and scary. I was terrified. My heart ached and I could hardly breathe. My heart cried out for my mommy.

Memories of My Older Sister

Gail Brady

I was sitting on the couch relaxing when the phone rang. I picked it up and on the other end was Jeff telling me that Linda was on her way to the hospital. Surprised, I asked why. He told me that Linda had a bad headache and went to lie down, which was very odd for her. When she got up her words were all slurred and he called for the ambulance. I called my sisters, Carol and Roxanne, to pass on the news. We agreed that we would gather some things and hit the road for Myrtle Beach. In just a short time Jeff called back and said that they thought that Linda had a stroke. My first thought was, "Oh, God no!"

We had just lost our mother and the thought of losing my sister was unthinkable. Linda had been the caretaker of our mom for many years—first due to her mental illness then through a long fight against cancer. The passing of our mom was extremely hard for all us girls but especially hard for Linda. She was very close to mom and was used to being with her when she got off of work. Linda had a three-story home and mom lived in the bottom section. Linda's world had revolved around mom. She would paint and grade papers as mom watched TV and they would talk. I thought that the stress of mom's passing was too much for her to handle. I prayed the whole way to Myrtle Beach.

Jeff called and said that the hospital was rushing Linda by ambulance helicopter to Charleston. He was calm, but obviously shaken.

We were filled with so much fear and anxiety I don't know how we made it to Myrtle Beach. I don't even remember the three hours of driving. We arrived at Linda's house and left our sister Roxanne to take care of our little nieces. We hugged them and comforted them then Carol and I left immediately for the three-hour drive to the hospital. When we arrived, we jumped out of the car and ran for what seemed like miles for the hospital. We were so afraid she would not make it. When we arrived inside it was almost like the world had stopped. The doctor met all of the family in the waiting room. He told us of Linda's stroke. I couldn't believe what I was hearing. She was young and healthy. How could this be happening? I remember praying silently, *Give me strength for whatever lies ahead.*

Another doctor appeared and told us that Linda had a massive stroke and aneurysm. In a matter of minutes we were able to go in to see her for just a few moments. She looked beautiful to my eyes, even hooked up to so many machines. We were distraught and filled with fear but we are a strong family and did our best to give each other hope. We rented a room at a hotel nearby and stayed in Charleston as long as we could. I visited the hospital and was able to go in Linda's room for a few minutes and say a prayer and tell her the time, date, who the president was, and what the weather was like outside.

Everyone at the hospital was kind and understanding. We would walk to different restaurants around the area and get fresh air. Out of such a tragedy, the unity of family was strong and we gathered in a semi-private waiting area. We were told that Linda would most likely not survive. I don't think one person among us truly believed it.

Agonizing days turned into more hopeful weeks that went by so slowly. When Linda finally regained consciousness we could only recognize a few words from her efforts to speak. What I remembered the most was her effort to talk about mom. She was trying to tell us that mom was with her the whole time. Mom would do anything for her daughters, so we absolutely knew that Mom was there to protect Linda.

Eventually, she was physically able to be transferred to a rehab center. She had to learn to walk and talk again. I went to visit as often as I could and French braided her hair and rubbed her feet and legs. I went up to get her favorite makeup and she would put it on herself after much effort. In her words, "I can **look** normal." She would not use a walker nor permit much assistance from others. Linda was and is an inspiration to me. Linda always loved learning even though it was hard for her. She used to say, "I don't understand how anyone can waste the opportunity to learn and use their brain."

She is very well educated. She worked so hard to get her masters degree and teaching credentials. Because of her passion for learning, she learned to read again. She began sketching almost immediately after the stroke. She continues to take classes and learn to this day. She does not want to waste her brain. She is an amazing sister and role model. She has worked relentlessly at gathering information and learning what caused her stroke. We talk weekly by telephone. At the end of every conversation, Linda says, "I love you." After being told that she would not survive or ever speak again, this is a wonderful way to end our conversations. Linda, I love you! Gail

A Grandma's Faith and Despair

Peggy Weatherspoon

My son called on Good Friday. He took a breath before he started speaking. I was immediately alarmed because there was a detectable quaver in his voice. He quickly told me that Linda had a life-threatening medical emergency, probably an aneurysm and stroke. She was in a coma. She was being transported by helicopter from Myrtle Beach to Charleston, South Carolina.

"Oh, my God, what happened?" was all I could say. Then he described the horrible scene at his home in the moments preceding the emergency call for paramedics. The conversation about her status was brief because he knew so little about her condition at this point. I remember telling him I loved him and that I would fill his father in so he did not have the trauma of repeating those awful words again. I put his father on the phone so that Jeff had the assurance and comfort only a father's voice can provide. He asked us to pray for her and said he would call again as soon as he knew something. We cried and prayed all evening for a miracle for our Linda and for God's wisdom for our son. My faith and trust in God are strong, yet I had an overwhelming sense of impending doom and fear. My heart filled with despair.

Jeff and Linda are both rock-solid with a good marriage and are good parents, but I knew Linda had been under terrible stress for a long time. She was struggling with the terminal cancer illness of her father, the recent death of her mother, and escalating concerns about her own health status. She was worried about getting cancer like both of her parents.

Linda was a multi-tasking mom of three young daughters. She had a very long daily commute and a new career in teaching art that was her lifelong dream. Jeff and Linda were also in the process of looking for a new home. From a psychological perspective, she was off the charts on the Holmes Ray Stress Scale. If only it had been so black and white. *Was this the catalyst for a perfect storm?*

For the next 48 hours, Jeff called us every few hours with news— and to relieve some of his tension. I knew that the sound of his father's reassuring voice was comforting. During a long stay in the waiting room, Jeff said that Linda had been to visit her terminally ill father in Tennessee that week before the incident. Her blood pressure had been very high and she was having terrible headaches. After coming home, she was exhausted and went to bed with a migraine-like headache. There was simply no warning. She woke up from a nap and started walking downstairs and in a flash their lives changed forever. Linda was incoherent. She was yelling and frantic. She was screaming obscenities and phrases that made no sense. Jeff tried to calm her down and realized she was spinning out of control. He instinctively knew they were in a major crisis situation and sent his ten-year-old daughter, Carmelita, to retrieve her sister, Elena, a few doors down the street. Linda went wild when Jeff tried to touch her arms she began kicking and flailing wildly. Losing the battle to gain control, Jeff called 911 for emergency help. With red lights flashing and sirens wailing she was taken away. I cannot shake Jeff's verbal portrait of Linda's behavior from my mind. I never will. This was to be the darkest night of his life.

This was an unforgettable scene for all of them. Within minutes, she was wheeled into the emergency room at the Grand Strand Regional Hospital. The doctors diagnosed a possible stroke or aneurysm, and said her condition was life-threatening. She needed emergency medical intervention and neurological evaluations they could not provide at a community hospital. She needed surgery immediately and was transported by air-ambulance to the Medical University of South Carolina, a world-renowned teaching hospital in neurology.

Always direct with us, he said we needed to prepare for the worst; she was not expected to survive the night. He was at the lowest point of his life. She was in grave condition. As a responsible husband and father above all else, he relayed the steps he had taken to secure care for his daughters, seeking help from Linda's sisters in North Carolina, notifying her sons in Florida and North Carolina, and calling us. He put his teenage daughter, Christina, in charge of the younger sisters until their aunts arrived from Fayetteville. He was paying careful attention to every detail, efficiently organizing his troops, and had his battle plan drawn – it was clear he was grasping for control over the uncontrollable. But the fear in a son's voice cannot be concealed from his parents. I knew he was terrified and shaken to the core. I told him I would be on the first flight whenever he was ready for me to come.

I will never forget the fear gripping my heart and my stammered explanation to my husband. "Linda's condition is so severe—she may not live through the night." We both cried in disbelief and our hearts ached for our children and grandchildren. We wept and prayed. I went to the fireplace, lit candles, and knelt in prayer. Between sobs, I begged God to spare her life, to hold her children in the palm of His hands, and to give my son the strength to handle the events that would follow. I have been taught to always pray for God's will, not mine, but I also begged Him, *Take me and let her live. Her children could not be without their mother. Her life is just beginning and I have already had a wonderful life. Take me.* But God had other plans.

That tragic night turned into tragic days and agonizing weeks. No news from Jeff was ever encouraging. Every phone call was heart-wrenching and we were powerless to effect change. He explained every medical intervention and outcome in detail, as if reciting it aloud would give him some control over his uncontrollable circumstances. Jeff had excellent instincts and was accustomed to managing in a crisis. He intuitively knew what to do at each critical point. Linda's sons were close to him and they all loved each other and functioned as a team.

Linda suffered a brain aneurysm and the swelling was severe. She was in a coma. Cerebral edema is unavoidable in most cases of brain injury. Jeff indicated that the doctors had to control the swelling to relieve the cranial pressure that was building; she could die if they did not succeed. Every possible measure was being taken to reduce the pressure. She required around-the-clock monitoring and control of every bodily function and remained in neurology ICU. Her breathing was controlled by a ventilator. She was given powerful medications. They were hoping to stabilize her to conduct more tests for a more definitive diagnosis.

Then the news worsened. A second brain bleed occurred. Each desperate intervention led to another life-threatening episode. Jeff was in lock-step with the surgeons. He explained to us that the damage to her brain was massive. Every imaginable test was sequentially performed, specialists were brought in to consult, and her case was triaged constantly by the multi-disciplinary medical team. Jeff was buoyed by the expertise at MUSC and the outstanding quality of care. He believed that no stone would be left unturned to sustain her. It was a big comfort to all of us knowing that she was in the best possible hands with world-renowned experts in the neurological sciences. It means a lot for the family to have confidence in the medical staff responsible for the survival of a loved one.

Despite the heroic efforts of the doctors, medical staff, and family members, Linda's condition continued to worsen over the following days. Ultimately, she was non-responsive. Then we received the most dreaded call from Jeff.

"She is in very bad shape. I need you to come back here now and help with the little girls and to possibly make funeral arrangements in Fayetteville." His dad and I were both sobbing and our hearts were breaking for the pain that our son and grandchildren were feeling. We were powerless to help them. We could feel his despair and our own. Parents always assume the burdens and pain of their children. My heart was so heavy I could barely climb the stairs to pack my suitcase. Then a phrase came to me from my friend, Sandy, "My God is bigger than her stroke." I kept praying for the miracle.

Jeff made arrangements for a close friend to pick me up at the Myrtle Beach International Airport. The somber plane ride and layovers gave me seven hours to walk down memory lane with Linda. I drank coffee, prayed, and started reminiscing from the beginning of our short time on earth together, just seventeen years of annual visits and brief intervals of time together. The most trivial incidents became precious memories to me that night.

Our first meeting was in Fayetteville. After Jeff telling us that he was quite serious about this relationship, I decided to stop and meet Linda on my way to a national conference in Hilton Head. I was not happy that she was older, had children, and lived more than 3,000 miles from us. I recalled sweet memories that night about Jeff, too. I adored my son and we enjoyed a fun and close relationship. His father has a powerful presence in our lives having had a career in the FBI, being a respected attorney, and as a superior court judge on the criminal panel. He was the ultimate authority in our home. He was the rock and the final arbitrator of all disputes in the home! Or so he thought.

Jeff was eleven years old and he and I were having a major argument. As usual, Jeff's father intervened. For the first time, Jeff and I looked at him and in unison said, "Butt out! We can fight our own battles." That was the beginning of a new relationship on our own terms. It grew over the years into mutual respect, courtesy, loyalty, and love. Jeff and I just had a way of being frank with each other. I felt I could just be myself with him. That is a great gift in life. I am glad I did not miss this chance to be his mother, a confidante and his friend. But his father was the lighthouse – always there in stormy seas. Jeff depended on him.

Linda was a beautiful, raven-haired woman. She had flawless olive skin and seductive eyes. She had a way of tilting her head back and to the side when she looked up at Jeff. Her eyes twinkled and she could not conceal her adoration for him. As a couple, they lit up the room. There was an obvious mutual admiration between them. She seemingly deferred to his intellect but I could sense the wisdom of Solomon in her. She was confident and self-assured. She had a lovely figure and took pride in her appearance. She regularly worked out at the gym. I enjoyed my time alone with her on that first trip. We became instant friends with slight reservations. I could see how much they loved each other but I hated that she was a seventh generation North Carolinian who would never leave her family roots for a condo in California. I also respected her for that.

I was impressed with her artistic talent. I remembered a large oil painting of polar bears on ice that hung above her bed. The primary color of the entire painting was white! White on white is not an easy for an amateur, self-taught artist. She achieved the effects of ice and fur with many subtle hues of color carefully blended with white. A hundred shades of white captured my attention. She was shy about showing me her work; she never thought it was good enough and pointed out to me how her work could be improved. She had the ability to critique her own work. Her face lit up when she talked about technique and pallet. When I left, she gave me a painting of six horses walking at an angle toward the artist. It was a perspective that showed all the forms and muscles of a horse. The manes were blowing gently, dust was stirring with the movement of the hooves, and there were three breeds. That oil painting still hangs in our den.

She was social and personable. She loved animals and shared that at one point in her life she wanted to become a veterinarian. She was careful, deliberate, analytical, and perfectionistic. She appreciated the beauty of animals and captured the feel of their environments on her canvas. She had depth. She was solid. Begrudgingly, I finally conceded "She would do for my son." I laugh out loud now as I remember that moment.

Over the next seventeen years, our relationship became more than a mutual love for Jeff. I often felt more like her mother or big sister. Even though our times together were annual visits of a few weeks, we always picked up where our last conversation ended. We also shared the bond of family, the birth of grandchildren, the trials and tribulations of child-rearing, and devastating family illnesses. The tapestry of our lives merged and we both cherished the bond of our history together. We walked the same road together – great distances and years apart. We have never spoken an unkind word to each other. We are equally opinionated and strong-willed and we intuitively knew how to avoid those minefields. Our desire for family unity was far stronger than our egos.

I can still close my eyes and hear the drone of the engines that night on the airplane as I remembered my life with Linda. They brought a lulling comfort to me. I was close to God up there in the heavens. Perhaps He could hear me better. I prayed to my Father over and over, and took comfort knowing people were praying for her from coast to coast. I prayed for the miracle of life for her. *My God is stronger than her fragile brain. My God can fix anything. Dear God, please let her live.*

I arrived on Friday morning and Jeff's friend, Rick, picked me up and delivered me to their home. Linda's sister, Roxanne, gave me an accounting of all the events of the past several weeks. She was a quiet, unassuming source of strength for this family. Roxanne dropped her own responsibilities in life and rushed to Myrtle Beach to assume every possible task that her oldest sister would want done. Roxanne did the cooking, cleaning, laundry, and shopping. She told me about Jeff's commitment to keeping things at home as normal as possible for the girls. She described Jeff's formidable weekly routine between the hospital and home. She was glad that I came. She managed to stay calm despite her own heartbreak. She was so reassuring to the little girls and they loved and trusted her. She took on the challenges of the rebellious teenager, Christina. She was a godsend for Jeff. He trusted her care.

Jeff and Larry traded off sleeping at the hospital in the waiting rooms, lobby, or wherever they could find a spot that was safe from the security guards. Jeff wanted his daughters to have some semblance of normalcy in their lives and came home every few days to spend time with them. They were frightened and they all piled up together and slept on his bed. He made their breakfast in the morning, got them up for school, packed their lunches, and dropped them off at school. Then he drove back to MUSC just in time for the first round of visiting hours.

Although Linda had very limited visiting restrictions, it was worth it to Jeff to be there for each of them. His daughters needed him and his wife needed him. Jeff has always gone the extra mile for those he loves. She was in a coma and could not see him but he needed to see her face every chance he could. He traded off with Larry and Nathan. They held vigil at her bedside 24 hours a day, seven days a week. They took their showers in the parents' room of the children's hospital adjoining MUSC. When they ran out of clean clothes, they went to Wal-Mart and bought the essentials. They were good men, a good team, and their love and concern for Linda and for the three little girls were paramount. There was never a visible chink in their unity.

Roxanne was exhausted, not sleeping, and running on frayed nerves. She needed respite from her 24-hour caregiving. She wanted to be there for her sister's children and I knew maintaining her own stamina was important for the long haul ahead. Whether Linda survived or not, she was invaluable to the family. With me here for a short time, she could go home and rest and come back a little renewed.

Jeff needed me to keep my granddaughters surrounded with love and kindness and to keep their lives as routine as possible. I am a restless soul, not one to sit by quietly and wait. I could not bear to wait around in Myrtle Beach for that next devastating phone call and I wanted to be there for Jeff when the worst came. More than anything else, I wanted to see Linda one last time. I had an amends I wanted to make to her; I knew she would hear me and know how much I cared. It is called the language of the heart—it transcends all forms of communication.

We decided to rent a hotel suite on the oceanfront near the hospital in Charleston. Jeff, Larry and Nathan could come and shower, change clothes, catch some sleep, and take a breath before returning to their vigil at the hospital. It would be good for my three granddaughters to get away from their routine, too. In closer proximity to their mother, just being in the same hospital would make them feel closer to her. They could at least visit the hospital where their mommy was trying to stay alive. Like little troopers, they had done their best to proceed as if everything would be all right despite the giant void in the house when their mother left in that screaming ambulance. Linda was the heartbeat of the house; they were so brave but understandably lost and confused.

Jeff was in favor of us coming to Charleston for the weekend. Once again, he drove the two and a half hours to pick us up and turned around and drove two and a half hours straight back to the hospital to ensure he was there for his five minutes with his wife at the next visiting hours. He said Linda's condition had just slightly improved, but only in small measure. I remember feeling that God had answered one prayer, that I be able to make those amends to her while she was alive. At that moment, I could also feel the power of prayer wash over me. Friends and family from all over the United States were praying for her and the family. My friend always says, "The prayer warriors are on it!" I believe in the power of prayer. God's presence is palpable when prayers en masse are shared on behalf of the others. A warm calm washes over me in those moments. I hear that small still quiet voice within strengthen me. I intuitively know we will be okay – no matter what happens – we will be okay.

We arrived at 8 P.M. at the hotel and visiting hours had passed. Jeff left the girls with me. We ordered dinner and a movie in the room. Emotionally exhausted, we all passed out asleep before we saw ten minutes of the movie. I woke up at 2 A.M. with the television still playing. I sat in a chair and studied the faces of each of my beautiful granddaughters. I thought about their unique personalities, their strength of characters still unfolding, and their delicate emotions. I thought about what might lie ahead for them if Linda died. I thought about their quality of life if she languished in a long-term care facility in a vegetative state. These were unbearable thoughts and I shook them off.

I loved their individuality and playfulness with me. Despite the distance in miles I felt close to them always. While Christina was in her rebellious teen phase, Carmelita was the little homemaker and organizer. Carmelita had unpacked her suitcase with amazing speed, organizing her little outfits in neat rows in her drawer, and following her nightly rituals. Elena dumped the contents of her small suitcase in the drawer. Carmelita reminded her little sister, Elena, to wash her face, brush her teeth, put on clean pajamas. Elena was the feisty little drama queen. The baby of the family, she held title to the Center of Attention Child. She could make me laugh more than anyone on earth. She was a stand-up comic who could light up a room. There I was in the middle of the night crying crocodile tears thinking about their innocence, shattered and scattered to the winds on that single Thursday afternoon in April. I had a different but special connection with each of those little girls. Only God knew what was laid ahead for them. I decided I would be like Scarlett O'Hara, "I'll think about that tomorrow." I had to stay in the present moment.

I thought about their lives until this hour of tragic circumstance. I could not bear the pain that they would endure if Linda died. Their little hearts would be shattered. There is an unbearable but illogical sense of abandonment young children experience when a parent dies, wondering if it was somehow their fault. This would be their burden for a long time. Their mommy would never leave them by choice, but they would still take responsibility for the loss of her. I asked God for guidance in my every thought and deed and to show me how I could be of service to the broken hearts around me. A meddlesome mother-in-law was not needed here. Living on the opposite coast, our times together were once a year. How much comfort could I be? What would God have me do, and be, and say? If I could just do His will I would have served my purpose in their little lives.

God sent me a quiet knowingness: *Be still and know that I am.* It reminded me that I was there to be of service. Comforted, I started to see our suite with different eyes. I smiled as I watched their sleeping antics. Elena kept trying to pull the covers up and Carmelita kept kicking them off. Christina kept kicking me and throwing her leg over my stomach. Carmelita held entire conversations in her sleep. Elena whimpered. I fell asleep smiling because God was in charge. All I had to do was show up and love them all. I could do that easily.

I adored Linda's sons, Larry and Nathan. They were remarkably fine young men who loved family above all else. I was so happy they were all there together supporting each other, hugging each other, praying for a miracle and trudging this road together. I was reminded of a phrase by Mother Teresa that went something like, "I can go anywhere and do anything if I have somewhere to go and someone to walk with." The boys and Jeff—the three of them were the embodiment of that expression. Linda would be so proud if she could witness this family in action on her behalf. They were her biggest success.

I was really nervous when we walked into the hospital the next morning. Linda's situation had slowly improved since my first day here. At least there was a glimmer of hope in the boys' faces. Jeff said that her eyes had opened – she was awake – but non-responsive. It was my turn to go in and I felt so apprehensive. I tried to picture what I might see to prepare myself. I felt like all the air had been sucked out of my lungs and I could not breathe when I opened the door. She was ghostly white and her skin was stretched taut from fluid retention. She looked like a teenager with the tight skin. She looked right at me when I walked in, a blank look with vacant eyes. I came right to her bedside and took her hand. It was taped, monitors attached, and needles stuck in for the IV. Her body was frighteningly swollen. Her hair was wild and uncombed. But it was my Linda. She was in there, all right. I could feel she was in there. I kissed her forehead and gently squeezed her hand. I wanted to crawl into bed with her but the tubes, machines, and restraints did not allow closer contact. I studied her eyes and face. I studied the environment – the bustling nurses, the unwanted noise of the machines. I knew Linda had kissed the face of God and I wondered if she would live to tell the tale.

Fearing I might never see her again alive, I leaned over and buried my face in the crevice of her neck, with my head on her shoulder. I closed my eyes and quietly told her all the things I wanted to say. I made the amends that were in my heart. Linda had always been wonderful to me. We never exchanged a harsh word over the seventeen years they were married. She adored my son and he adored her. She gave me three beautiful granddaughters and two marvelous grandsons. I wanted her to hear from my heart how much I admired her forthrightness, her dedication to her own mother who suffered mental illness and a long battle with lung cancer. I identified with her humble beginnings, her passion for art, and her long and triumphant struggle to achieve her educational goals and get an advanced degree.

I shared my pride with her that she and Jeff shared strong family values and I loved that she never dissed my son, despite his faults. I loved Linda's ability to stand up for what she believed in. She never seemed to sacrifice her principles. I thought of her as a daughter or a sister, not a daughter-in-law. To this day, I cannot think of anything I don't like about Linda. Albeit, she has an intractable streak of stubbornness!

I shared all those things I loved about her. I wanted to make an amends to her for my failure to act on a special reward that she deserved. When Linda graduated with her master's degree in art history, I planned to do something really special with her. I had walked her path myself and I knew the rags-to-riches life she led. I planned to take her on a great trip to a major city to visit all the art galleries. We could stay in a great hotel, go to the theater, eat dinners out, and spend quality time together. I just never got around to it. I never even talked to her about it. I let time slip by and now it was probably too late.

"Linda, I am so sorry. Please don't die. Please stay with us. If you will recover and get out of this bed, I will take you anywhere in the world to see your favorite art galleries and experience the works you love. Please hear me. Please recover and get out of this bed. Your girls are too young to be left alone – they need their mother."

I kissed her neck, told her I loved her, and asked God to wrap her in His loving arms and shield her from pain and despair.

As I reached the door, I was choking back sobs. I looked back and she followed me with her eyes. She was looking right at me. This artist's holiday with her was a promise I desperately wanted to keep. I cannot say for certain how much of it was to salve my conscience for failing to honor her achievements and how much was to give her something she profoundly loved to hang on to. But I took the right action. I lifted her up in prayer, asked God to surround her in His white light, and departed knowing the results were in His hands. I walked hurriedly down the hall and buried my face in Jeff's chest, shaking and sobbing. Instantly, I realized that this was not what he needed from me.

The whole family had been holding a vigil of hope for weeks. There was another family sharing the same anguish. We all settled into the family room marking the time until the next medical report. We visited with the family whose young daughter was in a coma following a tragic car accident. She was driving with her friends for a fun night out. She dropped her cell phone on the floor, bent down to retrieve it, lost control of the car and crashed. She sustained massive head trauma and her life was hanging by a thread. I prayed for her parents knowing the potential loss of a child is undeniably every parent's worst nightmare.

They were lovely, warm people who shared their food and snacks with us. They were so kind to the little girls. All of my grandsons and granddaughters have artistic talents inherited from their mother. Carmelita had drawn a beautiful card for Linda with a verse that took my breath away. She had drawn a colorful picture of a house, with hearts around it. The verse inside read, "Mommy, there is no heart in the house without you. Please come home soon."

Carmelita shared the card with the girl's mother, who read the card, and with great pride she proclaimed, "Carmelita, this is a lifetime treasure for your mommy. This is the kind of thing she would grab before anything else to take with her if the house was burning down. This is the best thing you could possibly give her." Everyone smiled watching Carmelita's smile slowly spread across her beautiful face. It was a lovely moment that warmed all of our hearts. This was one of those magic moments when all of God's children are connected.

A large box of tropical flowers arrived from Jeff's sister, Kelly, who lived in Hawaii. The flowers were magnificent and carefully packed to preserve freshness of the delicate orchids, bird of paradise, and tropical flora and fauna. There was a beautiful card enclosed and orchid leis for each of the nieces. They were delighted and grabbed their leis and giggled as they did the hula all around the waiting room. Everyone was smiling again. Inside the box, there were instructions and all the materials needed for arranging the floral. Nathan and I sat on the floor and assembled all the flowers. Following the instructions, Nathan created a masterpiece to the delight of everyone in the waiting room. It was also a joyful moment that broke the heavy load everyone carried. It is precious to recall that when twenty people are sharing the load, it isn't quite as heavy to carry.

Linda's condition improved bit by bit throughout the day. Everyone was breathing more easily. In a lighter mood, we spent a small fortune on Starbuck's Frappuccinos, loaded with whipped cream and chocolate. Just being out of the imminent danger zone was enough for a celebration. Larry and Nathan were young men but they sat on the floor and played Monopoly with their little sisters as if everything was perfectly normal. Their faces were still tense and they were easily distracted by foot traffic; they kept eyeing the hallway where the nurses appeared for updates. Such wonderful big brothers; they were suffering, but always put their little sisters first. The day continued to bring tiny rays of hope and the mood was getting a bit lighter with each passing hour. Maybe she will make it!

Jeff ordered Larry to take a break and get out of the hospital for some sunshine and fresh air. Larry took the girls to the mall, bought them each a new outfit, and dutifully critiqued the fashions they modeled for him. He and Nathan were the best big brothers and the girls loved them. More than anything, Elena wanted the wheelies I had promised her. They girls both tried them on and wheeled around the store on their heels. To their delight, Larry donned a pair and was "wheeling" circles around them. Again, that still small voice within told me, "They will come through this … they have each other … they will be okay no matter what."

Nathan and I took the girls back to the hotel, ordered a good meal and another video. The relief for the girls was evident and they were in a playful mood. As usual, Elena engaged in her stand-up comic routines and we laughed until our sides hurt. She did her entire routine standing on the bed and we laughed. It was a blessed miracle to see their little faces smile. But Nathan wasn't smiling. His burdens were heavy.

I chatted with him at the table for a while as the girls watched the video. He was morose and under a visible strain. His life was full of burdens at the moment and he was shouldering more responsibility than a young man can bear alone. We talked a while and he was uncharacteristically guarded about his present circumstances. We had always enjoyed an easy relationship and he called me Grandma Peggy. (I told him when he was little that there was no such thing as a step-grandma!) Nathan worshipped his mother and this crisis was taking a terrible toll on him. I don't think I helped him much. But at least he knew I cared. He took a long shower, fell into bed, and slept soundly on a real mattress for the first time in a long while. Even Elena's performances and the gales of laughter did not disturb him.

Jeff arrived in time for a great hotel breakfast and talked at length about the little improvements overnight. He hugged his girls tightly, taking turns with each one sitting on his lap and fussing over them. He took a real shower, changed clothes, and we headed back to his home-away-from-home – the hospital waiting room. The day unfolded with increasingly good news about Linda. She was slightly more alert, her vitals were improving slightly, and the doctors could not explain the miraculous turn of events in her favor. The extent of brain damage was severe and her functional capacity was a grave consideration. Her survival was still tenuous but extensive brain damage was assured. Like Larry said, we tried to ignore the negative and firmly grasp every straw of hope with both hands.

By lunch time, everyone was in a lighter mood. The signs of relief were evident, with smiles replacing the lines on tired faces. We decided a group lunch was in order for a little celebration and headed for the best beachfront restaurant Larry could find. It was a grand lunch hour, punctuated with laughter, hugs and kisses, photographs, high-fives, and smiles. Larry and Nathan teased their sisters. Jeff kissed them and hugged them one by one as they made periodic trips to his side. This was a valuable moment of comic relief. This was a Kodak moment—priceless!

The best part of the day came when I was allowed to go in with

Nathan and be with Linda. She was awake and calm. She followed me with her eyes. She could not move her right side. She could not speak. Occasionally she made guttural sounds and tried to move her left arm. I was able to look at her with clear eyes and see that her skin was so dry it was scaling and her hair was a tangled mess. I washed her face gently with a warm cloth and applied a small amount of lotion to her dry face. Her hands were bruised, battered, and taped with no space to apply lotion. I found my brush and began to carefully detangle her long black hair. As a woman, I intuitively knew that somehow she would feel better if she looked better.

Without being asked, Larry left to buy her favorite moisturizer and took the girls with him. He was so thoughtful that way. Then he took his sisters to the park across the street from the hospital for a little play time. I went in again to see her with Nathan. As Nathan put his head on his mother's chest, she was trying to lift her left arm – I thought to caress his bowed head. Instead, she suddenly began clawing her bedding and grabbing to find the PICC line and rip it out. Nathan was up like a shot, grabbed her left hand and summoned the nurses.

Linda could not be placated. Despite her limited ability to move and having been in a coma for a month, she fought like a hellion to get free. Now there were three nurses, a hypodermic needle, and more restraints with buckles. Nathan and I looked at each other and our pleasure vanished. Linda was in pure hell and we were powerless to help her. We wrapped our arms around each other and cried quietly as we walked back to the waiting room. Nathan was so kind that despite his own pain he was comforting me. I was worthless there.

Later that evening, the wonderful family we had been sharing pizza with got the dreadful news they prayed *not* to hear. Their beautiful young daughter was not going to survive. The parents were permitted to go in and say their good-byes to their precious child. Their anguish was oppressive and weighed heavily on every person in the waiting room. Jeff and the boys had been "living" with them all this time in one large room, sharing stories, sharing sofas, sharing food, and sharing every triumph and setback. Their battle was lost; their little girl would never come home. When they came out, wiping away tears and clutching each other, they were so gracious to their own family members. They praised and thanked the nursing staff.

They hugged Jeff and his children and offered their friendship and good wishes for the family. This is what people of faith do, even in their darkest hour. We watched with tearful faces as they slowly shuffled their way out of the place where hope lives. They were on a different path. Now it was harder to hold on to our faith. A waiting room is the place where faith is sorely tested.

Jeff, Larry, and Nathan wear their hearts on their sleeves. I could see them looking at each other, eyes darting from one to the other like they were searching for someone to utter a profound word. The muscles in their faces were taut and Jeff's jaws were set like steel. They knew they had dodged the bullet – for now. Again, they were reminded how tenuous the situation and that Linda's life still hung by a single thread.

It was Sunday afternoon and almost time to depart for Myrtle Beach. I needed to get the girls home, bathed, and ready for school the next morning. The girls wanted to see the room where mommy stayed. Jeff said he would show them the room, but they wouldn't be able to see her or talk to her. He was always honest and matter-of-fact with them about most things in life. He held tight reins on them, but he shared information appropriately and treated them like young adults. I think a lot of maturity came to them from that approach. They were more adult than their years in many ways.

Jeff bent down and met them at eye level. "Right now, mommy won't recognize you or know your name." They looked at him in wide-eyed disbelief. He gently reminded them that mommy was still critically ill, and they would not be able to see her or talk to her. But he would show them her room where they would see her the next time they visited. They were bewildered and so brave. He vanished around the corner, holding their hands.

Within a few minutes we could hear a loud wail in the hallway. It was Elena. She suddenly came charging around the corner sobbing and Carmelita was right behind her with tears streaming and agony on her face. Her plaintiff wail was, "That is not my mommy. That is not my mommy!" Jeff and Nathan had turned the corner to walk them by Linda's room. They were all stunned at the vision they saw. The nurses had moved Linda and her bed out into the hallway. Linda was elevated and semi-reclined, strapped down, swollen, discolored, and still connected to the monitors and IVs. The girls had not seen their mommy in weeks and this was an appalling sight for them.

This was one of those "hard right" lessons in life. On Good Friday 2007, these girls lost the innocence of their childhood. They were devastated, heartbroken, frightened, yet courageous. Their brothers scooped them up, hugged them, petted them, and soothed away their fears. At the end of the day, the only thing that matters is family.

It was time to leave for Myrtle Beach. Nathan went with me as I went in to tell Linda goodbye, praying it would not be the last time I saw her alive. I scanned her body and face again. Her legs and feet were encased in thick elastic stockings with only her toes exposed. Her toes were dry, swollen like sausages, and blue. Her face was beautiful, her skin stretched tight across her face, and her eyes were searching mine this time. I had no way to communicate with her other than to show her my face and do the things that I knew were important to her. I brushed her hair, massaged lotion into her cheeks and toes. Her arms and hands were black and blue and I was afraid to touch her there. Nathan took a picture of me brushing her long black hair. I stayed as long as I could until the nurses came. Again, I found Jeff and cried because I was leaving. "I should stay here. No one will take care of her like I will. No one will brush her hair, clean her eyes and the corners of her mouth, and massage her with lotion. You boys are wonderful, but a woman needs another woman's touch, especially Linda." He reassured me that they would take care of her, that her sisters would do that for her, too.

Nathan drove us back to Myrtle Beach on Sunday evening. The three girls were pensive and quiet all the way home. They were lost in their own thoughts, trying to process what they had seen and experienced with their mommy. Nathan dropped us off and drove himself all the way to Fayetteville for work the next morning. He was exhausted and weary; I was so proud of him.

I wasn't very good at doing what Jeff requested. "Try to keep their lives on a normal track, have them finish their homework, no junk food, eat nutritious meals, take their baths, lay out their school clothes and get them ready for school each morning. Help them make their lunches, get them to school on time, and pick them up from school on time." What about play time? He looked at me and laughed. "On school nights they know they are restricted on television time and they each know their hours on the computer. They know their cell phone rules. I will be in phone contact with you." After that week, I had a new appreciation for the joys and agonies of their life in Myrtle Beach.

The girls were thrilled with all the secret indulgences grandmas swear not to tell their parents. We laughed and played games. The little girls begged to sleep with me in their mommy's room and it was fine with me. The master bedroom was wall-to-wall portraits, pictures, and snapshots of family. Pictures of Jeff and Linda and their lives over seventeen years were depicted on all four walls of their bedroom. It was an eerie sight for me and I was still jet lagged and shell shocked. *Is this the end of their living collage with mommy captured in photographs?*

Emotionally drained, we turned off the lights and snuggled in. The girls could not go to sleep; Elena started to cry. Carmelita played mommy to Elena."It will be all right, just close your eyes and go to sleep." Minutes later, I could hear Carmelita sniffling. "Grandma, I can't go to sleep." And Elena, "Grandma, when I close my eyes I see my mommy and it is scaring me." When my words did not comfort them, it was time for diversion and distraction. I said a quick prayer for God's guidance. I could not bear making a mistake with these special little people. I began to share old stories of Jeff and Linda, their dating, their wedding, the birth of Christina, and stories of their own births. I described what ugly little babies they were, and they giggled. I asked them their favorite daddy memory then their favorite mommy memory. I told them secrets about their daddy, his report cards in grammar school and tales about his rebellious teens, not everything just some of the funny things.

Later, Christina came downstairs and crawled in bed with us, too. It was like my own childhood, four girls sleeping in one bed. The girls drifted off to sleep and I followed. At 1:00 A.M. Carmelita sat strait up in bed, reached across Elena, and slapped me on the chest as hard as she could and said, "That's my chair!" She lay back down and went right to sleep. By 2:00 A.M. Elena was whimpering and crying in her sleep. She began to repeatedly whisper, "no, no, no" and cried baby tears as she slept. At 3:00 A.M. I woke up startled by voices in the house. I was terrified something had happened and terrible news was about to be delivered. It was pitch dark as I made my way to the kitchen. I couldn't find the light switch, but I could hear Christina, talking on the phone and my heart stopped. "Who are you talking to, is it daddy?"

"Oh, just my friend, he lives in another state."

I was so mad at her I told her to hang up and go to bed. She did not want to hang up, then I ordered her to hang up, and she went into fits of tears and drama. She refused to go to bed and was going to sleep on the sofa. Within thirty minutes, I heard her on the phone again. Exasperated, I stomped out into the living room took her phone away and went back to bed. Teenagers! *Oh my Lord—how do Jeff and Linda do this every day? How on earth will Jeff be able to do this without Linda?*

I worried that I did not handle the situation with Christina very well. She was doing what all teenagers do and she was trying to cope like the rest of us. Perhaps I should have cut her some slack considering the grave circumstances. I felt miserable—and exhausted emotionally. I promised to do better tomorrow.

"Life is like an onion,
you peel off one layer at a time and
sometimes you weep."

Carl Sandburg

"A journey of a thousand miles begins
with the first step."

Lao-tzu, Chinese Philosopher (604-531 BC)

2
THE RECOVERY

The Pillow Ninja
Larry

It was the day Mom was being transferred to the hospital in Myrtle Beach. I was the happiest son on earth! I was happy to be riding in the back of a transport ambulance with my mom on our way to Waccamaw Surgical Rehab near Myrtle Beach. We were inching our way toward the next goal – getting her back home. I was super nervous about everything I had learned about aneurysms and strokes. We had researched and studied to comprehend as much as we could. The question that lingered was: "How could this happen to such a strong, passionate, healthy woman at age 48?"

The likelihood of Mom having another stroke was high. Among women, 25 percent have a second stroke and die within one year. Another 25 percent of stroke victims experience a fatal stroke within five years. The medical staff cautioned us, "There is no medical explanation for her survival, save a miracle! Be aware that she is highly vulnerable and could have a fatal stroke at any time." We were all determined to do everything we could to make each day count. We were all in agreement – do whatever we could do to restore her quality of life and increase her chances of survival.

I rode in the back of the ambulance to the rehab facility holding my mom's hand the entire time and intensely watching all of the equipment that monitored her condition. The ride was about two hours—but it seemed so very short. Time was now on speed dial!

The room at Waccamaw was much nicer and more family friendly than the hospital. No guards were trying to make us leave and the staff showed great care and understanding of the situation our family was in. My mom was not communicating at our arrival, but her eyes were open and the occasional "Who are you?" would be uttered very lightly as new family members or friends would visit. There was a recliner chair that I slid next to her bed. I slept there every night with my head on her arm. Jeff worked as much as he could and continued to keep life as "normal" as possible for my little sisters. We were the "A" team all the way.

Mom was on her third day without eating and we were all very nervous that she hadn't eaten. She had ripped out her feeding tubes and waved off any hint of consuming anything from the hospital. I knew what she loved to eat most. I went to the mall and bought her favorite pizza and her favorite yogurt with extra protein powder. I was hoping her favorites would entice her to eat. The yogurt shake was a winner! We breathed a sigh of relief because she had not eaten anything for two days.

Finally, there were no more tie-downs or strait jackets at the ready. She did not even require soft restraints at Waccamaw. She only had an alarm on her bed to signal her movements. She would get so mad when she rolled over and the alarm sounded. I would wake up, too, and the nurses always came to check. One very stressful part for mom was when the catheter was no longer needed, but she required an attendant to go into the bathroom with her. She wanted to do it herself and would not wait for the nurses. I went with her and Mom hated me for it. She used her most colorful language on me but I did not give in to her. The risks were too great. In my mind it was the only way I could make sure that she would not fall and suffer a fatal head injury. It was hard to defy the person you respect most in the world, but it was necessary.

Every morning at about 3 A.M. a nurse came in to give her a shot of Heparin to keep her blood thin and avoid clotting. There were frequent blood tests. Due to all her veins being "blown out" from all of the procedures, this proved to be agonizing for both of us. There was only one phlebotomist capable of hitting her veins with the first shot so he became the only one who was allowed to treat her. The very first words my mom said to me at Waccamaw, other than "who are you," was, "When that nurse comes in to stick me, I have a hammer right here and I am going to take his fucking head off." *Thank God she didn't actually have a hammer.*

The next day, the speech therapist came in to talk to mom and me. She asked me what games mom liked, whether she enjoyed any hobbies, and any other interests to stimulate her mind. "Bring us paint, paint brushes, paper, and more paint," I said. The therapist returned shortly afterward with paint brushes that had foam pads around them, water colors, and paper. I put the brush in my mom's hand that she used to rip out the PICC line. I held it in her hand as we dipped it in the paint. I moved her hand with the paint-filled brush on paper, then her arm went completely limp. She shook her head no and her arm lay there, lifeless. A hot stream of tears started streaming down my face. I was afraid to look at Mom because I was on the verge of sobbing. My mom's greatest passion in life was lost. It was another heart-wrenching moment on the road toward home.

A few days later, I took her to physical therapy. She still wasn't speaking but she was able to move her extremities a little. I pushed her in the wheelchair to the desk where we waited for the therapist to complete her session with the current patient. I left mom with the therapist and darted out to take a quick shower at home. When I returned, the therapist was just then saying goodbye to her other patient and my mom was still at the desk. I took a seat nearby and started watching them from the corner of my eye as I worked on a Sudoku puzzle. Approaching Mom's wheelchair, the therapist burst into tears and started saying, "Oh, my God!" I rushed over in a panic to see what was wrong. During her wait for the therapist, my mom had taken the tablet of paper I left in her lap

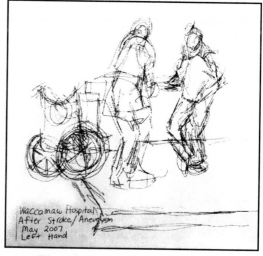

Waccamaw Hospital
After Stroke / Aneurysm
May 2007
Left Hand

and sketched the entire room. She sketched every person in detail. We all looked at Mom, at the detailed artistic sketch, at each other, and all of us were crying shamelessly.

*****

Mom's speech therapist was highly skilled and had good people skills. She knew her job well and performed with efficiency, persistence, and calculation. Nevertheless, Mom ignored her as much as possible. Whenever the therapist left, I would try to continue lessons throughout the day to help Mom get better. Each day that passed, Mom seemed more and more emotionally stable. After a week or so, Jeff and I hesitantly decided to bring my two little sisters in to see their mother. The girls had not seen Mom since their frightful experience in the hallway at MUSC when they saw her for the first time in ICU when she woke up from the coma. That was a tough scene to forget!

Thankfully, the experience this time was perfect. My mom's first response was a huge smile and then she asked, "Which one are you?" The girls did a great job of deciphering and understanding Mom's communication deficits. We didn't care about her aphasia, we were just so grateful to have our mother alive and with us just a few miles from home. My mom continued to mix up our names during her long recovery. In fact, she still mixes up our names and no one cares! We are just grateful to see her beautiful face and smile.

After the extensive brain injury she suffered, Mom started learning her basic skills all over again. Her most basic activities of daily living were all compromised. She could not eat, bathe, dress, toilet, transfer, or ambulate without assistance. Mom hates assistance and when she is afraid she can be downright hostile. She had to learn how to walk again during therapy. Although getting this far was incredible progress, it was very stressful for me. My mom did *not* understand that she had had a stroke. She did not comprehend the meaning of stroke, coma, or aneurysm. These were just words to her. In her mind, she was fine.

Without warning, she would get up from her bed and would fall side to side as she tried to walk toward the restroom. She had no sense of balance, her legs were weak, and her field of vision was blocked on the outer half of each eye. In effect, she had tunnel vision in the truest sense. She continued to get very upset if I tried to assist her. I would follow her with a pillow holding it right behind her head. I reasoned that when she got too close to the wall, her head would hit the pillow instead of the wall. *I am her pillow ninja.*

To her extreme displeasure I would assist her to the bathroom and seat her on the toilet. I would pretend to close the door, and stand at the ready with the pillow in the crack. I was ready to lunge with the pillow under her head if she began to fall. We could not risk another head injury.

Each day was a new beginning on the road to home. Each day some small victory of accomplishment was met with smiles and happy hearts. But the accomplishments were tiny and the road was long. Friends and family came and went all the days that followed at the rehabilitation center. My job was to stay close to mom and help her survive rehab without incurring another head injury. I don't know how Jeff juggled all the legal, medical, and insurance issues that he faced. He took care of the girls, the finances, found mom a new house that was safer, and took care of mom in between. I just focused on mom. I don't know how he managed it all and remained sane. I was and am so thankful for him.

Nose, Eyes, He, and She

The doctors were confident that my mother would never walk or talk again if she even made it out of the hospital alive. My mom is a very driven and stubborn woman, though. She also has a family that mirrors those traits. I knew without a doubt, if we could get her home, we could teach her to talk again. My mom would get frustrated within the first five minutes of her speech therapy sessions and would basically ignore the therapist. The therapist assumed my mom was giving up or was tired. My mom doesn't give up; I knew that she just didn't agree with how the therapist was teaching. The therapist would say "nose" and point to her nose. Then she would say, "Where is your nose?" My mom would sit for a minute then grab her ear. The therapist's response after the third or fourth time was "no." Knowing my mom, surely she heard this as a very condescending "no, no, no," and that was the end of that therapist ever having an opportunity to get my mom to pay attention to her.

I liked the therapist and would pay close attention to how she conducted the sessions. She provided me with information that I requested on aphasia and speech therapy. I studied all the materials and researched more. According to my research, mom's recovery didn't look promising. I decided at that point that instead of limiting her recovery to what journals and doctors said was possible, we would pave our own path and prove them all wrong.

My mom is an artist so I thought maybe if I drew everything we wanted to teach her, she would get it. This coupled with persistence, a little humor, and lots of love, finally started to get some positive results. I would draw exaggerated features of cartoon characters on a white board and then relate them to us. I would do funny things like draw a face with a huge nose, go up to her and touch nose, and then stick my finger up my nose and bounce around the room. I am usually pretty reserved so I made sure we were alone whenever I did things like this. I got a smile, occasional laugh, lots of head and eye-rolling, but it worked.

For the patient, speech therapy is very draining. I believed that we had to keep it fun so I could keep her attention longer without her getting tired. I also made sure that I never used any condescending thought, motion, or response. If she got something wrong, we just worked on it another thousand times. I was patient. I know I drew a hundred noses and pointed to my nose and hers well more than 1,000 times. This was repeated over and over for every word that we relearned together. The next day she would forget the word, but it was fine. We just started over again.

Names were impossible along with proper use of pronouns. My stepdad Jeff was always (and still sometimes) referred to as "she" and "Larry," and I am usually "she" and "Jeff." My little sister Carmelita is usually "him" and "Roxanne" who is actually my aunt. However, we all learned who and what she means to say.

Any threads of information were impossible for mom to connect together so we just stuck with the basics. All of our family members who visited would help. Whenever someone from outside the family would visit, we would try to make her condition seem temporary with expectations of a full recovery. I am a very optimistic person and believed it to be true. I still do believe that in time, mom will make a full recovery.

My role at Waccamaw was to protect my mom, learn as much as I could about her condition, and try to help her recover. I promised her that I would stay in Myrtle Beach when she was able to return home and would continue to help in any way I could.

It seemed as if we transitioned very quickly from Waccamaw Rehab to our home. When we first arrived I remember the staff telling us that Mom would be there for months. Suddenly after just a few weeks Mom's physical progress was astonishing. It wasn't long before the doctors told us they felt she could manage at home and continue outpatient physical, occupational and speech therapy. This was an exciting milestone for us, but one of the concerns was her existing home had stairs that she would have to take in order for her to make it to the bedroom. Jeff eventually found a new home with the master bedroom, kitchen, and living areas on the ground level. We moved everything in and welcomed mom to her new home. There was a small guest house that was attached to the home and I stayed there while my mom started her recovery. I would drive her to her speech therapy sessions and we would discuss her condition and practice words constantly. She still did not understand what happened to her at this point nor how fragile she was.

My girlfriend Kasia moved up from Florida and stayed with me at my mom's house for the first three months my mom was recovering at home. Kasia was great with helping me put together things to help my mom build her vocabulary. We cut out pictures from magazines and made a large binder full of objects with their names. We put post-it notes on all the objects throughout the house and reviewed them with mom constantly. Kasia and I found an apartment less than a couple miles away and continued our relationship for another year before we decided that it was best that we go our separate ways. Kasia was a great friend to me in the most challenging experience I ever had. Our relationship mostly consisted of her making a lot of sacrifices for me and not receiving anything in return. I will always be appreciative for her selflessness and for her helping my family and me through this period of our life.

I dove back into my career in the hospitality business in Myrtle Beach. I was working long hours and trying to catch my finances back up. I usually took one day off a week and would spend the afternoon with my family and the night going out with my friends. I met an amazing woman, Fabiana, who was on a study abroad program from Brazil and although the last thing I was looking for was a serious relationship, I quickly fell in love.

Fabiana was amazing and enjoyed spending at least every other day off we had with my family. My two sisters, Carmelita and Elena, would always compete with Fa to see which one of them would get the "Brain 1" award. Whenever my mom would talk, the girls would fill in the missing words mom would be trying to say. Fa would always get "Brain 3." We were all pretty good at it.

My mom's drive and persistence to get better is unyielding. She would sleep four to six hours and intensely focus on studying to recover the rest of the day. I would watch her read the same page of a news paper for half of a day. She would read and read until it finally made sense. She would study her book of pictures, her post-it notes, art books, and anything else she could get her hands on.

The doctors told us that her brain tissue was destroyed and what she didn't already have, she would never get back. Again, this never stopped her or even slowed her down. What if we all listened to the doctors and the medical journals? What would my mom be saying now?

I work in very high-volume restaurants and I see stroke victims being wheeled or assisted into our dining rooms occasionally. I always make it a point to spend time with the victim and the family if I can sense that they welcome the visit. There is one couple I met who told me about a stroke group in Myrtle Beach. I thought this would be perfect for my mom. These people needed someone like my mom to put a little hope and drive in their life. Almost every stroke victims' spouse or caretaker I have met says that their condition can't be improved. I knew that if I could get mom in there, she would be an inspiration to the other victims and it would add even more purpose to my mom's drive to recover. I gave my mom the address and that's all it took. She is now very active in the stroke group and is an inspiration to everyone there.

One of the restaurants I opened in Myrtle Beach is right on the Intracoastal Waterway. There is a beautiful view in the downstairs dining room overlooking the water. My mom's passion for art motivated me to host two art shows there. It turned out that my mom's art group also needed a place to paint on Monday mornings because their current location was not allowing them to continue there. I was very excited to be able to offer the space to them. My mom is the only student in the group having had a stroke, yet the entire group looks up to her work, drive, and spirit to inspire them.

My mom is very sad that she lost the ability to teach (for now). She wants to feel like she is helping out in the community and impacting lives. She had an idea to sell pastel portraits of people's animals and donate the money to the humane society, Mercy Care Hospice, and various other groups. I went and met the director of the North Myrtle Beach Humane Society. She invited my mom to set up at an event to offer her drawings. Mom set up at the event and it was a success. She continued seeking other avenues and opportunities to donate her work. She pays for all the materials and gives 100 percent of the proceeds to the humane society or one of the other charities she is compelled to help. She now continuously has drawings of people's pets to complete.

I am very happy that I was able to impact my mom's recovery. I shake a hand and my mom does all the work to make the world change. I believe the victim of a stroke has to still feel purpose to put the drive in gear. My mom never lost purpose and our family provides plenty of it. Even so, I make sure I try to add to it. I try to always be on the lookout for something new that I think will help her get back to where she needs to be so she can teach again if she wants. She always thanks me for saving her life. I always tell her, I would not be here in the first place if it wasn't for her.

A New Personality

I was born with love all around me. My mom wasn't so lucky. She grew up in a very tough environment. Her experiences definitely impacted who she was as a person and a parent. My mom was a strong-minded, strong-willed provider. She was in charge and listened to no one. It was her way or the highway with everyone except her own mom. I remember growing up in what I would describe as a tough love environment. I am currently 35 years old and I know that my mom did a much better job than I could have done at her age.

From a kid's point of view, my mom wasn't very friendly. I was the oldest of all of my cousins and they were all scared of my mom. When I was ten, I had eight cousins and a brother on my mom's side of the family. We were a very close family and my grandmother was the glue that never let us separate. Every family has their moments (although I remember a couple that are a little more intense than most), but nothing remotely near what my mom had endured growing up. My mom had thick skin and refused to take the least amount of shit from anyone, including me.

I was a good kid for the most part. Looking back, I probably seemed unappreciative to my mom growing up. She was raised with nothing, she provided me with everything, and I remember complaining about not having miscellaneous items that I thought were a necessity at the time. As an adult, I always try to put myself in her shoes and try to imagine what life was like from her perspective when I was growing up. My parents were separated and my dad would pick me up occasionally. I don't remember how often, but I know that it only seemed like a couple of times per year until I was eleven or twelve.

My dad would spoil me. I had two very different worlds. My mom's house was strict rules where all necessities and love were provided; my dad's world was a boy's fantasy comes true. My dad would take me everywhere, give me everything, and then after two days, drop me back off not to be seen again for months at a time.

I never felt really close to my mom. She always worked second or third shift and we did not get to spend very much time together. She remarried and I hated my stepdad with a passion. His name was Jose. He treated my younger brother great. I think that Jose saw my dad when he looked at me. I think he hated me almost as much as I hated him. I know that she never knew how Jose had treated me because he was totally different when she was around. He treated my mom well until she caught him cheating and she kicked him out. My mom was either happy or mad. I never really remember her being sad. I remember Jose crying and begging for forgiveness, but I never saw my mom shed a tear.

My mom was tougher than tough. Her way was the right way and she never stopped to question herself. If you were wrong to her, then you were wrong. If she felt like you screwed her over, there was no return. If you lied to her, it would take you years to gain her trust back (if ever). If she was ever hurt or sad, she did a great job of hiding it.

She was also very private. She shared nothing of her personal life or past with anyone.

Probably just like any boy whose parents divorce, my only wish was for my real mom and dad to get back together. I would pray and wish and hope endlessly for them to reunite. Instead, mom met Jeff and they quickly were married. Jeff was a very cool guy. He was in the military, had guns, a motorcycle, neat tricks, and knew how to fight. Jeff, like my mom, also parented with strict rules. I loved him and looked up to him. He treated my mom with a tremendous amount of respect but I still yearned for my mom and real dad to get back together. At 14, with my dad's constant nudging to come live with him where life was perfect and I could have anything I wanted, I moved in with my dad. I know as an adult that this had to really hurt my mom. I felt for years that she held this decision strongly against me. Jeff had come from a divorced family and he understood the dynamic of building up in your mind how life would be if one lived with the absent parent and he explained it to mom.

I never felt right going to visit my mom's as a young adult after that. I felt like I betrayed her and Jeff. I would choke back tears every time I would go visit. I took the easy road out. My dad loved me very much, but he was engulfed by business and success. I worked for my dad, went to school, and stayed at my dad's or grandmas. I always saw my mom for the holidays and felt like she disliked me for leaving her to go to my dad's.

My grandmother was diagnosed with lung cancer and Mom and Jeff immediately brought her into their home to live with them. This was the most vulnerable I had ever seen my mom. Our entire family pulled together as we always did in a time of crisis. We were all very scared, including my mom. I saw the range of emotions that my mom was capable of then. We all pulled together and I felt like she forgave me a little for leaving her to go to my dad's as a young adult. I felt the tremendous amount of love my mom felt for me. My grandmother lived through surgery and would spend the next six years with our family.

I was working in South Florida as a restaurant general manager. I called to talk to grandma like I would always do a couple times a week. She was always positive and had this little giggle that would light up my soul. She would always tell me that she loved me more "than the whole wide, wide world." She loved me unconditionally. It never mattered what I did wrong or what I did right, she was as proud as she could be and couldn't love me more. This time, the conversation was different. Grandma said, "I need you to come see me. You can't wait long, I need to see you now." It really bothered me and I knew something was wrong. I immediately booked a flight to see her.

Grandma seemed fine. She gave me the biggest smile and hug. She lived with my mom and had her own little mother-in-law suite right by the beach. She was very happy. We talked, laughed, and enjoyed each other's company. Grandma loved Waffle House. I used to take her all the time. She was hungry so I went to Waffle House to get her some breakfast. When I returned, I set us up the food at the table. We started eating and grandma was having a very difficult time swallowing her food. I got my mom and the next thing I knew, we were at the hospital. My grandmother passed away.

My grandmother was the glue and it was a huge hit to our entire family. It hit my mom hard and I am still to this day heartbroken and crying as I write this. What an amazing woman. My mom appeared to handle herself okay, but this would be only the second time in my entire life that I saw my mom cry.

I went back to work in Florida and my mom and the rest of our family continued on with their lives. About six months later, my mom had her stroke.

These days my mom isn't quite so thick-skinned. She considers others' viewpoints. She is still stubborn, but she will self-reflect. I don't know if she loves deeper now or she just shows it more but I feel her love and it seems like it becomes more like my grandmother's every day. She cries both tears of joy and sadness. She is an amazing woman and is full of wisdom. She is driven to help others and is relentless in her pursuit to become a more productive member of our family and society. She is open with her feelings and shares her personal stories with anyone she feels will be helped by them. She considers other ways than her own and accepts people who have views that differ from her own.

My professional life takes up a little more time than I would like these days. I feel driven to be financially stable enough that I can support my family better in the event of another crisis. I don't want to ever have a loved one suffer because proper health care could not be provided due to financial reasons. This wasn't the case for my mom, but it did teach me that it could have been. With all the tasks that life throws my way, the time between visits to my mom are increased. I talk to her often but sometimes only see her once every two to three weeks.

Mom's speech continuously improves. She goes to the gym almost every morning, reads every day, and is hopefully painting as well. She drives, she writes, she is a mom, a wife, a grandmother, a teacher, a motivational speaker, an artist, a survivor, and an inspiration to me and many others. She gave me the gift of life and I am very proud to be able to say she is my mom. She is my hero and I love her more than the whole wide, wide world.

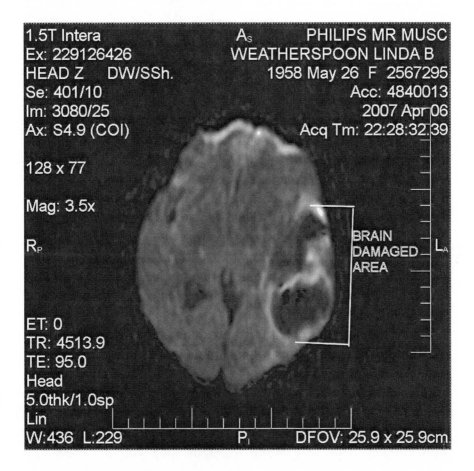

Awakening in Rehab
Linda

They say that after being in a coma, the patient doesn't just wake up and then remember everything within a few days. Brain injury and coma victims usually experience a gradual improvement in brain function. Sometimes the improvements continue over several months or even years; every person is unique. In my case, the "awakening" seemed like endless psychic pain. On the one hand I knew in my head that I could do anything I needed to do if others would get out of my way. On the other hand, all of my best attempts to do anything proved futile! There was so much confusion in my head. I had no mastery over anything in my environment. I thought that if I fought hard enough—I could will it to happen the way I needed it to. It would be two full years before I fully understood that I nearly died from the stroke and aneurysm. It was two years before I could comprehend and retain the definitions of those two words. But I do remember— and that is a good thing!

Day after day in rehab, I take baby steps toward recovery. I am seated on the patio looking at trees. *I never take time to just sit somewhere and look at the trees! I love trees, but damn! I don't want to look at trees ... I still cannot get my answers! How long has it been since I got here? Are they just drugging me up with pills for days so that I cannot protect myself? Why? Jeff would not let that happen! Please God, did I make the wrong decision again the third time and marry the wrong man? Jeff is so perfect! He is a wonderful husband and Dad. I don't understand what is going on but I have to trust that he is doing the right thing! My sons would have something to say if they thought there was a problem.*

I need to relax and try hard to think. It has to be my problem. I do not want to waste their time. I am sure they have things to do other than take care of my dilemmas.

What does this place mean? I feel fine. I am in a clean place; quiet with no one screaming with knives or guns. I am trying to think but I cannot think clearly about what to do. I always tried to think things through – even if I made wrong decisions, they were my decisions. Now, nothing is based on my thinking or decisions. I am not in charge of what is happening. Why can't I think? *Linda, stop letting yourself get all worked up like you are going off to war! Jeff and my sons know I am here, they are checking me. Why won't they just give me the answers? There has to be a reason they are not telling me the answers.*

I do not want to admit that I am not in charge of my situation. I believe in free-will and self-determination! I am asking them for the answers over and over, it seems like more than one hundred times. I am trying to ask the right questions as clearly as I can in English. *I'm not in another country, .am I? No, they would never agree with putting me anywhere but my country. Jeff and my sons know that. My sisters know that. Relax ... it must be something that happened and I just have a blank in my head. Will I always have a blank in my head? I am not sick ... am I? They did not say I was sick. If I cannot think then I should have gone to heaven when my mom was here. What good would I be, taking up space for nothing? I don't want anyone to help me. Someone to bring me food, medicine and my, my, my, my what is that called? No one should go with me to potty! Jeff married me as a wife, not a woman without a brain in a wheelchair. That is not fair to him! No, don't even try to put me in that chair! Get that away from me! I will crawl on my hands and knees. How long until I can figure it all out? I cannot paint tied down. I can't teach students and do my job!* My heart is screaming out.

Stop feeling sorry for yourself, Linda! Your mother would never feel sorry for herself in any circumstances. You know that! Look what happened to her. She didn't feel sorry for herself for six years of cancer killing her lungs! Stop crying and feeling sorry for yourself right now! Cancer killed her lungs but she held on to her heart! She would be so disappointed if you were sad! Get over it and figure out how to escape this prison! Think harder, maybe you are not thinking hard enough! Your head doesn't hurt, so think! They say you don't use all your brain, so use the rest of it, now!

No, I decide I was just going to go to Heaven. I am so happy because I miss my mother so much. I will see my older sister, the one I never got to see because I was not born yet. She had black hair, like mine, but blue eyes like the picture I have. She must have had my dad's blue eyes. My half-brothers have blue eyes, too, and they are so light and beautiful. My eyes are … I can see the color in my head but why don't I know the name of the colors? I gasp aloud. *Don't panic now, think, you will figure it out!* I could not find the words for green and brown: my eyes are hazel. *Linda, you might have to read again.* I am thinking and visualizing about what I am seeing but I cannot say it. *Stop saying "can't!"* I have to figure this out and think!

Okay, no more complaining. Get over it, Linda! You are the responsible mother of five children. You cannot give up or feel sorry for yourself. Do not think about that, change the subject and figure things out. You have got to do better than feeling sorry for yourself and crying! You have to figure out what happened, how it happened, and how to fix it. You have got to get a plan. Maybe that girl will tell me if I am nice and be patient. I like to smile but I want to have reasons to smile and I want to get on with my life.

I was outside with Jeff and I don't remember if we were alone. I think so hard to remember when I was in another world. Kind of like my mind when I am painting. The hours go by from the sun to the moon! *Do you think maybe God wants me to paint instead of teaching … would that explain it? What if I cannot paint? Well, this is scary! God surely would not do that to me.. .would He? Have I been bad? I don't remember doing anything wrong that would destroy my heart and soul?*

My thinking is so fuzzy and backwards. Looking up, I recognize a friend from Myrtle Beach, an artist from the other classroom. Oh yes, she was a teacher with me. I am glad she came to visit me and wondered why she is here. *We are not at school today?* Regardless, now I could ask her my art questions. I know she will remember but I just need to act like I am okay. I don't want to embarrass Jeff by being stupid. *Jeff has one of her paintings in a pastel?* I bought it for his birthday and he loved it. I cannot remember what it is. *Why? Just keep your mouth shut, Linda, and she will just think that you are sick but not stupid! You started the year at school and when you got sick … she finished it for you?* I am not sure that was her. If it was her, she will do a good job while I am out on leave. *See, Linda, you can relax. She needed a job.*

A flash of light in my brain – *"Yes, but I like my job … I miss … (Toby, the other Art Teacher at my school) … she just came to see me*

... is that why she cried when she was here?"   I see my mother's face and hear her words, "You cannot control that, Linda, maybe God has other plans for you ... and me ... maybe this is all part of *His* plan. You have just got to do your best like you always have and everything will be fine!"

At this point I am so glad I see my mother's face because my thoughts are scaring me and I definitely need to calm down. I do not want to be in heaven yet. She must have come for a reason. She is in Heaven and I am here. My girls are too young to be left by their mother. Jeff could handle it but we are better together as a team. *I am tired. I am so tired.*

The next day a nurse comes to take me to a place and I am not sure what she expects me to do here. There are other people like me here. She is a sweet young girl and does not seem to mind my attitude. They want me to play all kinds of games there, or write on paper, but I am embarrassed because everything I want to say or ask will not come out. I have never been in a situation like this and I do not like it. I am sure they wish I would just get better and get out! They have no idea how much I want to escape and get out of here. (Looking back now, I realize what an awful patient I was. If I was a nurse, I would avoid people like me! What a bitch! How did Jeff and my sons put up with me? If I were them, I would have just closed the door to my room and left town. Teachers, nurses, police officers and fire fighters, how do they put up with people like me every day?)

A nurse picks me up from my room. "Can I walk?" I ask.

"No, you can't. You cannot walk or talk," she says.

Did she say that and I understood or was I just responding by looking at her face? I tried to get answers every time I had the chance. How long have I been here? I am getting better but it is taking so long and I do not understand why. *"I have to hurry up and get out of here or I will lose my job or stay here forever! It is now or never will make a run for it!"*

Unexpectedly she says "you will hurt your head." That is what Larry said about my head. I do not understand because my head does not hurt and nothing else hurts except when I try to get up.

I will not tell them. *"I will show you I can walk."* With only one side of my body holding my weight I push myself up from the wheelchair. Using mostly my arms I push my body up, stand on one leg and put my left arm to the wall for balance. I do not twist or take a step. I stay here for a few minutes. *I will show them I will not be in a wheelchair.* The therapist is with me and she is so excited and lets me try a few times again. Every time that particular nurse comes I like it because I know she will not prevent me from trying. The other nurses never let me even try to stand up.

When the therapy sessions start, Jeff and Larry get to take a break from me. I bet they are glad to get away from me. I am glad Jeff is not there to see me in some of the therapy sessions. The pain is awful and it hurts worse than my knee surgery ten years ago. I want to scream but I don't want to get my physical therapist into trouble.

The next day I see the speech therapist for the first time. I ask her so many questions. *(Well, I thought I was asking questions!)* I feel she is giving me the answers but I cannot understand her responses.

"Write some words down," *she says, but everyone knows I cannot write.* I say in a way that I recognize, "I can't."

I look around the room for the first time. There is a much older man in a wheelchair a few yards away trying to move his right leg. He is hardly lifting it and is using what looks like very light weight. He has a male therapist with him. There are so many people with physical limitations. I think they must have had strokes, brain injuries, or real hard accidents. Maybe they have what happened to me. *I wish they would tell me what happened to me.*

She seems to have been gone a long time. My right arm is not moving spontaneously and neither is my right leg. I can move my left arm but it is almost like it is attached to something else. Raising my arm to my shoulder is almost impossible on my right side. *Oh no, I paint on my right side!* I am determined to try to raise my right arm, but it is an old slow raise. *It is rising so shut up complaining about it being slow! No one wants to hear you complain.* I don't feel sorry for myself. *What can I do? What did I do before, and what can I do now? How long have I been here?*

Larry leaves during my therapy to go home for a shower. The therapist leaves to get supplies for our session. Looking at the old man nearby, I see his trainer watching and waiting. The old man's movements are so slow but he continues to raise the weight. I decide to sketch the old man from my wheelchair. I cannot use my right hand, so I sketch him with my left hand, I think with a pencil. When my therapist returns about ten minutes later, she looks at me in disbelief and says, "Oh, my God!" She looks at me with tears and starts crying.

"What is wrong?" I say.

"You can draw, it looks just like him," she says.

"I didn't tell you I was an artist?" I ask.

I know that is not what came out of my mouth. I try to tell her it was just a sketch, just okay but not my best ... this left side of my body doesn't work very well. I need to sketch with my right hand."

She does not know what I am saying. Larry walks in and he is alarmed that something is wrong. He sees the sketch and he now is crying, too. *Did I do something wrong?* Then she smiles and hugs me. She asks if she can show it to everyone and hang it on the wall. I am not sure what she is saying but I see her showing it to everyone. I am embarrassed because it is pretty bad; I used my left hand and all. The drawing side of my body is like a tree stump. My right arm is like dead wood. *I am ashamed remembering what I was thinking about her!* I decide that she had no taste in art at all if she thought that was good!

Continuing My Rehabilitation

There are several people who come to visit me. They are familiar but I cannot remember where they are from or what their names are. I want to talk to them but I cannot remember how to say what I need to know. Sometimes they hug me and are so happy and sometimes they are sad and teary. At first, I have no thoughts at all about my appearance when visitors come. I do not think about whether my hair is combed or if I am wearing lipstick. That is not as important as having a visit and escaping my own thinking. Even though I don't understand much going on, it is a diversion. *At that time my hair, teeth and makeup were not in my head unless I saw specific items that prompted the memory. For example, when I saw a comb or a toothbrush, I knew what to do with the item. This was progress. At one point, I did not remember what to do with a spoon or fork. I knew what these items were, but I forgot how to use them properly.*

I love to see my girls visit. Their bright faces make me smile. Each time I have to ask them their names. My best visitors are my sisters because I am not embarrassed with my sisters! I am so glad to see them. I think this is the first time I have seen them since I got sick. *I did not remember them being at MUSC. The only thing I remember is talking to my mom and Helen on the fence of Heaven.*

With my sisters, I can finally relax and be myself. I try to say something to them and the aphasia keeps me from saying the right words. When my mouth doesn't work we make hand gestures. I try to ask Carol to describe what kind of game we play to get the information I am trying to express or understand. Carol said Charades. They try to guess what I mean and half the time I am not sure if that is true or accurate.

After several weeks, Jeff drives me back to MUSC for a follow-up appointment. It is first time since my coma that I have been here. The doctors and nurses are truly shocked when I speak to them and walk through the doors and down the halls. These are the halls where Jeff, Larry, Nathan, and all my family and friends prayed for my recovery.

Just being here again, my memory is triggered. I remember how they gave me all the personal items I needed without asking for them. They anticipated my needs. All those things I tried to go to the store and get ... they just brought me. They *knew* what I wanted. They were glad to see me and I was so happy to see them. I wanted to tell and ask them all kinds of things but my words would not come out.

Oh yes, they tried to help me as much they could. *This reminds me of a game called Pictionary.* Drawing pictures to communicate. I asked, "These are not my *(shoes). I wanted to ask who these shoes belonged to. I had to point to them because I could not remember the word for shoes. "Do* you know whose shoes they are?" They said they didn't bring them. *I haven't worn those before. I thought it had to be Jeff.* Later he told me Peggy left the shoes for me. They were like tennis shoes—but without backs. I could slide my feet into them without tie strings! Peggy knows everything. She must have been aware that those shoes were my size and very comfortable. I used those shoes at home the first year of my recovery. They were well-worn and I thanked Peggy every day from afar for leaving those shoes for me.

My sister, Roxie, comes and brings me some red-colored vegetables (tomatoes) and makes a picnic basket with bread and white mayo to put on a sandwich. She brings the best red vegetables, my favorite. She looks so pretty and does not ask me any questions. I am glad to spend time with her and I eat like a little pig. We do not talk much. She does tell me that she and her husband Arthur left Fayetteville, and came up to Myrtle Beach, to be with my girls so they could return to school after spring break. In her special aristocratic manner, Roxie turns those tomato sandwiches into what looked like a gourmet meal! That is Roxie's style. I had not been eating and she must have known.

She does not have to say anything. She just takes some bread out that she know I am watching…and learning…as she slowly spreads the mayonnaise carefully on the bread….cut the tomatoes…adds the salt and pepper just the way I like it! I do not remember how to do that. I do not think that I would understand if she told me. She has the wisdom to know that she has to teach me again how to make my favorite sandwich! She even has the reddest, sweet strawberries. It is a feast. That is a masterpiece in my damaged brain! My sisters stayed with our girls until I was "safe and out of the coma." Larry's girlfriend Kasia drove up from Florida. She stayed all month with my girls until I was released from rehab. I am so glad our family helped Jeff so he could *think* and try to save his business.

My dad comes and we just sit together and did not try to talk too much. He wears a suit and I am so glad to see him. I don't have much to say and I know it wouldn't make sense if I tried. Although there are so many things I want to ask him. I visited him the week before my aneurysm and stroke on spring break. He is still very ill with cancer and I am concerned about the distance he traveled to see me. I try to ask him if he drove or flew—but I can't say or remember the words to ask him.

My dad had chemo and was in no condition to drive there. I recognized he was sick. Although I could not speak the words, I could not thank him enough for the gift of his time and this commitment to his sick daughter.

Another friend of mine named Kimberly comes to visit and I am so embarrassed because I cannot introduce her to my dad. I cannot call her name. I know she lives in Raleigh. I think the last time I saw her was on a (cruise)…a…on the water…large water…we could not get off because the sand was there…you could not see except where we stayed for Linda Roney's … (wedding)…she got married. I want to talk to Kimberly about the things I could see in my mind but nothing is connected. She and Dad are talking enough; I am focusing on my mind trying to *see* the words but they are not fitting together. I know she has beautiful girls. I can see their pictures in my head but not the names.

The wedding memory triggers another wedding memory. I painted a picture of Linda and Rich Roney at their wedding. I can see the (portrait)….it is at their house in their…a… (bedroom*). I see the painting in my head. Can I paint like that again, the one I did for them? I tried to think about the colors, what kind I used, how to start? Can I even remember how to (frame) it? If I can't think to myself… does it mean I cannot teach children? What if I can't…I am missing parts in my mind…can they fix it, the doctors, what kind of doctor?*

Thinking of painting triggers the next memory. *I just (sketched) with my left hand because my right is not working. I have to practice it right away lifting my leg even if it hurts. It will get (atrophy). I saw people like that…I am not going to do that! I started right then from my shoulder down to my fingertips! It will not be like my friend in school…she grew up with a leg and hand smaller than her other side. I see her in my head. She had (polio). Don't even tell me I cannot try! There has got to me something better ahead.* I manage a (smile) to my (guests) so they would not worry about my strange behavior.

Do they know what is wrong with me? Will they tell me? How do I ask them? I have been here a long time and it does not make sense that I do not know. I saw the doctors and nurses but I cannot understand any word they say. Dad and Kimberly are talking to me again so I will try again to remember something that Kimberly knows so she will not think I lost my mind. It is important that I think about my job as soon as possible. My mind is going through an (inventory) what do I have to have? What is it called…you see the materials…I did not forget the important stuff but not remembering the names is really getting on my nerves. Dad and Kimberly are not like me, maybe they understand.

What about my best friend, Linda Roney? She will tell me! She will come to see me if she possibly can   I do not remember how to ask about Linda, which is my name. *What is my name (spelling?) Don't look at it on the board...think! She was getting... (married) ... they had a (ring)...I see it on her ...a ...a (finger) but I forgot what that is called...* I just let myself relax then I have so much fun listening to Kimberly and my dad. I understand a little bit and it is a sense of *deja vu* knowing I used to be a part of conversations. She gives me some lotion and some great books *(I don't think it was a book)* and magazines. That is perfect timing because I do not want- -nor could I--talk to anyone near me. *Why can't I say what I want to ask? I can get started and it runs away! This was in 2007. I finally realize I did not send thank you cards and finally sent them in 2009!*

Larry turns on the television and I think he is asking me if I wanted to watch a show. I try but it is frustrating because I cannot follow the reasoning. I am very confused. I can recognize the difference between a boy and girl most of the time. I am sensitive to lights and noise. It is irritating my nerves. Larry asks me questions and goes over to the white board in my room. He is asking me questions and drawing diagrams for me to show me what happened to my brain. This is the first time I understand what has happened to me—I remember very little of the past month. Now I understood why I was at the rehabilitation center at Waccamaw. I want to cry but I do not want to upset my son. I recognize that he must have been so sad and the time he must have taken to take care of me. He is always busy but must have dropped everything from another state (Florida) just to see me. I am sure Larry, Nathan, Jeff, and God looked out for me or I would not be alive. I do not retain the information Larry told me about the stroke. It came into my head—I understood it—then it left. I do not remember it again.

My head does not hurt anymore and I did not die...but that meant I would make sure I did everything possible to keep from being a (burden). There are so many questions I wanted to ask Larry but again I forget the words. I can recognize my brain and the damage he draws on the board. The pictures make sense! Doctors and nurses should show pictures to their patients. Maybe they did but I do not remember seeing them. The words and sounds did not make as much sense right now. Larry must suspect that the sketch makes sense to me. I immediately stop fighting everyone and understand Jeff and my sons do not want to be here anymore than I do. It would be so selfish to keep them any longer! I become as helpful as I possibly can until they try to wash my hair!

I remember we have parts of our brains that we don't even use. I will just have to use that part that I have not used. *"Here I come brain...move over so I can fill up that brain!"* For the first time I have the thought I might not be able to teach again.....I cannot think like that.....my mother never would feel sorry for herself.....maybe for a moment...I was alive.....don't people usually die when this happens....I have always been proud of my sons....and looking at them now....I wonder how could I have created such wonderful sons.

The next day Jeff takes me back down to the chair place outside to sit in the sunshine. I ask him about his school (he was getting ready to start medical school at MUSC in Charleston) but I do not understand his answers. Why is that hard? He speaks English. I speak English and...and...*(Spanish).* I used to say both! I do not like this place and they probably don't like me either because I complain or have so many questions they're not answering. I have to be smart... I have an advanced ... (degree). Why can't I stop and remember the names and how to do anything? I need to get better and fast! What can I do? I feel like crawling under that a ...a... a (rock). See, I am looking at a rock and I can't even remember what it is! It looks like they could answer the simple ones....why?

I think I understand Jeff when he says some of my family and friends will be visiting. I am happy to hear that. Maybe I can figure out the right questions to ask them. Maybe they know why I was ready to scream! I continue to control my anger for my family. I feel like I was insane. If I didn't know what happened, how the hell was I supposed to solve my (dilemma)? Everyone seems to be fine and happy! I am the only one who is angry. I had to control that when I was a manager!

The anger I felt as a manager led me down another trail. I escaped in my mind back to Kelly Springfield (Goodyear) where I was a production manager. There were a few people working for me who I could not stand but they never knew it. The rest of the people were like my family, especially the ones I worked with for fifteen years. Now I feel like I am out of control and can't think! Just how long do they expect for me to sit in this chair? I will crawl until I can walk. I will not turn like ...like....my *(history)*...where is it? I cannot even remember her name! She is in my brain but how can I forget her name? I see her paintings, her eye brows that .... connect over her eyes. This is so sad! How can I teach art history if I can't even remember the name of a famous painter? Damn it!

My students would never forget her on exams—but not because of her art. I always tried to find something about the artist that was interesting and *(unique)* to help them relate. High school students never forget how her eyebrows look, especially teenagers. Now I can't even think what that is called...the name of her paintings.... the name of her husband!! That is a simple name and I cannot keep my job! I need to start right now and learn again...again....again? That sounds so....so.....impossible. *See there you go again being negative! Do not let that happen. Think of Jeff, your kids, and your family....they love you....they are happy...you have to be strong like your mother was.*

(Writing this today, I know I was trying to remember Frida Kahlo (1907-1954). I looked at my study plans for my class. I used her work in my classes because I wanted the Hispanic students to know about a very famous female Mexican artist to make a cultural connection. She had such a wonderful body of work and colorful life. Mexico's most famous female artist, she led a turbulent of physical and emotional pain following a tragic bus accident and the inability to have children. She married another artist named Diego Rivera—he was a famous muralist and they had a turbulent relationship. Only forty seven years old when she died, she painted over two hundred self-portraits, mostly from her bed. Today, she is ranked one of the top artists of the twentieth century. *She portrayed herself as a peasant in her work. She did not like the idea of being referred to as an expressionist. Most artists I have talked to or read agree that her paintings are expressionist and focused on the folklore of her country.* I believe her works have realism but have dimensions of emotions and intensity. There are distortions of line, shape, and color. She reminds me of Edvard Munch—evoking powerful emotions. Now I have to re-read

95

this slowly but I still have trouble telling you what I just wrote.)

Yes, I feel like screaming—I am frozen in my body and my brain is not working right. I can barely move. I have to practice it right away lifting my leg even if it hurts. I do not want to atrophy. I saw people like that...I am not going to do that! I start right then from my shoulder down to my fingertips! It will not be like my friend in school...she grew up with a leg and hand smaller than her other side. I see her in my head. She had polio. Don't even tell me I cannot try! There has got to be something better than this for me. I manage a smile to my guests so they don't worry about my behavior. *Do they know what is wrong with me? Will they tell me? How do I ask that?* I have been here a while.

Speech Therapy—or Not!

Shortly after I return home, Larry takes me to another speech therapy session. I cannot drive. My vision is missing the picture of the whole car. I can only see the center of the car but not the sides; I have field of vision damage, (some of which persists to this day) and I cannot understand or read. I hear my family and the nurses talking. I only pick up a few words of a regular conversation they are having. But I cannot comprehend. I asked her again. "Why didn't they tell me I had a stroke?" I am upset when I look straight at her. She says "we *have been telling you* that but you did not understand it." I have to stop and think about what has been happening. Some of the pieces in my mind start to fit together. I start to understand for the first time I had a stroke and that was the only time that I felt sad. I start treating people better. It is my problem and I believe they are trying to help me. I do not comprehend aneurysm but I do understand stroke and see other people who had *strokes. I apologize to her that I did not understand. She said she knew and she had doing therapy speech for thirty years. I felt sad and stupid.*

I keep going to speech therapy. After a month, she tells me how my brain is working—and I do not agree. I know how my brain is working—and she does not listen to me. She says it again, "Your brain does not work like that." She asks me questions and I remember the second part of the answer but not the first. When I tell her how I can see the second part in my head—but not the first—she continues to tell me my brain does not work like that. We are playing Scrabble and I see the second part and put it down on the board. Like a child she takes the letters back and only brings the letters out and I have to make a word. I do not know why my mind sees the second part of the word first and then I figure out the first part. I cannot understand. She stops playing that game and I took it as a (punishment). I am not sure what she means but I am fair and not hard to work now. She starts playing solitaire. She says to do it at home every day but not on the computer. I do not like that game….I would rather continue with the Scrabble.

When I get home I tell Jeff, "There must be a reason she wants us to do this every day—but I am only going to do solitaire once a week and the rest of the time I will use the Scrabble. Jeff tries to encourage me to stick with it. But he knows me well enough to know I am going to do what I thought was best for me. He does not try to make me change my mind. He knows it would be futile. I keep going to therapy, but about the third time she tells me that "Your brain does not work like that" I make a decision. When I get home I sent her a card to thank her for all of her help but I believe I can (accomplish) my own mind.

Larry quits his management job in Florida and moves to Myrtle Beach to help Jeff, the girls, and me. We have a 1 room "guest house" on our property I am to use for an art studio. Larry and Kasia stay in the guest house to help out. They are planning to take care of me in a wheelchair, drive me to therapy and to doctor appointments. I refuse the wheelchair and tell them where to put it—in the attic! Jeff has to get back to work because the business is sinking with the economy, the medical bills are mounting, and my salary is going to be discontinued. Jeff does everything he can, keep a roof over our head, food on the table--and holds us all together.

Larry makes a series of books in 3 inch binders he thinks will be helpful to teach me names of household and food items. He cuts pictures out of magazines—using vegetables and furniture first. These are words I need to learn to function! I cannot remember the words—but I can remember the pictures. That is the best thing he could have done. I study it every day…oranges, apples, cake, chair, and table. How smart and simple—and the little book helps me learn those words without using a kindergarten book. Jeff and Larry do not think I should stop therapy but I am the one in those sessions with her and I am the only one who knows how I think. I think the last half of the word first! I cannot explain it but that is how I think. Had she not handled it the way she did by scolding me or talking down to me— I could have tolerated it. Maybe that is the way her books taught her— but that is not how I see words. She disrespected me. Maybe it would have been better if I just asked for another therapist—but I could not think to do that at the time.

After a while, I am able to go out of the house for dinner, or walking around. I call Carmelita and Elena "Brain One" and "Brain Two." Whenever I need a brain for an answer—they pop up and answer for me. They do an excellent job and never make me feel stupid. Any word I cannot remember—they say it for me. It is as if they could read my mind—what little I have left! They are, in fact, my brains!

Even after six months, they always have to speak for me when I am ordering off a menu, or we are going through a drive-through to pick up food. My vocabulary and speech improve, but I am very slow formulating questions and answers. Being so slow is embarrassing because the whole line has to wait for me. The speech and language condition is called "aphasia." I have to visualize the word to picture the letters in my mind. Then I sort through the alphabet to find the right letters to drop into the right places. This helps me recover the first half of the word. Once I capture the last part of the word—then the first part comes more easily. I usually have a problem with the first word. When I am out socially and go silent, then one of the girls with me will finish my sentences. Jeff seldom finishes my sentences. He does not want to humiliate me. He just listens and waits to see if I can figure it out. If I ask for help he answers for me. He is very patient.

It is annoying and embarrassing when I need to go out in public and cannot communicate properly. I hate to explain to anyone that I cannot remember my answers because I had a stroke. Being independent by nature, it is hard to accept that I have a significant communication disorder. People who work with the public are usually so helpful— but they become impatient or confused when I cannot give them my zip code, or my street address without handing them a piece of paper and pointing to the words.

I have good days and bad days trying to remember conversations. I try to figure out why this occurs. Is it better in the morning? Is it better before or after going to the gym? Is it better before or after a meal? Do any foods I eat make the condition better or worse? I would love to know from someone how to prevent the *aphasia pause!*

It is almost two years before I can fully realize and make sense of what had happened to me. There are still gaps in my knowledge and Jeff says I have misperceptions about some of the facts surrounding the causes of the stroke. At times I think I am losing my mind. There are times I want to give up. I have to accept the fact that I may not be the teacher that I used to be. My son, Larry, and my husband, Jeff, frequently try to tell me this in the most caring way they can. They try to tell me that I may not be back in a classroom—but I can still paint. So just paint! I retort with anger, "You mean **just fail!**"

We have some hard days after that. I intend to teach again and that is all there was to it. This is before I find out that I had brain damage from the stroke and cannot remember most of the names of the basics of art history but I refuse to accept failure. No one can tell me different! I insist to go back to the high school and talk to the principal. Jeff is wonderful. I guess he knows better than to tell me I can't even though I can't drive. He knows the principal will understand the situation and talk with me. I just think I am sick and I will get better…but I do not know what is going on in my brain…and what is left for me to function with! They realize I was not ready to accept defeat. They understand that it will take time for me to make peace with my situation. The principal from North Myrtle Beach High School visited me in the hospital but I didn't remember it. Some of the teachers I worked with visited me, too. I have no recollection of their visits.

Teachers are amazing people. My daughters' teachers at Seaside Elementary made cards and comforted Elena and Carmelita the best they could. I tell everyone I am going to start back to school. I know if I don't go back I will lose my job and I absolutely love North Myrtle Beach High School, the students, and teachers. I had planned to be there the rest of my life. My friend Toby Brenizer taught art with me. I realize now that she knew I would probably never come back and that is why she cried. At the time, I could not understand why she was crying. I was happy to see her and I knew I would get better. I had no idea about the extent of my brain damage or any awareness of the long struggle ahead of me to relearn basic activities of daily living. I could not comprehend the length of time that had elapsed since I had the stroke—much less how much time it would take to be functional again.

Linda's Recovery
Jeff

The long weeks in MUSC had us all ready to be near home. Linda transferred to Waccamaw Surgical Rehabilitation Clinic by ambulance, which was only a few miles from our house. Larry rode with her in the ambulance and Linda was assigned a room. My friend Brian, a certified physician's assistant, and his partner Dr. Wilkins ran the rehab facility. I knew that Brian would go the extra mile for Linda and he absolutely did everything in his power to help her while she was there. In the beginning, after reviewing her MUSC medical records and conducting an initial examination, Brian told me that I should prepare for Linda to be in the rehab facility for a long time.

It was an understandable assumption. Linda still wasn't communicating verbally although as each day passed she seemed more cognizant of events around her. She couldn't walk and the right side of her body was only just beginning to wake up. Larry and I were scared to death that with Linda's stubborn nature she would try to get up and end up falling and hitting her head so one of us was within arm's reach of her almost all of the time.

The focus at Waccamaw was therapy: physical, occupational, and speech for Linda. The therapists kept meticulous records of even the smallest amount of progress. In the beginning Linda mostly did group therapy with other stroke survivors. They seemed to constantly try to keep Linda busy with different activities and tests.

- Looking back now, I can see that Linda's recovery occurred in several areas: Physical – from paralysis as well as visual and hearing impairment on her right side, Linda has improved to the point to where she is able to work out several times weekly. There is nothing visible to the outside observer that would

100

indicate Linda suffered a severe brain injury and stroke.

- Mental – Linda's mind was very cloudy and confused when she got to the rehab center. Aside from her language difficulties, she processed information very slowly and didn't understand many basic things. Over the six years since the injury, she has had amazing improvement in this area. Through the course of writing this book, Linda got progressively more focused and effective with her writing skills. Linda's emotional control has probably been the slowest part of her recovery; today, she is quickly and easily moved to very strong displays of emotion.

- Verbal Comprehension – In the first years after the stroke, Linda could only follow one conversation and her comprehension was limited. If there were multiple speakers, around a dinner table for example, Linda would be overwhelmed and wouldn't get any of the conversation at all. Today, Linda participates regularly in any single- or multi-person conversation. Occasionally she has to concentrate or work out a specific word, but it is generally seamless.

How was Linda able to make such a comeback? A quick look at her brain MRI shows massive damage; however, today people who didn't know her before are surprised to find out she had a stroke.

Linda's recovery began with the doctors and therapists telling us that due to the extent of the brain damage she would have a very limited recovery of speech and movement. We were told that Linda's recovery would peak at about six months from the injury. In other words, they told us that the vast majority of her expected recovery would already have taken place at the six-month mark, and then there would be very slight and gradual improvement for a period of one to two years. After that, the window for improvement would have pretty much closed. In a few weeks they sent us home from the inpatient rehab center with a walker, a cane, and a potty chair.

Linda took one look at these and shook her head. She made it clear she wasn't going to use any of those items. As she began taking outpatient speech and physical therapy classes, Linda came home with copies of the words and definitions they had worked on that day and slowly built up a large file folder. She kept every piece of paper they gave her and spent hours puzzling over an individual sheet.

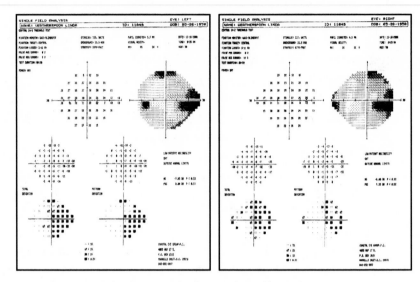

Black spots indicate the affected areas

Her vision was terrible; not only did she have significant field of vision impairment, but there was a delay in seeing part of each image. As Linda explains it now, she would see an image, and then a fraction of a second later another part of the image would fade in and suddenly appear. The doctors told us that optic nerve damage accounted for the delay of a portion of each visual image. This went on constantly for her and continues to this day, although over the years it improved somewhat. Linda also improved in her ability to interpret the confusing images her eyes showed her.

Larry put together several large photo albums with pictures of everyday items cut out from dozens of magazines. For example, he would cut out a picture of a cookie, put it in the album and label it with a piece of paper that said COOKIE on it. He Then we took post it notes and covered the house with them, labeling each item. They were everywhere!

Linda studied all day, every day. When she improved and began to learn her ABC's again and tried to spell and read words, Linda began to realize something had been changed in the way that her brain processed written words. She had become dyslexic! (Linda, of course, didn't know this word yet, and it was some time before she could effectively communicate it to us.) Linda would always say "I see the second part, but not the first."

The speech therapist, a very nice older lady, vehemently disagreed with Linda about how her brain had changed. "That's just not how the brain works," she told Linda. Frustrated, Linda eventually told me she didn't want to continue with the speech therapy.

Linda set herself up study periods every day. She would get up in the morning, try to help out with basic housework, and then settle into a daily routine of study. She had me make copies of all of her speech therapy paperwork and she filled in the blanks on them daily for hours at a time. We went out and bought basic children's study guides and flash cards and she studied them endlessly. Previously a high school art teacher with a bachelor's degree in studio art and a master of arts in teaching, Linda had tons of textbooks and art dictionaries. She was fiercely determined to someday teach art again and she studied those books constantly.

Linda also sketched and painted on blank greeting card stock, and did small paintings in oil and acrylic. We called this art therapy and believe it had as much to do with Linda's recovery as anything. In essence, Linda was in recovery school all day, every day.

I thought that over time Linda's devotion to study and her determination to recover her mind would diminish, but it never happened. To this day Linda studies for hours. I remember she started trying to read basic words out of children's primary school books. She made many copies of her speech therapy handouts and went through them endlessly.

Eventually she transitioned to the daily newspaper. At first Linda struggled for hours to try and read the headlines. Over a long period of time (a year or two) she began to try to read selected articles within each day's paper, mostly front page articles. Then after another year or two she could read most of the newspaper each day. She spent time focusing on areas in which she knew she was deficient. Written or cartoon humor and idiomatic expressions were (and still are) very hard for Linda to understand as well as she used to. Each day she would read the editorial cartoons and the horoscopes to see if she could puzzle out their meanings.

Once her reading comprehension was at a basic level, Linda went back to her school books, art books, and lesson plans. She quickly realized that re-learning terminology would be very difficult considering her current state of abilities, but she didn't let that stop her. She spent hours every day going through materials and then trying them out.

Linda got almost manic about her studying. Even though it became nearly impossible to see daily, weekly, or even monthly improvement after the first two to three years, it was still obvious on a yearly basis that Linda's recovery was continuing. This was fuel for her fire. Many times I went to bed to the sight of her sitting in a chair with her glasses perched on her nose and woke up in the middle of the night to find Linda had fallen asleep in the chair studying.

Today as I write this, more than six years after her brain injury, Linda has graduated to study on the computer and the Internet. I came home today from work and she was laughing to herself and looked at me helplessly, "I spent an hour putting together an email with some pictures for Larry and then I deleted it ... I don't know why I deleted it." Her response was typical, she sat at the computer for another hour, redid everything, and sent the email.

This is my Linda. The most determined human being I have ever met, she is also one of the kindest, sweetest souls one could ever hope to be around. It is an awesome privilege to be her husband.

Recovery at Home
Linda

Putting the sequence of events in order is impossible for me without medical records in front of me. I lose new information quickly—even when I spend hours memorizing, drilling, and repeating it. In April of 2007, I experienced the nightmare of an intra-cerebral bleed from the ruptured aneurysm. I developed a venous thrombosis from lupus anticoagulant with severe neurological consequences that I cannot begin to describe.

I remained in a coma for almost a month. Significant damage occurred in one-third of my brain. I was on life support for weeks and the various doctors were not enthusiastic about my chances for recovery. They pronounced that should I live by some miracle after removal of the life support; I would live in a vegetative state. I can only imagine their heartbreak and fear. My husband was faced with the loss of his wife—the love of his life. I do not doubt that he would have given his life for mine. My children were losing their mother, and my little girls were too young to lose their mommy.

As I have shared through the chapters of this book—I survived. After all the agony my family endured—I was released. I was transported by ambulance to rehab in Myrtle Beach—I was getting a step closer to home. My mind was not functional. I was disoriented as to person, place, or time. I could not speak coherently. Obviously, I had no capacity for critical or abstract thinking. Despite the bleak situation, my husband, five children, family, and dearest friends remained hopeful and determined to help me recover. I was frightened, confused, and non-compliant. I relied more on my impaired thinking than on anyone else. I intuitively knew that I could trust myself but could I really trust the knowledge and motives of others? I knew my husband and children loved me—they wanted to take care of me—I simply could not put the recent past into perspective. I could not let go of the few things I could still control.

Indeed, I survived rehab "my way," and pleaded to return home as soon as possible. My welcome home party was bittersweet. My thinking was fuzzy and distorted. I had no physical strength and very little stamina. I could not give myself any slack for having been in bed almost two months!

My family could worried that another stroke would take my life during the first year—the odds of that happening were very high. They initially walked around me on eggshells. In his infinite wisdom, Jeff instinctively knew that *"I was in there—somewhere"* and that he needed to treat me with all the respect and patience he could muster. My children followed his lead. They could not do enough for me. I appreciated it and resented it. I could no longer do things for myself. That was a hard pill to swallow.

I continued to focus on the recovery of my cognitive and physical deficits. It was slow, painful, and frustrating work. My physical deficits were restored relatively quickly, with the exception of speech and vision. My family did their very best to create a rich learning environment for me. Elena created mobiles to hang above my bed showing the names and faces of my family members. Larry pasted flash cards on every item in the kitchen. I resisted the speech pathology sessions. There was a clash of wills between me and the therapist on teaching methodology—at least that was my belief. In truth, I thought she was patronizing and dismissive of my efforts to describe the way my brain was working. I soon refused to attend those sessions.

Despite good progress in physical functions, the progress with cognition was very slow. In addition, my health status seemed to be deteriorating. I was taking up to fifteen medications daily. Blood pressure monitoring was recorded hourly for several weeks and three times daily for months. My legs itched and burned unmercifully. My extremities were painfully swollen—my ankles and feet looked hideous. I tried to relearn words and names, but when writing or reading with concentration I fell asleep. I began walking like Frankenstein, my hair was falling out, and I was clinically depressed. It was the perfect storm for a second stroke.

2008 Recovery - Adrenal Gland Surgery

In April of 2008, it was time for a repeat CT scan on the adrenal tumor. I was anxiety ridden, afraid that on top of everything else that was happening to me I would be diagnosed with adrenal cancer like my father. Because of the stroke the doctors had placed my concerns about the tumor on the adrenal gland on the back burner. It had been thirteen months since the last scan rather than six months. During that time, the tumor grew significantly. Various doctors treated my symptoms of weight gain, hair loss, abnormal fat distribution, and uncontrollable blood pressure without finding the reason for my problems. I felt that most doctors believed I should be glad to be alive rather than complaining about my 'minor' symptoms.

Oddly, I was never given a referral to an endocrinologist. Today, looking back, this is inconceivable to me knowing that I had a tumor on an endocrine gland and all kinds of symptoms that were pointing to an endocrine problem. Eventually, I was given a referral to a urologist. On my very first appointment the urologist told me he felt I had a clear endocrine disorder. The results of a dexamethasone suppression test were positive for Cushing's Syndrome. This diagnosis set off an immediate flurry of activity. The tumor on my adrenal gland had evidently interfaced with my adrenal gland and was causing abnormal production of the cortisol hormone. It had to come out immediately! Surgery took place as soon as it could be scheduled. It was a long, difficult surgery and because I needed constant blood thinners I was forced into recovery for quite some time in the hospital. The good news was that the pathology report on the adrenal adenoma evidenced no malignancy, and over the next few months most of my Cushing's Syndrome symptoms abated.

Looking back, I am somewhat bitter and angry about what I feel are missteps in my medical treatments, both before and after my aneurysm and stroke. The blood pressure spikes in all probability caused the ruptured aneurysm in my brain No referral or follow-up was ordered by my doctor. I was a walking time bomb for another stroke—and it would be fatal. Instead of an immediate referral to an endocrinologist, I went through several doctors before I ran into the urologist who diagnosed my condition. I am confident that an endocrinologist would have diagnosed Cushing's Syndrome *before* I had the aneurysm. These missteps had life changing ramifications for me and for my family.

To my *God in Heaven*, neither Jeff nor I were made aware that the adrenal gland tumor diagnosed four months before the stroke *was likely the underlying cause of my stroke.*

2009 Recovery - Medication Madness

I was doubly motivated to improve my physical stamina because I hoped to take a trip with my mother-in-law. I still experienced so many side effects from medications that affected my cognition, mobility, and balance. I was walking like Frankenstein due to the side effects of one of my medications—with some spasticity. I redoubled my efforts at the gym and worked out harder to grow my strength and stamina. I took kickboxing and exercises that helped with balance. I had the strength of an ox by the time we left on our trip, although I still experienced dizziness and confusion.

I desperately tried to improve my memory of art history. I studied several hours every single day without exception. Despite hours and hours of study and note taking, it was frustrating and demoralizing that I could not retrieve the information the very next day. I could remember historical data, identify paintings and artists, but not "at will." The memories just "appeared" in my thoughts. These bits of information came to me in free thinking but not when I needed them to make a point or share the information with another person. It was during this period of time that I gradually realized that I would not be able to return to the classroom. I had lost the ability to respond spontaneously. *How could I answer a student's question?* I also lost the ability to speak extemporaneously. *How could I teach effectively if I had to standup and read the entire lecture?* I did not want to be a robot instructor. I would despise being inadequate in the classroom more than I ached to return to my profession. Like Scarlett O'Hara—*I will think about that tomorrow! I must focus on what I CAN do or I will lose my mind.*

By this time in my recovery, my grammar and enunciation were vastly improved. The aphasia pause was frequent resulting in poor syntax and most often I mixed up my pronouns. At times people just looked at me quizzically as if I were speaking in another language. On the surface, it was difficult for people to know during a short conversation that I had suffered a stroke. *When* questions were posed—I had extreme difficulty answering. *What is your address? What is your phone number? What is your date of birth?* Although I could not answer the questions, I could produce the information by handing them my driver's license or other written sources. I stopped being embarrassed and often replied, "I am sorry I cannot answer you I had a stroke." I tried to avoid situations where I would be put on the spot.

Aphasia: I wrote this down from the dictionary and put it in my own words so I can remember. Then I study the meaning again and again. I understand it at the time—but I cannot retain it. *"Aphasia is a medical condition in which you are unable to use or understand some words, caused by damage to the brain."* I notice it most when I remember exactly what to say—but aphasia prevents it and does not allow my sentence. Sometimes I can see the words when I close my eyes.

I hated feeling like a loser. I realized that I had to shake that attitude. Without taking the risks of humiliation I would continue to be dependent on my family members. My ego was costing me my independence. I would rather be embarrassed than be an albatross around the neck. I also discovered that most people are kind and helpful when I explain the problem. I no longer hesitate to say, "I'm sorry, I had a stroke. Can you help me?" It was hard at first and more than once I had to call Jeff and hand my cell phone to the person asking me questions. Jeff always took the time to help me—always. No matter what he was doing or where he was, Jeff was there for me at the other end of the phone. Not normally the most patient of men, he most often showed the patience of Job.

To the consternation of my entire family, I began driving when I felt my vision had improved. Although I was a very careful driver, I frequently got lost. I guess you could say I was "directionally challenged." A GPS was not helpful to me. In fact, I was more confused because I could not confirm what was being said to me. As usual, I called Jeff and he directed me home. He must have memorized every street in Myrtle Beach because his response time was immediate. *How does any man have that much patience?*

It was not until 2012 that we were fully aware of the consequence of the misdiagnosis back in 2006. I saw an endocrinologist, who reviewed my medical records. I thought my heart would explode with grief. I could accept a genetic or environmental health crisis. I could not accept that I was tested, the results and diagnosis were recorded in my records, but my doctor failed to refer me properly for treatment. While there is no guarantee that being referred to an endocrinologist in 2006 or early 2007 would have prevented my injuries, it is very hard for me to wonder how different things might have been: *If—if only*—if I had been referred to the proper specialist—I might still be in my classroom. *Oh, my God, I cannot believe this could have happened.*

"In the beginner's mind
there are many possibilities—

in the expert's mind
there are few."

Zen Mind—Beginning Mind

3
LIFE AFTERWARD

Italy 2009
Peggy Weatherspoon

Linda's recovery from near-death was a humbling experience for everyone who loved her. We take so much for granted—like missing those golden opportunities to share the gifts of time with someone we care about. We lose so many opportunities to make new memories. After two and a half years, she had recovered enough for me to deliver on my promise to take her on the art tour of her dreams. She chose the Italian Masters—we were going to Italy!

Before we could go on our trip, Linda had a long road of recovery ahead of her. Jeff was my main source of information for the next year regarding Linda's progress. Thus, much of what I am writing is filtered through his eyes. In the first months of her recovery, the family was quite aware that Linda was high risk for a second stroke. They were cautioned that the next one would be fatal. Strokes are still the leading cause of death of individuals over age 45 in the United States, especially women. For the first year, her blood pressure was erratic and uncontrolled despite medications. She was taking up to fifteen medications daily and the side effects often led to additional prescriptions. The aphasia and her communication skills were significantly impaired. The prognosis was promising with the help of a speech language pathologist. With intensive effort and therapies, more rehabilitation was possible with any hoped-for improvements peaking at two years post-stroke.

Her language disorder was embarrassing for her and she tried to overcome the deficits. She was unable to speak or write in a coherent manner. I believe this was called "receptive aphasia" characterized by her inability to comprehend language or speak with appropriately meaningful words. Her comprehension was hit or miss. She seemed bewildered much of that time. Jeff said at nine months post-stroke, Linda addressed every Christmas card and wrote a personal sentence in each one. It took her more than one hour to write each card. She asked Jeff or one of the girls to proof her writing for errors. If she made a mistake, she would painstakingly rewrite the entire card rather than crossing something out. She was still partially blind in half of her visual field.

When Linda sent me notes or cards, her careful penmanship was good. Her written expression was a bit confusing with syntax, phonetic spelling, and word placement errors. But I could always understand her meaning and loved getting her drawings and notes that year. I was also humbled by her tenacity and the amount that she cared enough to make the huge effort. That was the essence of Linda—she would do her routine come hell or high water.

About a year later, Linda developed profound restless leg syndrome and skin lesions on her lower extremities. She experienced extreme swelling and stiffness in her joints. She would say, "I walk like Frankenstein!" Subsequently, she became severely depressed, which is common following a stroke. Emotionally, she could not accept depression as a medical consequence of her brain trauma. Her quality of life was suffering and I know that she held so much inside to protect her family. She firmly believed it was secondary to all the medications, but she realized at some level that she needed help. She did not understand the concept of reactive depression. Except for family, she lost everything that was important to her. Of course she was depressed. When I talked to her, she seemed to think of depression as a weakness of her character. I had the sense that she was also comparing her short-term condition to her mother's life-long condition. She absolutely refused anti-depressant medication. She suffered months of internal anguish.

Linda was always independent and capable. When she first came home, she needed help with her most personal activities of daily

112

living—bathing, toileting, dressing, grooming, and transferring. During the first year she improved rapidly in self-care, but she had significant limitations with the instrumental activities of daily living—cooking, shopping, transportation, light housekeeping, laundry. It was humiliating for her to be reliant on others. Knowing Linda, I cannot imagine her internal hell.

Linda was also unable to lose any of the excess weight she gained in the year prior to the stroke. Despite going to the gym, rehab, and a healthy diet of less than 1,000 calories per day, she was 75 pounds heavier than she had ever been in her life. Her doctors attributed the excess weight to medications and middle age. Her appearance was not on their radar screen, but it was hard on her. Regardless of the cause, Linda's sense of being an attractive, desirable woman was shattered. It was completely demoralizing for a beautiful woman who always wore a size eight—even after giving birth to five children—to weigh almost 200 pounds.

She was more ashamed that she was experiencing hair loss hid it from others—she was completely demoralized. Life was so painful at times that she almost gave up the battle. I don't know all the forces at play, but surely from the love and support and encouragement of her league of supporters Linda managed to trudge through those awful days.

It was two and a half years before Linda finally reached a level of functioning conducive to international travel. Her doctors cleared her to go and we began planning our two weeks in Italy!

Once all the hurdles were cleared, tickets purchased, bags packed, I was terrified. *Holy crap—what am I doing?* I thought. *I am taking a woman to Italy who is recovering from a stroke and aneurysm who cannot communicate her phone number or home address, who takes more than a dozen medications daily, and who has such a profound fear of flying she suffers panic attacks! Are you crazy?*

I had a million questions for Jeff about her abilities and tried to plan for every contingency. Jeff dripped with self-assuredness. He had walked through so many phases of her illnesses that he was on happy street with her current condition. He was completely relaxed and comfortable that she was physically and mentally up for the trip of her dreams. "I haven't seen her so happy since she had the stroke! This will be great for her! Stop worrying!" he said. *Easy for him to say!*

She traveled alone from Myrtle Beach to Atlanta, where I met her plane. We were happy and excited to see each other and both in disbelief that we were really taking this trip. We boarded our flight to Milan and settled in two aisle seats across from each other. She never uttered a word or smiled after we boarded. She closed her eyes during takeoff and I braced for a panic attack that never came. She ate dinner inflight and closed her eyes to rest. I decided that God was in charge—He would be awake all night—so I could go to sleep!

Each time I woke up during the night, I saw her sketching with pencils. She sketched all night long. She frequently rubbed her legs and knees. I noticed her legs sporadically bounced up and down from the ball of her foot to her knee. She tried to explain it was a form of restless leg syndrome. She finished one sketch and started another throughout the flight. The only thing I remember her saying is, "I can't believe we are doing this."

For two weeks our communications were hampered by two things: her aphasia and my deafness in one ear. We repeated ourselves a lot to understand and to be understood. When Linda wanted to tell me something, she looked down at the floor, held her arms out from her waist and made hand gestures as if she was filling in the blanks of a word. She would say, "It ends with *n-c-e* and it has an *r* at the top." Then I tried to think of the context and throwing out possible words until one stuck. She was so happy when I got one right. She was trying to communicate "renaissance." We engaged in a lot of charades and when that didn't work we went into gales of laughter. Somehow we managed with good humor! When she really wanted me to know something and she didn't succeed at it, she would say, "That's okay, Jeff will fix that."

Having worked as a professional gerontologist for thirty years, I knew a lot about people with physical and mental impairments. I taught courses in dementia and helped develop numerous programs to serve individuals who were at risk of institutionalization due to physical and mental illnesses. Although I had the expertise, most of my confidence went out the window when I realized I was handling precious cargo that belonged to my son and grandchildren! My anxiety would soar and I would pray for right thinking and right action. All I had to do was enjoy this gift of time and trust God to do the rest.

A number of things come to mind related to her recovery on the trip that are both comical and groundbreaking! I was impressed by her strength of character. She was willing to take risks and step out there despite her apparent anxieties. She overcame her fears with a lot of positive self-talk. ("If I died right now I would die happy! Well, I just can't sit at home like a loser all my life!") The first two days, she smiled a great deal and shook her head a lot. Every hour or so she would say, "I can't believe we are doing this—is this real?"

She had a lot of trepidation the first day and evening. I could tell she was tense and didn't know what to expect next. We went for a long stroll around Lake Como and I treated her to her first gelato. She loved it. She was a little unsteady on some of the cobblestone streets and pathways, so we pretty much walked arm-in-arm. It is the sweetest memory for me. I was as nervous as she was in the beginning. I worried about something happening to her and me not having the knowledge to help her. I caught myself getting fearful and watching her like a hawk. I remembered the saying, "To the extent you have faith—there is no room for fear." The solution is always the same for me—prayer fixes me—my fears and anxieties are always quieted. I think when I finally relaxed—Linda relaxed. Funny how we sense things without any words being spoken.

In Milan, we drove through the bustling city of narrow streets, rail cars, miniature automobiles, and hundreds of motorcycles zipping by in every direction. The speed and excitement made her dizzy. She could not look down from the coach to the street level without turning green so she would close her eyes or look at the ceiling of the tour bus. No matter how bad she felt, she always looked at me and tried to smile. Money was a major challenge for Linda. Jeff had mentioned before left that she could not manage her money well. That news was a real thriller when we converted dollars to the euro! Now we were both impaired! My math is dreadful and Linda had no idea how to adapt to the exchange rate. When she was making purchases I tried to stay close because she would hold out her euros and let the cashier take the desired amount.

When we arrived at the famous Galleria in Milan, Linda became a different person when she set foot inside. She was grinning from ear to ear, animated and wide-eyed. I took pictures of Prada and the designer showrooms and she took pictures of the floor tiles and the architecture and glass ceilings. Built in 1867, the Galleria is an enormous glass-roofed shopping arcade lined with elegant shops and high-end restaurants—just my style! Linda was awestruck with the amazing architecture. The intricate floor mosaics depicted each of the cities that formed the united Italy. Built in a cross shape, the Galleria links the squares of the Duomo and La Scala. When she saw the towering Gothic Cathedral, she broke out in a huge grin and said, "We weren't going to see this I thought! Did you know I didn't know?" She knew a great deal about this magnificent structure. It is the largest Gothic cathedral in the world and took 500 years to build. There were more than 3,000 statues and I think she photographed every single one. She was so excited.

In that moment, witnessing this palpable transformation, I knew that something magical was happening inside her. She was pointing and chattering like a magpie and she knew what she was talking about, although I couldn't understand most of it. I just smiled a lot and tried to help her explain by supplying a list of words or just being patient. It was worth the entire trip to witness her epiphany.

Linda was walking in the clouds by the time we reached La Scala Opera House though perhaps a little jet lagged. She loved the magnificent architecture and elegant interior. She just plopped down on a large red velvet chair and studied the room. She was smiling ear to ear and I knew she was thinking about the Gothic Cathedral. She finally said, "I think it is heaven and I have died."

We had a fantastic trip that afternoon to Lugano, Switzerland. We landed in the heart of the village known for Swiss chocolate. We enjoyed our chocolate at a sidewalk café. We noticed the most beautiful women walking their dogs. The ladies wore designer coats and amazing purses and boots. I loved the chic apparel and Linda loved the dogs! The breeds were exotic and I knew some of them from the AKC dog shows. But Linda knew *all* of them. We saw about 25 breeds! In her element, she started testing me on the breeds. "Do you know what that one is?" I would guess. When I was wrong she would say "No, no, that's a _____, a _____ a _____." She would try to spell it with her hand gestures. When she couldn't find the name in her brain file she frowned, so I took a picture of the dog for us to look up on the Internet. She had a lot more brain working in there than anyone knew about. I could see her eyes light up and her expression of delight, if not a little superiority! She loved that she recalled these breeds. When I guessed incorrectly and she couldn't find the right words to correct me, she slumped her shoulders and laughed, "Well I know you are wrong but I can't tell you what is right, so I guess you win." Neither one of us took anything too seriously.

One of the stellar moments in Milan for both of us was a surprise last-minute visit to see "The Last Supper" by Leonardo Da Vinci. Linda could not contain herself! She tried talking about the history of the work and telling anecdotal stories to me to supplement the information from the tour guide. Linda had retained her knowledge of da Vinci and she could retrieve it but she could not verbalize it well. When we left she said, "I could go right now to home and be happy. I have seen the thing best I could possibly see!"

Another symbol of her indomitable spirit was the afternoon ferry we took into Venice. Linda experienced vertigo on dry land and on the water she was green from motion sickness. I felt so sorry for her and hated watching her. She took medication and just pushed herself through the ride in silence. When we reached the city landscape she lit up again, grabbed her camera, and started snapping pictures. Still seasick, she held the camera with one hand and the railing with the other hand. She was excited by the city of so many separate islands, the cathedrals on every other street corner and the architecture. We had an amazing hotel that had murals in the alcoves and ceilings in every guest room. We could just lie in the bed and look at art! Linda often said, "I think heaven is here and I died."

On a rainy afternoon, we sat on the quaint hotel veranda near the beach in Venice. This was when we first talked about Linda writing a book to tell her story. I told her, "Linda, you kissed the face of God and lived to tell the tale. You have a message of hope for survivors and their families." She looked so puzzled and said, "How could you say you know this before I got a way to say it?" I realized she had already given some thought to this. I told her I would try to help her. She said things she would like to include. Then she started discussing patriotism and the saluting the flag in the classroom and so on. I suggested we go get a delicious pastry and latte! Whew...

She bought postcards to send home to family. She wrote for about two hours one evening. I asked, "Did you get them all done?" She said, "No, but I almost finished one." I smiled. Throughout the trip, Linda was quiet during transit. I knew she was suffering anxiety, motion sickness, and restless leg syndrome. She rubbed her legs with cream to stop the itching. She never complained and she never wanted to stay in the room and let an excursion go by without us on it. "I can sit sick when I get home and here I am not sitting!" she would say. She would smile and keep trudging and take medication as needed.

Linda had difficulty communicating on demand and responding appropriately. She could talk and engage in conversation but her responses did not always match the question. She would just smile and tell people, "I had a stroke and my brains are not here. They are at home in South Carolina!" Watching the faces of our companions, I wanted to fall out of my seat laughing. She was so charming and happy and engaging—everyone just loved her and watched out for her. I was quite happy to learn that there were two doctors and two nurses among the members of the tour group because I had no idea what I would do in a medical emergency.

There were so many instances of a miraculous awakening of her memories of art history. It seemed with each passing day, her intellectual capacities increased. This was most apparent in Florence. We visited an art shop and I bought Linda a book about four inches thick covering all of the works contained at the Uffizi Gallery. Every page was a picture of the work inside the gallery with only a small amount of text. She devoured the pictures with her eyes and I could see the excitement in her eyes. Linda has a very expressive face that turned "flat" after the stroke. I was standing there gawking at her as I witnessed the caterpillar turn into a beautiful butterfly. I still get goose bumps when I recall that vision of her. She just came to life!

The gallery was not part of our tour and I was unable to get tickets in advance. At the least I wanted her to have a book which she could study at home. Strolling around, we met a young couple on their honeymoon. They told us the art gallery had just opened for walk-ins but the line was very long. I showed Linda the book of the collections in the gallery—it was magical for her and her eyes were darting around the pages like fireflies. Mesmerized, she was adamant that she wanted to go and could easily stand in lines that long in the heat, on hard cement, without shade, without benches, without public bathrooms, without food. "No problem—let's go, Linda!"

We got into that waiting line and inched our way up to the gallery entrance for the next three hours. Linda was thumbing through the large tome and getting more and more intense. She started tearing up pieces of paper and rapidly slapping them into the various pages of the book. She turned every page and knew in an instant whether she needed a strip of paper to mark the work. She occasionally stopped to thump a page with her index finger and recite the piece to me, then she would say, "You can't understand me can you?" I would shake my head and say, "Not a word, Linda, but its sure fun watching you!" We enjoyed so much laughter in our unique way of communicating.

Linda also suffered from frequent urination syndrome. When she needed to go, she needed to go *now.* There are few public restrooms in Florence. We were in that line for more than three hours. My feet were numb and there was no place to sit down. Linda just kept turning the pages of that book, pointing, tapping her finger, thinking, and marking the pages. By the time we got to the ticket booth we had only two hours until our next appointment with the tour group. She marked what she wanted to see and I used the floor plan inside the book to chart our course to cover as much ground as possible in two hours.

We were finally inside! I said, "First, we have to go to the bathroom." Unbelievably she said, "No, no, not enough time," and took off at a trot! I caught up and grabbed her arm, put my arm around her waist and led her to the bathroom. Walking out, she giggled, "Thank you—we probably needed that." I was relieved she wasn't mad at me. We started off and maintained a fast pace. Her eyes were wide and her wheels were spinning. She knew exactly what she was looking at and doing her best to articulate it to me. I shook my head "no" a lot and she rolled her eyes to the ceiling and shrugged. Her recall was fully intact and I was amazed, but saddened she could not put the words together to share her knowledge. We had an amazing time there and stayed until closing time. Well past our scheduled time with the group, we missed our next tour and dinner with the group, but we were totally happy.

Another minor deficit Linda experienced was something like "black and white" logic. Jeff tells me that this persists to this day. There were no shades of gray—only black or white, yes or no, right or wrong. For example, she needed a special adapter for her hair dryer. The European adapters we brought did not function in many of the Italian hotels. When Linda asked for the item at the front desk— she did not understand that it was not an item provided at this hotel. She would question the clerk—"How will I dry my hair if you don't give me that piece?" This was followed by several more attempts to get the clerk to recognize she needed this item. She kept asking the same question, expecting a different response. She stubbornly stood her ground until I found a way to intervene. Another example was tipping clerks for special services, like bringing coffee to the room. When I tipped a clerk she would be flabbergasted. "Why do you give them money for doing their job? *That is their job*—I don't understand." For Linda, pure logic trumped customary practices every time.

The Uffizi was hard to beat, but the nighttime tour to see Michelangelo's "David" was spectacular. Linda discussed the work at length and pointed out things the casual observer would miss. She knew the details of most of Michelangelo's impressive body of accomplishments, but she was on fire about "David." Undaunted by limited vocabulary, Linda did her best to communicate the things she wanted me to know. We had a marvelous young docent who wrote her doctoral dissertation on Michelangelo's "David." Linda commented that the young lady knew exactly what she was talking about and her love for this work was contagious. Watching Linda study the piece, walking around it, pointing out techniques was one of the highlights of the trip for me. This woman with damage to more than one-third of her brain was trail-blazing a return to her intellectual roots with me. I felt like a proud momma!

She was quiet most of the day but couldn't stop talking when the lights went out.

"Peggy, am I talking too much and keeping you from sleep?"

"Yes, Linda, we have to be up at 6 A.M." Silence for two or three minutes.

"Peggy, do you remember the name of......?" After three or four episodes, I burst out laughing and so did she. But even the laughter did not stop her if she had a question on her mind. I decided she could think when it was quiet, the lights were off, and there were no distractions. She also hated that I would not get up in time for 6

A.M. breakfasts—I could eat an apple on the coach and be happy. She really wanted me to get up and go with her and resorted to her own strategy.

"Peggy, don't you want breakfast?" I was silent.

"They have the best food there!" I was still silent and tried to ignore her.

"I hope Jeff remembers to brush their teeth!" I would try hard not to say, "Linda, be quiet!"

"I wonder if they miss me or glad I am here." I mashed my pillow over my ears. When all of her dialogue failed, "Peggy, could you fasten my necklace hook?" Yup, she was dumb like a fox!

The crowning glory of the trip was St. Peter's Cathedral in Rome. She was mesmerized by the *Pieta* and I was able to understand her captivation. Linda enjoyed that day so much but she was unimpressed by the tour guide. She proudly whispered, "I think I know more than she does and I don't have a whole brain!" Inside the Sistine Chapel she educated me again. She said Michelangelo painted the breathtaking art on the ceiling for money. His preferred medium was sculpture. Thus, he created this world-famous artistic feat to earn money to support his marble masterpieces, like "David." I realized at that hour that I wished I had been present for one of her lectures three years ago. I also had no doubt that this Linda would return to the classroom one day. I still think so.

On our final tour day in Rome we had one extra day to rest and reflect on our wonderful time together. Many aspects of her personality, character, and recovery stood out in my mind. She took an amazing risk to do something she was terrified of doing to experience something she loved more than life—an international flight to personally experience the greatest art treasures of the Roman Empire.

She took a blind leap of faith in trusting me to get her there and get her home. She told me several times not to worry. If she died, she would die happy. She was determined to push the outer limits of her abilities and try to recover as many of her losses as she possibly could. She never complained—not one single time. Despite anxiety, nausea, periodic incontinence, vertigo, agoraphobia (both motion and heights), and many other maladies, she kept going and did it pleasantly. *Who can do that?*

She tried to learn something new every day and took painstaking notes at night.

She didn't know the meaning of the word "brothel" when we toured one in Pompeii despite reading all those books without covers as a child. She could not comprehend why the others in our group thought that was humorous. She was a trooper anyway—undaunted. She recalled so much more about art history than she thought she could and it was a major confidence booster.

She never stopped smiling and was so easy to travel with—I would go with her on another trip anytime. (I would just take earplugs for bedtime!)

She is by far my favorite daughter-in-law in the whole wide world and I love her very much.

Reaching for My Dreams
Linda Weatherspoon

It is Christmas 2008 when Jeff's mom calls me from California. "Linda, I know you do not remember this—and neither does anyone else except me—but I have a surprise for you." She tells me about praying over me when I was in the coma, and that she had whispered from her heart, "Linda, if you get out of this bed and recover, I will take you anywhere in the world to see your favorite art history. Please do not die."

I am still very slow with comprehension. The moment it sinks in, I realize she is asking a question, "Linda, where do you want to go with me to collect on that promise?" I still don't quite understand. "Linda, where are your favorite artists and where do you want to go? France? Spain?" Before she finished the sentence, I blurt out, *"ITALY!"* I had forgotten—my favorites were the Italian Masters from the 14th – 16th centuries. I feel more ecstasy than anyone can get from a mother-in-law! *Italy?* I am speechless—partly due to the aphasia, and partly due to the thought of the trip of my dreams. I say, "There was no way to hear you so I didn't know and you do not have to."

I do not remember anything about Peggy talking to me in my coma. (Later, when I shared this dream-come-true with my art friends, they teased me about it. They said, "the reason you didn't die is that you wanted to go to Italy before you went to heaven! Linda, you are crazy if you really are going to Italy with a mother-in-law! No one takes a vacation with a mother-in-law!")

Jeff tells me later that Peggy really did make that promise, and after the first eighteen months of my recovery, she had begun asking him about the possibility of travel. She wants to keep her promise before anything else happens to me or to her. He encourages me to go and assures me he thinks I can handle the trip medically and cognitively. My brain is still very slow, and my language and communication skills are minimal. Still—what is stopping me? Two things come to mind immediately.

First, it hits me like a heavy brick—*I am terrified of flying!* And secondly, I have forgotten so much of my art history and the ones I remember are mixed in partial visions in my brain. I sit down to think. *I can figure this out.* Is this *another dream? She wouldn't do that for me ... would she?*

I fill up my head with fear and doubt. *Why am I getting so mad at myself? Well, you better get over it. How can you refuse to even consider not going to Italy? You had to do it to get your degree ....and flying didn't stop you then! I have to think for a while.*

I talk with Dr. Susan Slavik—my mentor and advisor in college—and tell her about the chance to go to Italy. She is thrilled for me and begins outlining what I must see and where. She is so excited and gets me excited because I cannot follow her thoughts so quickly. If I can't stay focused mentally with her sitting right next to me—how could I stay focused during a tour of the Great Masters? What am I going to do? She sets up an appointment with my art history teacher so I can audit another art class and brush up on my history. Still, I feel too slow, and thick, and a bit like a loser compared to the way I was before. Dr. Slavik says, "Linda, you can go to Italy again when your memory is better—but you cannot miss spending those special days with a woman who loves you so much and is willing to make a dream happen for you." It takes a while for me to realize that she is right—everything takes me a while to comprehend. Still, I think to myself, "over two weeks is a long time and Italy is far away."

Eventually, I realize that going to Italy with Peggy is a "no-brainer," no pun intended! I have to spend that time with her, no matter what. I am slower in every way but I will keep up. I am not going to be a burden and I will start saving my money. I am taking a lot of medication and have so many side effects—but we just accept it all as best we can. My personal pharmacy included:

- Cymbalta 60mg once a day
- Klor Con M20 once a day
- Crestor 10mg once a day
- Lyrica 50 mg twice a day
- Warfarin Sodium 5mg on M, W, and F; all other days 2.5 mg
- Ropinirole 1 mg four times a day
- Neuropamax Cream as needed
- Xanax as needed for stress and fear of flying
- Asthma inhaler as needed

This is medication madness!

Periodically, I suffer with panic and too much excitement about the trip. I suffer anguish about my mother's condition and that she would die while I was in Italy, until I remember that she has already passed away. Then I worry I might miss a requirement to get my degree until I remember I have already earned my degree.

I am worried about the cost of the trip. When I started working at the high school, the human resources manager had told me about salary continuance. It had cost another deduction from my paycheck, but I thought it was important and I am so glad I listened to her. I remember that lady's face when she told me, "You never know when something could happen and that will not be enough money for the rest of your life." If you have a stroke like I did and are unable to return to work, a paycheck during recovery is critical. Jeff has it rough trying to pay the bills, the mountain of medical debts, and my car payments. Then they had to pay back $10,000 because they said I didn't pay my extra insurance in case something catastrophic happened. I am confused about this. I took that deduction—I was sure of it.

Peggy is learning Italian for the trip! She is so smart. She will do all the speaking because if I have to I will have problems. There are twenty of us and Peggy has made friends with everyone. By the time the trip is over they will all know exactly who she is. She is gracious but not afraid to confront someone, either! (For example, I remember a lawyer was telling stories about obscene cases in the courtroom using graphic language. Peggy was livid that he was inappropriate and using foul language with young children present. She was not afraid to "take care of that situation" but keep her dignity! This is part of why I felt safe with her—she could take care of business and take care of me!)

I have nine months to learn again before the trip. Peggy sends me a video of Italy and some tour books and marks the things important to me in yellow ink. I have so many art history books about Italy that I studied and mastered in college—now I can only look at the pictures. I cannot understand the text. I think part of it is in Italian? Most of it is due to my inability to *receive* information. Looking at the pictures, I can *retrieve* some of the art history I have forgotten. She sends me a map and marks in yellow highlighter all the places we will be going. She has arranged for us to travel from the top of the "boot" to the bottom. Jeff has to show me on the map what Peggy means by "the boot." I think it is exciting to go on a trip with twenty people who love Italy. For some reason, I feel more safe that we have a knowledgeable guide and a group to be with.

I still have to look at the notes I kept from Peggy and our guide as I write this. I can understand more when I study it and have time to look up the right meaning of words. It is slow but I am doing a lot better than when I first started this book. I could not have done it without Peggy, my angel.

Walking is still a strange experience for me. At one period after the stroke, I began to walk like Frankenstein—swaggering stiff-legged from side to side. My muscles ached and so did my joints. Initially, when the doctors said I was paralyzed on the right side, I knew I would not spend my life in a wheelchair. When I was walking like Frankenstein, it was so agonizing that I entertained the idea of a wheelchair—but just for a second! The therapist told me to walk with a book on top of my head to regain balance and posture. But I was so slow and constantly stubbing my feet and my toes on the walls and doors. I was just slow and leaning a lot—like that "Tower of Pisa." I kept reminding myself to push my shoulders back; sit up straight. I wanted to go to Italy like "Linda" not like "Frankenstein!" Peggy had excellent posture and I intended to walk correctly without swaggering. I didn't want to embarrass her.

On October 3, 2009, I meet Peggy at the airport in Atlanta. I fly there by myself from Myrtle Beach—miracle number one! I am sure she made this arrangement to get there first to meet my plane so that I won't get lost. (Remember, my hospitalization was just eighteen months earlier.) I am getting better but the aphasia delays or prevents me from asking questions and remembering a lot that I don't know I have forgotten! I am not sure how much of my medication attributes to my impaired mental activity and "grogginess." (I am so happy I can remember enough today with the help of my pictures to explain our trip!)

Peggy is an angel and keeps me pretty close to her everywhere we go in Italy. She doesn't even let me go to the restroom without her nearby. We leave Atlanta and take an overnight flight to Milano. I don't remember the flight very well and believe I took anxiety medication to keep me from having a panic attack.

When we arrive in Milan the next morning, I cannot believe that I am in another country! This is only the second time I have been out of the United States in my entire life. Everything is a mystery to me. We take a shuttle from the airport and take a beautiful drive. I look at everything in disbelief that it is really me, in Italy! We drive along the western shore of Lake Como and stay at the Grand Hotel Di Como, only thirty minutes from Milan.

We go to Lugano, Switzerland, and have a wonderful time in the Italian community village. This is where we can get the best Swiss candies and chocolate. We could have taken a private boat to see the home of George Clooney—and the gem of Bellagio—but we shop instead. Peggy is an expert for shopping! She also know I get seasick on a small boat.

The next day is exciting. I am glad Peggy loves art, too. She knows exactly what is the most important and awesome thing for me to see in this city! It is very hard to find the right words to tell Peggy, "I want to see this, or this, or that!" But she knows what I would most dream of seeing as an artist—although we did not discuss it much. The work of da Vinci is everywhere in Milan and many statues of the Master himself. Personally seeing Michelangelo and Leonardo da Vinci's masterpieces is too incredible to describe. Like most people, I have only seen them in books and videos. There are historical details of these masterpieces that I discussed with my students but they are missing in my mind. I can only grab bits and pieces from my memory. I am sure Peggy enjoys the beauty and we really don't have to say anything else. (I am writing this in 2011 and I hoped I would be able to discuss and explain the works of the Masters better by now but I can't.) I am so happy that I can see the beauty firsthand. I taught the history of these sculptures and pictures to my students—but I could not fathom the depth of the beauty. It would make you speechless even when you already cannot talk!

The treasures of Milan are so many. I did not expect the fast pace of the city and the tiny cars and speeding traffic. From my window seat on the bus the speed of the cars and motorbikes makes me dizzy. And I am always a little dizzy anyway. At the center of the impressive *Castello Sforza* is the first huge area. There is a guide to explain the *Pieta* by Michelangelo the sculpture of Mary and Jesus. The guide gives us very important information. I am glad to hear her knowledge about the *Pieta* and think of additional sections to include in my classes. Even though I have worked hard to relearn lost information, I still cannot retrieve it without notes. But suddenly the memory returns hours later or in the middle of the night. (I often woke up Peggy to tell her the memory I had forgotten). Although I am improved, read faster, and comprehend more, I still cannot teach or answer questions that my students may ask.

The most significant comparisons of Michaelangelo's *Pieta,* the famous sculpture of Mary and Jesus, is the different perspectives and proportions of Mary and Jesus by Michelangelo at St. Peter's Cathedral in Vatican City in Rome. Michelangelo's Jesus was painted *after* the crucifixion. Some of the artistic interpretations of Mary appeared larger in comparison with her adult son. She also appears a lot younger than what most artists paint. It is believed the artists created Jesus to appear "feeble" after his death.

In Milan, there are many incredible paintings, sculptures, and cathedrals. We continued to the *Church of Santa Maria della Grazie* (which means Holy Mary of Grace). We take an incredible private tour of the church and Dominican convent. It was there we see Leonardo da Vinci's most famous painting "The Last Supper." Again, luck is on our side and our tour guide is able to reserve enough tickets. The famous painting was the final meal Jesus shared with his disciples before the crucifixion. *I am in the same room where da Vinci painted this historic work on the wall!* The wall was almost destroyed by soldiers who had used the wall for target practice. The wall is being meticulously repaired to restore the original colors. Much clarity was lost over the centuries due to the type of paint used by da Vinci. I am so happy I have a chance to see the real work, thanks to Peggy. They only allow a few people in the room at a time, and we go through a decontamination chamber first. It was worth it.

After experiencing the work of these two master artists, I could have just gone back home because they are the ultimate—the closest an artist can get to heaven. What if I had died or had so much damage in my brain that I couldn't acknowledge the beauty and comprehend what these artists created? I am so happy that I came here with Peggy.

There are so many times I wish I could tell Peggy more information about the art we are seeing. She is very knowledgeable about art and so happy she shared with me. The guides are doing an incredible job with the basics, which we find fascinating. But I want to tell her the "juicy stuff" that I taught my students to help them remember the history; the secret stories about the people and the artists made the students listen and become more interested. I am so sad because I remember parts of what I want to say but then when I get ready to tell her, nothing, absolutely nothing, comes out of my mouth.

Then my mother comes back to me with her wisdom: "You are not going to appear sad and Peggy could not have done anything better than what you dreamed to do … so get over it, and be happy even if you fake it." I do not fake it but I understand exactly what my mom's voice was saying and I taught my children and students the same way. You can shake out of your own attitude! My mother did not have an attitude … I do. I recognize that and try to improve.

(Right before my stroke when some days were so draining at school, and I was so exhausted and having headaches, my inner voice would say, "Your school is paying you and they expect you to teach students in a way that they will not forget, even on the days with headaches. No one wants to hear about that. These are students … the students want to hurry and see someone in the hall so make it positively memorable in that classroom." Unfortunately, I do not remember most of their names but I sure see their faces. I still recall their struggles and their successes with applied art.)

In Italy, I think more broadly about art history. I feel secure with Peggy, and the environment is stimulating my brain and my heart. In quiet times I think about how hard I had to train for my degree. The flash cards, hundreds of applied art projects, immersion in art history all ran through my mind. This knowledge is not there now. *Where did it go?* Even with all the medicine they are giving me, I don't quite feel like myself ... is that normal? Why didn't I get to finish the second school year teaching when I just got started? That is just not fair ... why did God do that to me?

Teenagers get bored quickly and teachers have to compete with so many external factors to hold their attention. The cell phones, texting, the computer, the iPod, and their friends all occupy their minds during the one hour I have to teach them. I tried to teach by engaging them with relevant stories and facts that would connect them viscerally with the artist. Art history was an immediate attraction to about one-third of my students. I discovered unless I could feed their little hormones with relevant anecdotes, I could not hold the attention of the other two-thirds of the class.

As a teacher, I had to be able to beat the competition or the students would day dream, text, or fall asleep! It is not their fault. As a teacher, I wanted to capture their attention to appreciate the history and meaning of art. This dream was not to be ... at least not at this juncture of my journey.

I had no idea or intention of asking Peggy for another wish! Yet here we are—writing my book that will help me share my experiences, my determination, and my hopes with other stroke victims and their families. How incredible is this? I have a desire to tell people that the principles of learning and preparing for a career are the same principles that influence recovery. We have to work for what we want—with all our being—to succeed in life. It is so critical that stroke victims and their families maintain a vision of recovery and hope.

Today, I will focus on Italy! There is so much to discover here. We are only on our second day and took the tour to visit the famous La Scala Opera House in Milan. This is the center of famous art, sculpture, and the world's most renowned operatic artists. Built in 1776, the architecture is fascinating. The theater was one of the largest in Italy, holding more than three thousand patrons.

The next day is relaxing and I begin to feel more at ease. We visit the Swiss frontier. We buy the best candy and chocolate! The Swiss version of hot chocolate is amazing—so thick you can drink it or eat it with a spoon! At the lakeside resort of Lugano, we do a lot of window shopping for watches and eating exotic desserts! Their coffee is very different than ours—much stronger and served in tiny cups. It is fun to experience the differences in our culture and theirs. In the end, we vote to drink café Americano but to eat Italian ice cream! The gelato is so smooth, creamy, and fattening! Although Peggy's brain is pretty much all there we manage to get lost the second night trying to find the bakery and creamery we had visited the night before! It is so beautiful at night just strolling around Lake Como, the deepest lake in all of Italy, at night. Drinking in the history, beauty, and hot chocolate is intoxicating!

Venice

October is a wonderful time to visit Italy. We tour the City of Shakespeare—Verona! We take pictures with the statues of Romeo and Juliette and climb up to the famous balcony. We visit the ruins of the 2,000-year-old arena! We love the shopping in the open courtyards but warned to watch out for gypsies who are notorious pickpockets. In the Renaissance City of Venice, we have three memorable days to experience life on this waterbound city. Everything in Venice is delivered by boats and gondolas are a primary mode of transportation, especially for the tourists. The weather is perfect and I love the history and romanticism of Venice!

One interesting trip is taking the boat, which causes my panic and seasickness to increase, to see the famous Murano glass factory. This is an art form I have not studied and I find it interesting. They actually demonstrate glass blowing in the kilns with their amazing artistry. Owned by the same family for centuries, the secrets of the methods used are shared only with successive generations of the men in the family. The women are not privy to the secrets of the art. They are only allowed to work in the gift shops. The artisans work in a large warehouse with enormous kilns and many craftsmen assist the master glass blowers. We sit in bleachers to watch the entire creation from start to finish! The blown glass is crafted into expensive and colorful vases, elaborate chandeliers, museum quality jewelry, dishes, and almost anything else you could imagine! It is an unexpected treat to learn another art form. I am glad they offer smaller items that I can purchase and take home for my family. I buy small animal figurines which I manage to get home without breaking them.

In the evening, most of our group opts to take the romantic gondola ride through the Grand Canal before dinner. I think Peggy would have loved it—and I would have gone if she really wanted to—but I am so relieved when she says she does not want to. I just feel better with my feet on the ground!

The most unforgettable experience in Venice is the trip to St Mark's Square! It is impossible to describe the awe and emotions I experienced here. The pictures below help me remember what I saw—and the names of some of the most historic scenes of Venice!

The Doge Palace is fascinating with the works of Titian and Tintoretto—I studied their work! We take pictures of the statues at the top of this staircase because neither one of us can remember the names of the subjects of the sculptures! We even call Jeff in Myrtle Beach to have him tell us or to look it up because we are without a tour guide!

Florence

Over the next three days we cover a lot of ground! The longer rides are very hard for my body. I must be making Peggy crazy. I am *itching from my ankles up to my knees. On top of that my legs are numb ... I am so swollen ... I feel like a pig sitting beside Peggy. My clothes are at least two sizes bigger than hers ... I have to stop eating. You already tried that before and you got sick ... I am so ugly ... how can Jeff still love me when I have all these problems ... little does he know other things I am keeping to myself. I can't even help myself and now I have a whole set of new problems ... what about my insurance coverage going away? It must take a lot of money to pay for me and I am not even teaching ... some employee that the principal chose has my job ... I only worked one and a half years and I am sitting on my ass! Well, you are sitting on your ass in Italy with one of your favorite people ... Peggy. Why do I want to cry? ... It is so breathtakingly beautiful here.*

We are moving south to the tip of Peggy's "boot!" We visit the Leaning Tower of Pisa and travel on to Florence. One my favorite nights of all is our unexpected luck of getting last-minute tickets to the Fine Arts Academy in Florence to see one of the four sculptures of Michelangelo's *David*! I am so impressed by the depth of knowledge shown by our college-age tour guide! Her enthusiasm and expertise are so stimulating I think my brain might overload! I have so much knowledge about *David* and remember so many historical facts that it is invigorating to compare my knowledge with hers. (This was one of the major highlights of the trip.)

Florence – Uffizi Gallery

I am happy I had practiced and improved my walking. There is so much to do in Italy and all of it involves a lot of walking. The tour guide did not make arrangements for our group to tour the Uffizi in Florence because there were no available tickets but Peggy makes sure that I do not leave Italy without going through that gallery! (I remember telling Peggy there was no way I could see everything. Our time was limited so I put small pieces of paper in my Uffizi book to mark the portraits and sculptures I most wanted to see.)

Our time there limited, we move fast so that I can see the most critical works of art. I taught the Italian Renaissance history to my students—now I was *living* it in person. Some of the ones I am most impressed with are the ones that are easiest for me to remember. I am excited by my brain's ability to actually remember facts!

Workshop of Cimabue c. 1290 (triptych): The babies still looked like adults with Madonna and Child and the perspective was flat—not dimensional. It was so different.

We also saw *Cimabue Maesta of Santa Trinita* c. 1280 which was tempera on wood as well as Giotto's tempera on wood. Giotto was the principle master and painter of Venice. I also see several Leonardo da Vinci paintings I had never seen in art history books and that is so exciting. The works were completed in 1472—showing incredible aerial perspective. *It is exciting to me that I remember these experiences two years later!*

The Piero Della Francesca – Diptych of the Duchess and Duke of Urbino c. 1472, was another work in my class. My students

132

remembered this artist when they were tested on exams because the appearance of the subject's hair line was unique. When the ladies pulled their hair back, the hairline receded extremely far back. I used that example because I knew the young girls would relate to the unusual hairstyles. It showed their skin but I do not remember how they actually took the hair off ... it seemed painful! The artist painted Federigo's broken nose which was actually broken during a tournament. *(I remember things like this unexpectedly!)* The pale skin tones were thought by artists to be desirable and beautiful—my students remembered the comparison with the trend of getting the best tan possible in Myrtle Beach. These were the types of comparisons that I used to help the students remember. I think it helped me, too!

Two of my favorite paintings in the world are by Sandro Botticelli—and both are housed at the Uffizi in Florence! Painted on linen canvas, "The Birth of Venus" shows the goddess Venus has emerged from the sea and arrives at the shore as a grown woman. "The Primavera" (also known as the Allegory of Spring) is a group of mythological figures in a garden with Venus in the center under the arch. Both of these works are believed to be wedding paintings—probably commissioned by the Medici family. The "Primavera" and "Birth of Venus" in my opinion, were probably the most famous works in the Uffizi. I introduced students to both of them, but did not want to let them know these were my two favorites.

When I see the real paintings, they are even more beautiful. Many recall the painting of the naked Venus standing in a huge seashell. You see it everywhere today—on coffee mugs, stationery, purses, and umbrellas. It is very interesting to read the various interpretations of this artwork over the centuries. Most colleges and art historians usually follow the meanings described by Vasari.

I have only a little time to look at the work of Raphael. He is considered the youngest of the three giants of the Italian High Renaissance. He was orphaned at eleven and his genius was tied down by the demands of his rich patrons. I think he was masterful in the way be painted babies. He died when he was thirty-seven. Many believe if he had lived, he would have achieved the status of Michelangelo and Leonardo da Vinci. Here, I also see the famous self-portrait of Raphael. *(In the Vatican: "Painted by himself looking in a mirror...it is a youthful head of very modest aspect, accompanied pleasantly and gracefully by the black beret he wears.")*

Another of my favorites was the self-portrait of Albrecht Durer. He was an excellent draftsman and engraver. He was one of the outstanding personalities in the cultural world of his time. It is just plain awesome to see the oil on wood self-portrait of Rembrandt, too! There are about 80 self-portraits of Rembrandt with the three most famous ones on display in the Uffizi. There are many other artists that I am so glad to see in the Uffizi. Some of them are Titian, Pieter Paul Rubens, Francisco Goya, and El Greco.

I especially love seeing Michelangelo's Doni Tondo "The Holy Family." *Tondo* means round and the painting is in its original frame in the Uffizi. The beautiful and young Madonna is the dominant figure in the painting. The colors are vivid and beautiful.

When I first painted years ago I tried to study and capture the yellow and blue in the Doni Tondo. Michelangelo did such a life-like painting with tempera on wood ... that was amazing! I had only seen these paintings as pictures in a book. When I taught high school I dearly loved working with the advanced students. I remember lecturing and showing them the styles of folds in clothing and draperies and how to achieve these using a brush. The draped cloth of Virgin Mary in the Doni Tondo is a good example. The students were more intimidated by painting people but relaxed more by learning to paint the folds of fabric. I remember thinking, *if they can get this right, they will grow their confidence and painting people will be less challenging!*

I remember quickly going through the different cultures and styles including Eastern and Western, Classical and Romantic periods. In Renaissance, like the fabric on Michelangelo's Doni Tondo, the fabrics were more "form-fitted" and emphasized the human figure. The Baroque and Eastern artists showed the fabric reduced to straight and curved lines—which was more boring. For the Doni Tondo I used actual fabrics to teach the advanced students. When I saw the real fabric that Michelangelo used it was even more fantastic than I had ever seen. I can tell you since I saw the actual work, I have a lot more to practice, especially now!

Throughout the time I am in Italy I recognize things and try to remember what I did or did not do when I was teaching. It is distracting and a little sad for me. I say to myself, *"Don't think about it ... enjoy it ... and you can think later."*

134

There are so many things I have mixed up or forgotten about my trip. Some of what I am writing, I found in my notes that I used when teaching. I taught before I actually saw the masterpieces, they were just pictures in my mind before my stroke. Now seeing the "real" thing, I could better explain to my students the depth the artists have created. Yet, I still have questions that I cannot research because my reading and comprehension are agonizingly slow. *I wonder if I will ever be in a classroom again.*

After the stroke, I tried to study Giorgio Vasari on the Lives of the Artists of Oxford. I was sad I had to put it away after six months. I just could not understand and I knew I was not ready for it. I will continue to refer to it because my art teacher at Coastal Carolina said that it was recognized as the most accurate source of artistic interpretation. I was tested on it considerably. Now, it will not sink in to my brain. When it does and I can retain it, I will feel competent to teach like I did.

I look back at my lecture notes for those classes. In many instances, I still do not understand what I meant in more difficult concepts. I remember I was careful about not giving my personal opinions, which would influence their thinking rather than thinking for themselves. I used famous quotes a lot to reinforce important concepts and to emphasize the power of art. For example, I thought this quote was critical:

"...I'm interested in working with pictures and words, because I think that they have the power to tell us what we are and who we aren't." – Barbara Kroger

I wanted them to think and use their own brains—allowing them five minutes for reflecting on the meaning. Then they would answer questions expressing their own points of view.

Arthur Miller, in his notes from *Death of a Salesman,* said "I write as much to discover as to explain." I have never been disappointed by my students' sharp, unique questions and opinions. I think it is the best way to draw out their ability to create their own work. I show them techniques from other artists and ask if they need more examples. It occurs to me today that Arthur Miller's quote has more meaning to me personally now   because it applies to me—I am *"writing as much to discover as to explain"* what happened to me. This is one of my own quotes and my basic philosophy of teaching:

> *"The best way to motivate students is to help them think more deeply and inventively than anyone else about any subject."* – Linda Weatherspoon (2004)

I cannot tell you how proud and moved I was when a student wrote this response:

> *"It's very personal. I tried to bring myself and the feeling I was having to my artwork when I was drawing and painting. This is the first time I have made an artwork that shows my feelings."*—Student (2005)

We do not have enough time in a high school class to teach technique and history! There was so much subject to cover and so many choices of what to include in my lesson plans; it was challenging to select the major important works. I tried to expose them to the major artists from each of the historical periods. *I loved my job.*

The Uffizi is a major stimulant for me and my brain! I hope to go back one day with my husband. We walk so much that day around the City of Florence, then through all the chambers of the Uffizi—from sunup to sunset—Peggy develops a huge blister on the ball of her foot and will probably never let me forget it! When we are through for the day, she shows it to me. I take a picture of it! We choose to get a taxi back to the hotel and miss dinner with our group. But it is all worth it. *I wish I would have gotten the blister instead of her!*

On October 10, our entire group has a gourmet dinner at a magnificent villa and working vineyard in the hills of Tuscany. That night is Peggy's 62nd birthday. I am able to think this one out for myself! I ask the tour guide if Peggy can have a cake to celebrate the occasion. After dinner, the lights in the massive dining hall are dimmed and the entire group of twenty tourists, the owners, and all the staff sing to her. Everyone likes Peggy because she is friendly and kind to everybody she met. *Well, almost everybody!*

We leave Florence across the Veneto Plains and drive over the Apennine Mountains—which are very steep! I take more medication to control the motion sickness and my legs are numb, itching, and restless. Some of the most familiar memories are Michelangelo's *David* and the golden mosaics and Byzantine architecture. When we left, I had no idea I would get to see Ghiberti's *Porta del Paradisco*— the amazing double doors to the cathedral with inset panels sculpted to tell the story of the Old Testament. It was one of the art forms I made sure the students were aware of when I taught. The doors were immense. We take a lot of pictures of those doors—and each individual panel depicting another story. Most people of that era could not read the scriptures, and the art work was used to tell stories visually. When Michelangelo saw it he said, "These doors are fit to be the Gates of Paradise."

I will stop writing about my favorite things about the paintings I saw at Uffizi because I can see it would become another book just about history to use when I get better! There are so many things that are mixed up in my head ... thank God I kept my notes I made when I was at Coastal! At least I can look through them and start thinking and remembering ... that is so exciting! So many times I almost threw them away for a move but I just could not part with them. Hanging on to them was painful when I could not comprehend the words—now I can understand sections of my writing!

The Amalfi Coast – Isle of Capri

After seeing the Bay of Naples, we stay three nights on the magnificent Amalfi Coast. Our home base is in Maori, and it must be one of the most beautiful places on earth. I think my heart will stop beating when I see the width of the road and the height of the mountain we travel down to reach the coast. On our descent to the Mediterranean, there are so many switchbacks, curves, and twists I am afraid I will die from the panic. Remember, I have a fear of flying, fear of heights, and I don't trust many people behind the wheel. And this is a large luxury tour bus with twenty tourists on board from all over the world. I am so relieved when we finally reach our hotel that I don't mind carrying our luggage up four flights of stairs because the elevators are too tiny to hold a person and a suitcase! I carry some of

Peggy's luggage, too!

The lady who guides us in our trip was born in Italy but educated in England. I do not have a problem with her English. Peggy does an outstanding job speaking in Italian! I trust the tour people and Peggy.

Once we are settled we walk along the seafront to experience the beautiful blue waters of the Mediterranean and I feel at home. If only I had a canvas and a paintbrush—I would be in heaven.

Our next tour is to visit a famous artists' colony. Peggy sweetly cautions me that the route from Maori to the scenic City of Ravello will be steep and scary for me—she tells me to take extra anxiety medication! She knows it will be worth it for me to see the picturesque artist's colony. Situated on the mountain top far above the city, it really is a treacherous drive. Had I known the road conditions and that the same large bus would be taking us up to the top of that mountain—I would have taken more medication before I got on that bus! At every turn, it looks like the front of our bus is already extended beyond the road and teetering over the cliff—and if anyone in the back of our bus stood up—we surely would plunge into the ocean and rocks below. There aren't enough pills on the whole bus to quiet my stomach!

Our bus just keeps climbing the terraced hillsides until we reach Ravello at the top. This is the city that is also famous for its annual music festival, Lemoncello liqueur created by the nuns at the turn of the century, and colorful lemon pottery—another art form I admire. The views are breathtaking. Our guide takes us to visit the 11th century Cathedral and the manicured gardens of Villa Rufolo—which inspired the works of Wagner! Imagine how the majesty of this view gave birth to some of Wagner's great compositions.

This is a place of majesty and inspiration. There are so many places in the world to stimulate the artist's creativity, but this is definitely my favorite place. I see so many things I want to paint. An artist could paint forever and still not finish. I definitely want to come back here with Jeff.

After this tour bus trek around the roads of Amalfi, I think I am cured of getting panicky and car sickness. I have almost no problems with driving or flying the rest of our trip—including on the long flight home. My eyes only close a few times. It is amazing how our driver never touches the branches of the closest trees, or scrapes the steep embankments of solid stone, or another car.

I love the little town of Maori, too. We walk along the shoreline, eat delicious foods and pastries, and sample all of the local fare. We had been so busy from the moment our plane landed in Milano that this is the first afternoon that we can relax and breathe in all the beauty of southern Italy.

We take a mini-cruise to the Isle of Capri but it is a motion sickness nightmare. We had just eaten breakfast, and I am so seasick in that small boat that is rocking and rolling in the turbulent waters. Peggy says I might feel better if I it outside the cabin in the fresh air. I am too afraid to move. To make it worse, we come ashore and have to ride a funicular to the peak of the mountain to Capri town. When we get off the boat, the ground is full of potholes and rocks. Peggy steps in a hole full of gravel and falls down really hard, hitting her head on a big rock. She is stunned and very dizzy. One of the doctors talks to her and she decides not take the walking tour with the rest of us. Instead, she orders a Café Latte Americano at an outdoor café. The rest of the group does the walking tour of Capri, including the glorious Caesar Augustus Gardens—which I would love to paint! The magnitude and unusual formation of the Faragloni Rocks in the waters below the gardens is breathtaking.

After the long walking tour of the mountain side and markets, I am glad she did not go along. When I find her again, she is in Prada shopping. She sees me through the window and comes out of the boutique laughing. I didn't really understand at the time why that was so funny to her.

That evening we finally have a little time to relax before dinner. I take a couple of hours at the hotel and sketch some pictures of an Irish setter dog. (I could not remember the breed at the time! That is significant because many things I forgot. Even after I study again, and again, and again, it takes a long time to imprint the information in my brain. It encourages me that there are some events that I can now remember—like right now, I see the dog in my mind and remember the breed. I didn't have to look it up! How does that happen? If I only knew the secret, I could retain and retrieve more information and be more like myself again.)

I am so proud of myself that I survived the ferries and boat rides in Venice and lived through the bus rides above the Amalfi Coast. Now I am ready for anything.

Pompeii

The rest of our trip is Pompeii and Rome. We drive to Pompeii, the city that was covered in molten lava and ash when Mt. Vesuvius erupted. It is spectacular and eerie. We join an elderly tour guide who has lived in Pompeii most of his life. It is a lot colder than we expected and the icy winds are blowing hard. Everyone on the tour is bundling up, trying to stay warm. Pompeii has the richest artistic and cultural importance. The preservation of the artifacts is mind-boggling. The chariot ruts are still carved into the stone streets, the marble counters are still standing in devastated kitchens, the intricate mosaic designs on the floors in the remains of the homes, the bath houses, and the erotic frescoes in the bordellos are still intact. I cannot understand what the guide meant by brothel. I ask him to explain it and everyone in the group starts laughing. I ask again, and more laughing! Then Peggy quickly steps in and uses several discreet phrases to describe the meaning—like "bordello" and "house of ill repute." I still cannot figure out what it means. She finally leans next to my ear and said "whore house" and I get it! (I guess it was a remote memory from those books without covers that I read in childhood!)

Peggy is so aware of other people she takes off her beautiful warm coat and wraps it around one of the elderly ladies who doesn't even have a sweater. We are all moving very slowly but Peggy keeps her eyes on me—like she has done throughout the trip. Today she is aware of the wind and the smell of ash and soot that surrounds us. I have breathing problems and she is aware of that without me saying anything. She tells me to wrap my scarf over my head and mouth to help me breathe easier. The smells of the eruption of Mt. Vesuvius are pungent in the damp, cold winds. She does not want either one of us to trip on the cobblestoned road and we walk a lot arm-in-arm. All of Pompeii was carved in rock and stone.

My favorite part is the architectural ruins. There is more than we have time to see, but I especially enjoy the murals and the petrified remains of the inhabitants. There are remains of a woman in childbirth, an old man still sitting in a chair, and hundreds of other artifacts of the life in Pompeii in 79 A.D. We look in the gated storage areas and see actual petrified people; eerie! There is even a petrified dog in there and incredible pottery.

Rome

And then—there is Rome! The bustling contemporary population speeding about in tiny cars, motorbikes, and traffic jams. I am shocked to see the city so full of graffiti. This is a mixture of the modern world and the ancient Roman Empire. It is hard to keep the city in perspective. There is so much graffiti, and so many people in the streets, stores, and cafes. Yet the antiquities are seemingly undisturbed. We are at the end of our trip—and the best is yet to be.

We start early in the mornings in Rome. We take a driving tour of the city then observe the Seven Hills of Rome, finishing the morning with a walking tour of the catacombs. This is another eerie and moving experience underground. There are more than forty catacombs in Rome—underground burial places for Christians and Jews. They are thought to be open mass graves with tiny cubicles to hold each of the dead. The underground tunnels are barely high enough to stand up. The walls also contain Jewish and Christian artworks of great historical significance. Their art depicts the lives and times of the most persecuted in Rome.

We go into amazing Sistine Chapel in the Vatican Museum that contains the frescos of Michelangelo which is critical study for every art history student. Artists understand why this is a masterpiece and see the ultimate beauty. This is a day of my dreams. I am actually seeing The Vatican, the Sistine Chapel, St. Peter's Basilica, the Cathedral, and St. Peter's Square—and best of all is the *Pieta.* This is the home of the Pope and the Catholic faith and the heart of the Roman Empire. Artists know these works and their importance by heart. Every teacher wants students to be aware of Rome and all its artistic and architectural treasures. I am seeing the ultimate beauty. A person could stay there all week to look and still not see everything.

These walls are sixty-nine feet tall and the vaulted ceilings are decorated with frescos by Botticelli, Ghirlandaio, Pinturicchio, and Signorelli but what makes the masterpieces here known all over the world is the work by Michelangelo. He was commissioned by Pope Julius II to create the work. Around the nine episodes taken from the Book of Genesis were Michelangelo's gigantic prophets and five Sybil's. It is amazing how he raised his neck and arms for so many years to paint the barrel-shaped panels. Many say he lay down and looked up to create the paintings on the ceiling.

We probably spend more time here than anywhere else in the Vatican. I am so happy I get to see the real Caravaggio, my favorite master artist. I am so mad at myself that here was my third favorite artist of all time and I can't remember the first part of the name. I still can only think of the second part of his name. My favorite painting is not in that museum but I do see one of his other works. His are incredible because the light and dark colors and lighting create his unique perspective. I have to look up his name to write this and it was Chiaroscuro. *I can remember the visual work—but I cannot always remember the names of the artists—or I can only remember half of the name.*

I have so many favorites! I love the oil painting by Caravaggio called "Conversion of Saint Paul." It tells the story of Paul on his way to kill the Christians in Damascus being blinded by piercing light from God. Paul is on the floor with a horse in the back almost on top of him. His arms are spread almost the length of the animal. It is very difficult to paint a dark scene and make it realistic. There were no photographs to help the artists, either! I wonder in person things I did not think about as a student. *How long was this picture down, who was the model, how did he get the perspective and lighting right?* The vision he painted is incredible, in my opinion. It is sad that we only have 80 actual paintings and he died when he was 38. He was recognized as "radical" and they know he killed someone. There are several stories how that happened. Michelangelo and Leonardo almost lived to be a hundred!

We go to St. Peter's Basilica and it is amazing beyond words. Afterward, we cross the Tiber and enter Ancient Rome. We go to the Forum and see the ruins of the Circus Maximus—the world's most famous and largest arena for chariot races. We take a walking tour of the mighty Colosseum—one of the seven wonders of the world.

Our trip is ending on a high note. We are tired—but both of us could have kept going for more. This is a glorious learning and enrichment experience for an artist, and more, it was a dream come true for me! I am impressed by the months of planning and organizing that made this trip possible. I will be forever grateful for this gift of time and love from my mother-in-law. *Who the heck goes on vacation with their mother-in-law?* If there were any problems or concerns I was not aware of them. However, Peggy was responsible and dealt with all of the details. It is a good thing because I was like a child! I couldn't think too much or express much of anything so I just enjoyed the art!

Looking back, I think my self-image changed due to the trip to Italy. For the first time, I was able to focus on some of my strengths, not just my deficits. Knowing that Jeff supported me taking the trip boosted my confidence, too. He would never let me leave if he thought I could not handle it. Reliving my career was sometimes very painful. But immersed in the art treasures of the world I was reconnecting with something I had lost. I thought a great deal about art history and struggled with the concepts. With the stimulating environment and being steeped in my favorite art period, I thought I would explode with excitement at times.

Touring the Renaissance Masters at the Uffizi Gallery in Florence and standing close enough to *David* to reach out and touch him—it felt like a new pathway opened in my brain and shed light into the darkness in my mind. I began remembering the tools, colors, sources of marble, and how paint was made. Prompted by the tour guides who were walking art books, I could feel the electrical excitement in my brain. My heart actually swelled with pride when I realized what I had done. I had actually taken a huge step in my recovery of "self." I could put my life into a little more perspective again. Loss of self was the missing piece to the puzzle. I had been thinking that I needed to get back to the place where I had succeeded in my career. In reality, my "self" is not a place at a high school in Myrtle Beach. My "self" is not a place—it is a destiny.

Peggy and I were in Italy for just longer than two weeks. That is when we first talked about me writing a book. We were in Venice on the veranda of our hotel. She said I had an important story to tell and I should write about my illness and miraculous recovery. People needed to understand how a stroke impacts the patient as well as the family. She said she would help me even before I asked her. She is a professor, does a lot of things in her community, and lives in California. I did not want to bother her, but I felt safe saying anything to her. Like with my sisters, I can be myself with Peggy and she will not judge me. I started making notes that very night in October 2009.

I made notes every day to remember what I wanted to include in my book. I was so slow in the beginning. My memory is better for the past and not so much for the present. I can remember things that happened ten years ago but I cannot remember what happened this week. I had a lot of notes by the time I started writing my story. My first notes were memories from that trip. I wrote when I got home. I try to write sometimes but fall asleep. I don't like to sleep too much. I think when I cannot sleep I try to write. I can see several times I was writing a sentence and the words dropped an inch below the line from where I intended them to be.

When I started trying to write the book, it was frustrating that my thoughts did not match what I tried to write down. It was the same problem with my speech. My spoken words did not match what I was thinking. How would I ever get my thoughts on paper? No one will even understand what I am saying because it is "stuck" in the pathways of my brain. I decided that the medications were at fault and I began to decrease all of my medications gradually. I did not want to be a zombie falling asleep and I did not want to walk like Frankenstein. Some of these drugs were addictive and I think I experienced a lot of the side effects of withdrawal from the Ativan. But I did wean myself from more than half of my medications and I felt better. I also functioned better. Maybe I could write my book after all.

Giving Thanks 2009

Today is Thanksgiving. I am thinking about all the things I am thankful for. I am happy to be alive at my second Thanksgiving since my stroke. I am so excited to see my oldest daughter, Christina. She is expecting her first son in March 2010. She lives in Mississippi with her husband who is in the Air Force and about to be deployed to Iraq. I do not know him well. Or at least I don't remember knowing him. I just trust my instincts. When I meet someone who I suspect is not a good person, the hairs on the back of my neck raise up. I did not have that with him. I am not doing a very good job explaining how I feel but I have improved since the last time I tried to explain. I hope my children find the most special husbands or wives. I am glad that

I am older than Jeff. The chance for me to die first is good because I do not want to live without Jeff. I would not want to be alone every day with my mind, either.

I am still taking the same amount of medication except for allergies. One of the main things I want to stop doing is falling asleep. How can I learn anything again if I cannot stay awake to see the words? I am like a grandma—always falling asleep! I am trying to keep notes on medications and find out what I use, what time I take them, and how each one affects me physically and mentally. I believe my body will work fine without those drugs. The doctors keep giving them to me and do not want me to stop taking them. I try to tell Jeff and my doctors but (aphasia) won't let me say it the right way. I am trapped in my head much of the time.

Aphasia: I wrote this down from the dictionary and put it in my own words so I can remember. Then I study the meaning again and again. I understand it at the time—but I cannot retain it. *"Aphasia is a medical condition in which you are unable to use or understand some words, caused by damage to the brain."* I notice it most when I remember exactly what to say, but aphasia prevents it and does not allow my sentence. Sometimes I can see the words when I close my eyes. I have the most problems on the telephone or ordering at Wendy's or McDonald's. My daughters are Brain One and Brain Two because they are familiar with my condition and speak for me. This is embarrassing and frustrating unless I can just read it. But if the clerks ask me questions I cannot answer. I do not attempt to order without someone to help me say what I want to say. I study every day for hours. Improvement is slow and retaining what I learn again is out of my control. I have improved but not enough.

The months are going by. I have a hard time sleeping and I think it is the medicine. I just make notes and study in the middle of the night. I am trying to learn everything again and retrain my memory. God has provided me with the most special person for a husband. He remembers how hard I worked to help him make a good life for us and for our kids. We made three beautiful girls together. I went to school to get an advanced degree. I took care of myself physically. I always watched my weight, took vitamins, and Jeff cooked the most nutritious meals for our family. I have been part of a gym since I was seventeen years old. I never dreamed of smoking or using drugs.

Yet I had a near-death experience. My father has adrenal cancer. My mother died of lung cancer. My Aunt Jean, Mom's sister, had breast cancer and had two radical mastectomies. Now she is seventy and has Alzheimer's disease.

My healthy lifestyle did not prevent the aneurysm and stroke that nearly killed me. However, Jeff said the neurologist said my age and healthy body were the main reasons I survived.

I took Christina to get a hamburger. I did not trust myself to be driving alone with my new grandson, Jaxon. I am doing everything I want to do—except teaching in a classroom. I am driving myself to appointments, driving my girls to school, working out at the gym, going to therapy, shopping for groceries. However, I can make a mistake and I do not want any harm to my grandson due to my lack of care. When we decided Jaxon could stay with us a while, I tried to read *America's Bestselling Childcare Series: What to expect The First Year.* I had the hardest, slowest time trying to understand it. I could never live with myself if something happened while Jaxon was with me. Babies are helpless. No one would ever forgive me.

While Christina and I were eating lunch, there was a television elevated on the wall. I tried to look at it while we ate. I told Christina I was concerned about my neck because I could not hold my head up that high very long. My neck was so swollen with a large globule of fat at the top of my spine. It was like a camel's hump and I could not bend it. I instantly wished I had not told her. By late that evening, my neck was more swollen extending up to my right ear. *I hate getting old and fat.* I do not want anyone to take photographs of me. Jeff does not seem to understand and he loves me the way I am. I am miserable and always swore I would never let myself "go" this way.

My sister Carol came to visit us and we went out to a nice restaurant to eat. I wanted to talk to her about my book and my need to share the story of our lives while we were growing up. I wanted to be forthright about our childhood I want to tell my story—my whole story. I want to remember everything I can about my life. I want to understand what my life meant. *I care about what you think, Carol. There is nothing good that I can say about your dad, I am sorry.*

I told her about some of the worst parts of my childhood that I intended to include. These were awful things that Felton had done to us—things she may have been too young to remember. Her husband

and daughter were with us—and she asked me to share some of the stories with her that I wanted to include. She was fine with my decision and said she was looking forward to reading my book.

My sister Gail came to visit with my sister Roxie. We went to the beach and had lunch. Gail is a special education teacher and has been for many years. I know the children's parents feel so fortunate to have someone like Gail working with their children. I know the kids fell in love with her. Gail and Roxie did most of the talking because I did not talk that much at the time. They knew Peggy was helping with my book, and they started teasing me about being on Oprah with my story!

Cushing's Disease
The Discovery from Hell

It was not until 2008 that a physician finally identified the suspected medical cause of the aneurysm and stroke. The doctor (a urologist) made the initial diagnosis within ten minutes of my first visit with him. He was relying primarily on my physical appearance and self-reports. He requested my medical records and conducted diagnostics to confirm his suspicion. The doctor confirmed that I had Cushing's Syndrome—which could have been treated with a resection of the adrenal gland when it was first discovered in 2006. That is, the presence of the adrenal gland tumor, coupled with the Cushingoid physical characteristics, and the unmanageable high blood pressure—were classic symptoms. In fact, I had ten of the twelve classic symptoms of Cushing's Syndrome.

Until that day, I had no idea that my adrenal gland was causing my blood pressure and the core cause of my stroke. Why didn't any of my doctors recognize that all of my symptoms were the physical manifestations of an endocrine system disorder?

It was the discovery from hell! My stroke could possibly have been prevented with proper diagnosis and treatment. The failure was not from my neglect of my symptoms and health. I relentlessly pursued answers. The medical system failed me. I was traumatized by the diagnosis. I was also speechless, except to say, "Do you mean my stroke could have been prevented?" When he answered in the affirmative, my mind exploded in racing thoughts. My face was hot, my heart was pounding, and I could not process the information. By the time I reached my car—I was hysterical. Sobbing, I called Jeff. I was crying so hard that he could barely understand what I was telling him.

I lost most of the really important things in my life that day when I was transported by helicopter to Charleston. The stroke ended my career as an art history teacher. My children lost the innocence of their childhood. My husband suffered the loss of a partner in raising our daughters and managing household affairs. All of my five children lost their functioning mother and their roles reversed—my children became my parents. They were taking care of me. It disrupted the lives of my sons and their families. My oldest son quit his job in Florida and relocated to Myrtle Beach to help Jeff provide care for me. My little girls could not rely on me for their homework, or listening to their problems. I could not clean their rooms or lay their clothes out for school. Instead, they were doing those things for me and they weren't even ten years old yet.

My salary continuance benefits finally expired because it was deemed that I could not return to work. My medical insurance coverage from the school district was discontinued. My husband was paying enormous health insurance premiums just for major medical and he could not afford the premiums for regular coverage. The fees were simply not feasible with the failing economy and his downturn in his business. Everyone suffered because I was uninsured and uninsurable. Jeff paid for my essential medical care out-of-pocket. The financial burdens of twelve to fifteen medications a day and out of pocket expenses for critical diagnostic tests were escalating with each passing month. The medical debts were a crushing weight on him and impacted our entire family.

At times, Jeff had trouble making ends meet. The most simple amenities and opportunities our young daughters deserved were not economically feasible. My girls could not take cheerleading lessons or attend special events with their friends after school. They didn't have pocket money for treats when they went to the mall with their friends. It was embarrassing for them when their friends offered to pay for their sodas. Their grandparents continually provided help to give them the things that young teenagers can't live without. It was humiliating for Jeff and he felt bad for his daughters. In every way, our quality of life was forever altered. I could not perform the most basic activities of daily living, dependent on others for many of my physical needs. The only thing we had an abundance of in our home was unconditional love. *We must be the luckiest people on earth.*

Our entire world had been turned upside down and the weight sat squarely on Jeff's shoulders for the years that followed. He was the rock of Gibraltar. Needless to say, when one doctor noted in my records: "This is an unfortunate story," I welled up with tears. It was far more than "unfortunate," it was earth-shattering. Learning that it could have been prevented was heartbreaking. I progressed quickly from sadness and reflection to outrage. Over the following months, I was determined to find answers as to why and how this diagnosed was missed. Not by *one* doctor—but *several* doctors. Where was my safety net of second and third opinions? Why were my physical symptoms ignored? Was I stereotyped and ignored as a middle-aged woman who overeats and turns into a couch potato? Why wouldn't those male doctors believe that I worked out at a gym, lifted weights, ran on the treadmill, and enjoyed kickboxing classes? Why were the most simple, inexpensive but essential diagnostic tests unperformed? Why? Why? Why? The shock and pain was unbearable.

I suffered so much physically and emotionally due to the failure of medical doctors to recognize my symptoms and make a proper referral. I had a disease of the endocrine system and never received a referral to an endocrinologist. I was referred to a nephrologist, urologist, gynecologist, internist, and surgeon; I had a hormonal imbalance that nearly took my life, yet I never received a referral to an endocrinologist. As this new information sank in, I felt victimized all over again. I had made so much progress to recover some brain functions and then learned it was a misdiagnosis. It was too much for me to absorb.

I was overwhelmed by this new truth. When I finally stopped crying, I took on finding the answers as my personal mission. I wanted my doctors to admit they had made a mistake and to explain their reasoning to me. My husband stood by me and attended the appointments. He fully understood my hurt and he was supportive. He is articulate and well versed on my medical conditions. He was an excellent spokesman for me. Jeff was adamant that he felt that the medical team at MUSC had saved my life and provided stellar care. He also understood my heartbreak and anger with the primary care physician in Myrtle Beach. This shocking revelation about Cushing's Disease was a major setback in my psychological recovery. Simply put, a basic screening and inexpensive blood test, in all likelihood, would have prevented the stroke and its aftermath. Jeff is also a pragmatist. *It happened, it's over, we can't change it, let's move forward with our lives.* I was bitter that he felt that way. I reasoned that *he* did not have a stroke—*I* did! *Well, Jeff, if you feel that way— fine! I will fight by myself!*

Instead of answers from the doctors I trusted for years, I received the silent treatment and lame excuses. One physician who recognized the failure of cortisol testing and proper referral to an endocrinologist actually referred me to an attorney. That attorney visit was the beginning of a long and frustrating journey into the wastelands of the legal system.

I learned as much as I could about Cushing's Disease and Cushing's Syndrome in preparation for appointments with the attorneys. I took copious notes from the most respected web sources and spent countless hours with a dictionary to help me understand the disease, diagnosis, and treatment. I spent six to eight hours a day studying and reading and trying to comprehend the materials. I simply could not retain the information without notes in front of me. Again, Jeff went with me to meet with the attorney and speak on my behalf. He is an impressive and well-educated expert on this topic today!

Researching the most respected medical books and websites, I found the Mayo Clinic definition of my clinical diagnosis of Cushing Syndrome:

"Cushing's syndrome occurs when your body is exposed to high levels of the hormone cortisol for a long time. The most common cause of Cushing's syndrome, sometimes called hypercortisolism, is the use of oral corticosteroid medication. The condition can also occur when your body makes too much cortisol.

"Too much cortisol can produce some of the hallmark signs of Cushing's syndrome — a fatty hump between your shoulders, a rounded face, and pink or purple stretch marks on your skin. Cushing's syndrome can also result in high blood pressure, bone loss and, on occasion, diabetes.

"Treatments for Cushing's syndrome can return your body's cortisol production to normal and noticeably improve your symptoms. The earlier treatment begins, the better your chances for recovery."

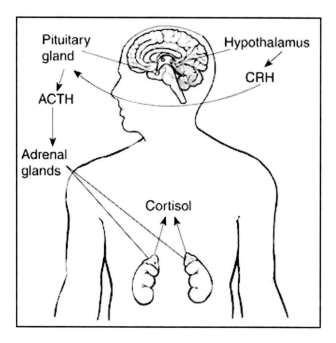

According to the National Institutes for Health, Cushing's Disease is a form of Cushing's Syndrome. _

"Cortisol excess produces significant and serious change in the appearance and health of affected individuals. Depending on the cause and duration of the Cushing's Syndrome, some people may have more dramatic changes, some might look more masculinized, some may have more blood pressure or weight changes.

"General physical features include a tendency to gain weight, especially on the abdomen, face (moon face), neck and upper back (buffalo hump); thinning and weakness of the muscles of the upper arms and upper legs; thinning of the skin, with easy bruising and pink or purple stretch marks (striae) on the abdomen, thighs, breasts and shoulders; increased acne, facial hair growth, and scalp hair loss in women; sometimes a ruddy complexion on the face and neck; often a skin darkening (acanthosis) on the neck. Children will show obesity and poor growth in height.

"On physical examination, a physician will notice these changes and will also usually find high blood pressure and evidence of muscle weakness in the upper arms and legs, and sometimes some enlargement of the clitoris in females.

"Symptoms usually include fatigue, weakness, depression, mood swings, increased   thirst and urination, and lack of menstrual periods in women.

"Common findings on routine laboratory tests in people with Cushing's Syndrome include a higher white blood count, a high blood sugar (often into the diabetic range), and a low serum potassium. These will often reinforce a physician's suspicion about Cushing's Syndrome. Ectopic Cushing's Syndrome tends to present with less impressive classic features, but more dramatic hypertension and loss of potassium, sometimes in the setting of weight loss from the underlying cancer.

"If untreated, Cushing's Syndrome will cause continued weakness of the muscles, fatigue, poor skin healing, weakening of the bones of the spine (osteoporosis), and increased susceptibility to some infections including pneumonia and TB." http://endocrine.niddk.nih. gov/pubs/cushings/cushings.aspx

These were all the symptoms I complained about for almost five years prior to the discovery of the adrenal gland tumor. I pleaded for diagnostic testing of the adrenal gland to determine whether I might have adrenal cancer, which my father was dying from at the time. The tumor was finally diagnosed in December 2006. My doctor felt that the tumor was small and monitoring at six-month intervals was determined. I did not make it to the six month mark—I had the stroke four months afterward. The removal of the tumor and left adrenal gland could have changed the catastrophic outcomes that nearly cost me my life.

To be fair, the incidence or frequency of Cushing's Syndrome in the United States is relatively rare—about 30,000 cases diagnosed annually—or approximately 2 percent of the population of adults. However, I was diagnosed with a hormone gland tumor—protocol should have been automatic referral to an endocrinologist. An endocrinologist would have easily been able to diagnose my physical manifestations of the disease and follow up with the necessary testing to confirm it.

I wanted to understand what testing *should* have been done to confirm the diagnosis. The National Institutes of Health Endocrine Society of Clinical Practice Guidelines suggest testing as follows:

Initial testing Recommended:

3.4 For the initial testing for Cushing's syndrome, we recommend one of the following tests based on its suitability for a given patient (1⊕○○○):

3.4.1 Urine free cortisol (UFC; at least two measurements)
3.4.2 Late-night salivary cortisol (two measurements)
3.4.3 1-mg overnight dexamethasone suppression test (DST)
3.4.4 Longer low-dose DST (2 mg/d for 48 h)

3.5 We recommend against the use of the following to test for Cushing's syndrome (1⊕○○○):

Random serum cortisol or plasma ACTH levels
Urinary 17-ketosteroids
Insulin tolerance test
Loperamide test
Tests designed to determine the cause of Cushing's syndrome (*e.g.* pituitary and adrenal imaging, 8 mg DST).

3.6 In individuals with normal test results in whom the pretest probability is high (patients with clinical features suggestive of Cushing's syndrome and adrenal incidentaloma or suspected cyclic hypercortisolism), we recommend further evaluation by an endocrinologist to confirm or exclude the diagnosis (1⊕○○○).

In my case, missing this protocol is significant because I was diagnosed with an adrenal gland tumor (adrenal incidentaloma) in 2006. Tragically, I was not referred for adrenal gland resection until August of 2008 and the connection of Cushing's Syndrome to my stroke was not revealed until that time. In incidental findings of the adrenal gland tumor, a dexamethasone suppression test is used to detect cortisol excess. *Prevention was possible in 2006 or 2007, months prior to the stroke.* I am appalled and angry that the stroke could have been prevented. I am angry that after the stroke my symptoms continued; I tested positive for Cushing's Syndrome and still did not receive a proper referral to an endocrinologist! Only divine intervention prevented a fatal stroke. When I finally did see an endocrinologist it was after specifically requesting a referral in 2012.

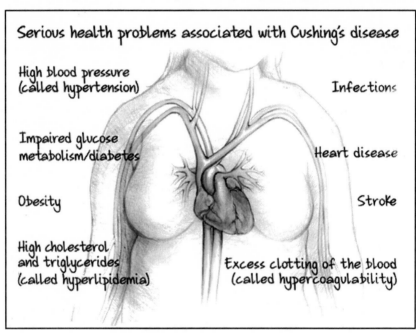

Serious health problems associated with Cushing's disease

High blood pressure (called hypertension)

Infections

Impaired glucose metabolism/diabetes

Heart disease

Obesity

Stroke

High cholesterol and triglycerides (called hyperlipidemia)

Excess clotting of the blood (called hypercoagulability)

Seeking Justice 2012

Some may say that I am obsessed with seeking justice for my catastrophic illness. I believe I have every right to unleash my heartache and anger on the medical system that failed me. Doctors I trusted failed to listen to my explanations of why their "diagnoses" were incorrect. The stereotypes for a middle-aged woman—I believe—got in the way of proper a medical diagnosis and referral to a specialist. Medical opinions are sometimes like "nailing Jello to the wall." I accept the complexities of medical science. I understand that diagnostics can render false negatives or false positives. I also understand that these complexities are the reasons for seeking second and third medical opinions. I

154

have been seeking definitive answers for my symptoms for more than seven years. My symptoms were unchanging, not the whining of a middle-aged female hypochondriac. My presenting complaints were unchanging. I believe the issue of "weight gain" to my doctors overshadowed the other major symptoms. That is, Cushing's Disease is characterized by weight gain, round moon face, fatty hump on the neck, HBP, swelling of extremities, and ballooning of the mid-torso.

Regardless of my own thoughts, the presence of an adrenal tumor in 2006 and the cortisol suppression finding—coupled with my presenting complaints and physical appearance—were more than a red flag for immediate referral to an endocrinologist. I trusted my doctors. I tried to find answers. I kept my doctors informed about my worsening symptoms. I have experienced untold suffering with the losses in my life and the traumas visited upon my family. Our lives are in shambles because of the failures of the key medical doctors who had the diagnostic evidence at their fingertips and they failed to act. With my physical characteristics, presenting complaints and the clear diagnostics—there is no justification for this failure to render proper medical care.

When my trusted doctors would not give me a satisfactory explanation, or even proclaim that they made a mistake, I must confess that I was even more devastated when they refused to talk with me honestly. I was kicked to the curb, so to speak. Now they had failed me twice. First, they missed the diagnosis and failed to act. Then they refused to take ownership of their mistakes.

Yes, I was and am angry. I want to be made whole. I want to drive to the grocery store and not have to call my husband for directions to get home. I want to order takeout food from a restaurant without stuttering and faltering and apologizing because my words don't make sense. I want to remember the names of my daughters and their best friends and the route to drive them home. I want to teach again. I just want my life back.

I want this mountain of medical debt to go away. I want to teach in a classroom again. I want to have the ability to send my daughters to college. I want to earn a living. I want to live

155

without the fear of another stroke or suffering early dementia. I want to write my own story without an editor. I want to go one whole day without asking someone else how to do or say something. I want to have one full night of restful sleep. I want to be able to balance a checkbook and pay a bill. I lost all of those privileges in April 2007.

I tried seeking justice through the legal system. It has been as frustrating for me as seeking medical answers. At the advice of a medical doctor, I sought legal counsel from a medical malpractice firm in Myrtle Beach. Jeff went to the appointment to speak on my behalf. We took my medical records. Jeff was not in favor of litigation. He felt strongly about the high quality of care and caliber of the doctors at MUSC. He credited them with saving my life. I respected his opinion, but I was the one who had the stroke, lost one-third of my brain function, and suffered all the consequences! I was adamant that this was *my* decision—not his. Jeff is no pushover—but he cuts a wide berth for allowing me to recover my "self." He never finishes my sentences or gives me the right words. He knows I will not learn and grow if he does.

At the very first appointment we were advised that regardless of the circumstances—which would take considerable time and expense to gather the evidence and analyze the findings—it was a moot point. The lawyers advised that the statute of limitations had already expired. In South Carolina, the plaintiff has only a few years from the date of the injury to file an action. Despite their sympathies for the tragic situation we were in, legal counsel offered no hope of a successful outcome and declined to take my case. This was a crushing blow.

More than anything, I wanted to be "whole" again and knew that was an impossible dream. But I was furious that my husband and children suffered the consequences of the doctors' failures to read my damn tests and refer me to the specialist that could have prevented my "tragic circumstances." I was not going to take "no" for an answer.

I proceeded to research my records, study the chronology of events, and poke holes in the first legal opinion. They were wrong about the date of discovery and I was sure that the statute of limitations had not expired. I proceeded to contact three other prestigious law firms in the surrounding area. Each time, the response was the same. One law firm conceded that the statute of limitations might be extended by six months, but that was not an adequate amount of time for preparing a successful malpractice suit. I contacted more law firms and became increasingly hostile. By now, Jeff was growing weary with my defiance and anger. We had a lot of heated discussions about litigation. He flatly refused to be part of any cause for action against ____. I think he said, "Not no, hell no, no way." As usual, I said, "That was just fine, Jeff, I can do it by myself."

I proceeded to contact law firms in the surrounding counties without success in finding a willing attorney to take my case. I began contacting law firms in nearby states because I thought the local doctors and lawyers were in bed with each other and I was at a big disadvantage. For months I collected information, picked up my medical records from all the doctors who evaluated me, and pursued every avenue possible for legal remedy. In fact, I contacted many more lawyers to take my case. With each rejection, my defiance and anger escalated. I was becoming obsessed and consumed with winning my point. Won't someone just agree with me and say, "Yes! You were screwed by a doctor who did not read the test results, who did not see the red flag waving, and who blamed my symptoms on middle age." I wanted them to pay for my suffering, admit they were wrong, and to stop this from happening again.

My Medical History Summary

To help me discuss my case with the lawyers I was contacting, my husband wrote a detailed summary of the progression of my disease. Like he always does, even when he disagrees with my approach, he supplies the information I need to make my case. He knew I was engaged in a quest for legal remedy and nothing would stop me.

Here is what he wrote:

In 2004, my wife complained of continuing hip pain (we now believe this was an early symptom of her Cushing's Disease). Dr. _____, her regular MD, found no results on her hip scan. Other symptoms began to appear. Dr. _____ found a tumor on her adrenal gland in 2006 based on an MRI. She developed high blood pressure while the doctor waited until her tumor grew. A second doctor also waited until it grew—without treatment. A CT scan was to be taken every six months. Linda consistently told me that she knew something was wrong. She continued to discuss her concerns and symptoms with her primary care physician: she was losing hair, gaining weight, displaying edema in her feet and legs, consistently spiking blood pressure and headaches. Dr. _____ prescribed various high blood pressure medicines. They would work for a short time and then her blood pressure would begin spiking again. She could have three normal readings and then one would spike to 200/135 or a similar crazy number.

In April 2007 she flew to Tennessee to visit her ailing father while on spring break from school (Linda was a high school art teacher). Just prior to leaving, she saw Dr. _____ and they discussed her erratic blood pressure spiking and the increased headaches she had been having. Throughout March of 2007 Linda had been going to the school nurse to have her blood pressure checked when the headaches got worse. The school nurse was shocked at the blood pressure spikes and told Linda something was definitely wrong. Dr. _____ kept changing the blood pressure medication, which would bring her down to a steady BP level, but would not prevent the spiking.

Linda saw Dr. _____ on April 2, 2007, and then left to go see her dad. She came back on April 4th and acted very absent-minded and disoriented. I called Dr. _____ office repeatedly on April 5th when Linda's disorientation was continuing. She had a vicious headache. The doctor told me that he felt she was reacting to a recent increase in Clonidine, a blood pressure medicine she had been taking. Her symptoms worsened throughout the day. After waking from a nap—her aberrant behavior led to a major crisis and my decision to call 911. On the way to the hospital I spoke again to Dr. _____ and he told me he was virtually certain this was a reaction to the Clonidine. However, at the hospital (Grand Strand Medical Center)

158

it was quickly determined that Linda was suffering from bleeding in her brain. The hospital flew her to MUSC in Charleston by medical helicopter.

Linda spent thirty-four days in the hospital at MUSC in neuro-intensive care followed by inpatient rehab at Waccamaw Hospital in Murrells Inlet. I was told she has suffered from a ruptured blood vessel within her left brain hemisphere. Linda lost roughly thirty percent of her brain mass due to this hemorrhage. At the time the doctors at MUSC could only speculate as to the primary cause and suggested it might be due to birth control pills or some sort of blood clotting factor that Linda might have.

With intensive rehabilitation she learned to walk, talk, and function on her own. She began to have many questions about her condition. She still felt that something was wrong and displayed all kinds of symptoms, some of which we attributed to her various medications. She was still on medication to control blood pressure as well as the blood thinner products she will have to take the rest of her life. She began to gain a significant amount of weight and had various aches and pains that we attributed to nerve damage. Some of the medication helped for a while and then stopped working. Throughout this time, the tumor attached to the left adrenal gland remained untreated. She did not talk well due to the aphasia but continued to complain that something was wrong. Instead of referring her to an endocrinologist to treat the glandular issue, Dr. _____ constantly changed her medications. He directed her to wear compression socks to combat the edema. He never referred her to an endocrinologist. Dr. _____ sent her to a neurologist who reviewed the medical records and diagnosed her with primary hypertension. She was referred to a nephrologist who finally gave up trying to control her HBP and referred her to a urologist, Dr. _____. His initial observation of her physical presentation caused him to immediately tell Linda and that he suspected Cushing's Syndrome/Disease.

The urologist conducted a preliminary Dexamethazone Suppression test (a test Linda had never been given) and was able to quickly confirm the diagnosis. This meant that the tumor on Linda's adrenal gland, which has been neglected since 2006, was the cause of her Cushing's Disease and, in all probability, her brain hemorrhage.

The urologist immediately scheduled surgery and removed the tumor and the left adrenal gland. There were various complications during and after the surgery but many of symptoms receded in the months after the tumor was removed. There were some intense episodes that required some hospital visits along the way, most of which we now believe were probably endocrine system-related. The urologist seemed satisfied very quickly that her other adrenal gland would produce enough cortisol to make up for her left adrenal gland being removed. Dr. _____ evidently agreed because I am not aware of another cortisol test being performed on Linda, which I find strange. I would think it would have been monitored more closely now that I have educated myself. Linda and I both feel like this has been a long rollercoaster. We felt all along all we could do is trust the doctors because we had no way of knowing that Linda's treatment might be incorrect.

Linda has been unable to return to work as a teacher as a result of her brain injury. When the Cobra Insurance expired we could not get any health insurance for her due to pre-existing conditions. Because Linda returned to college for her master's degree in her mid-forties, she did not have the required number of concurrent social security 'credits' for the previous five years as stated in the regulations. Linda was in her second year of teaching after college, and the gap in service caused Social Security Administration to deny her disability claim. In turn, this disqualified her for medical insurance. We did obtain the school system disability insurance which provided her a percentage of her original teaching salary. No health insurance company will touch her.

Upon completion of five years working in the school district, Linda's school loans were to be forgiven. All of Linda's student loans were suspended while she was in the hospital, but because we could not show Social Security disability status, the district revoked her suspension of repayment and added the entire amount back, which has ruined her credit.

Financially, we have been hanging on by a thread. I work six to seven days a week in the construction industry and own a small business. Linda cannot manage her financial affairs and I handle things around the house with the help of my two high school-aged daughters.

In June 2011 Linda went to a doctor, an MD here in Myrtle Beach who specializes in weight-control issues. This doctor is very well educated when it comes to Cushing's Syndrome/Disease and was shocked when he found out how Linda's adrenal tumor had been treated. Linda called me after the meeting and was extremely upset. The doctor told her that the adrenal gland tumor should never have been left in place with a watch for growth every six months. The adrenal gland controls the cortisol hormones, or metabolism, etc. The doctor told Linda he believed that lack of appropriate treatment for the tumor caused the spike in blood pressure which eventually caused the brain hemorrhage and stroke. He recommended that she contact a lawyer.

I told Linda then that I would help her talk to a lawyer but that it would have to be between jobs. Linda then went back to the urologist, the surgeon who removed her tumor. She got copies of his medical records and asked him lots of questions. Specifically, she asked "Why did I have a stroke and how did this happen?" The urologist told her that he believed her adrenal tumor caused a blood pressure spike which caused the brain hemorrhage. He said the doctors did not use the correct test to check her cortisol. He said that the required test was not a <u>cortisol level</u>, but actually a <u>cortisol suppression</u> test. Only the suppression test would show that her adrenal gland was producing cortisol when it was not supposed to.

We believe that the various doctors that Linda was referred to only treated her symptoms and not the core cause. Dr. _____ should have referred Linda immediately to an endocrine specialist when he realized the adrenal gland was involved with the tumor. Instead, he waited for the tumor to grow, and then after the brain hemorrhage he sent her to various doctors to try to treat her Cushing's symptoms. She was referred to neurologists, nephrologists, etc. These were referrals that cost thousands of dollars and did not address the root cause of her symptoms and problems. We believe that after the brain hemorrhage Dr. _____ deliberately avoided referring Linda to an endocrinologist because he thought he had made a mistake. He wanted to wait until the statute of limitations might be up.

I have researched the statute. It appears to me that Linda was not made aware of the misdiagnosis and malpractice until June/July 2011. It seems to me that the two- to three-year clocks should start *from that point. After trusting the doctors all along, we had no way of knowing until one doctor told us he believed the treatment had been inappropriate. Subsequently, the urologist confirmed the weight-loss doctor's opinion. We are at a loss to understand why the urologist failed to share this finding in 2008 when he performed Linda's surgery*

I do not know if this is a case that is too complex, too long, in or out of statute. What we do know is that we trusted our doctors. We now realize that Linda probably did not receive the correct treatment. Now she must live with this disability for the rest of her life.

Learning about Aneurysms

It is highly likely that the spiking high blood pressure caused the aneurysm to rupture, according information provided by the Aneurysm and AVF Foundation. The major causes of brain aneurysms are listed on their website. It is important to note that brain aneurysms may be caused by genetic or acquired factors. In my case, it appears to have been an acquired factor due to Cushing's Syndrome as discussed below.

Causes of Brain Aneurysms

Genetic Factors
Family History and Genetic Factors
Ehlers-Danlos Type IV
Marfan's Syndrome
Neurofibromatosis Type I
Autosomal Dominant Polycystic Kidney Disease (ADPKD)
Acquired Factors
Traumatic Brain Injury
Sepsis
Smoking and High Blood Pressure
Miscellaneous Factors – Cushing's Syndrome
Prevention
DeNovo Aneurysms

While the relative incidence of traumatic brain injury and

sepsis-caused aneurysms and subarachnoid aneurismal hemorrhage (SAH) are low, smoking and hypertension represent a much greater threat....There appears to be a relationship between IA & SAH and hypertension. The American Heart Association reports one study showing the frequency of hypertension to be 8.3 times higher among SAH patients as compared to a control group.

At this point, the only preventative measures are screening, controlling high blood pressure and smoking cessation. A secondary type of hypertension can be caused by:

Renal (kidney) disease
Pheochromocytoma
Cushing's Syndrome
Dysfunction of the thyroid or pituitary
Pregnancy

There are numerous resources that discuss causal factors. In one recent case study, researchers found, that the Cushing's Syndrome caused a cerebral aneurysm in a forty-five year old female. The study conducted in 2010 by Japanese researchers Tanaka, Kuroda, etal, at the Department of Neurosurgery in Gifu, Japan, found that overproduction of cortisol caused by Cushing's syndrome may be related to the development of cerebral aneurysm. The abstract is presented below:

Abstract

45-year-old woman presented with subarachnoid hemorrhage of World Federation of Neurosurgical Societies grade IV. Cerebral angiography showed a dissecting aneurysm of the right vertebral artery (VA). Internal trapping of the right VA with coils was performed. The postoperative course was uneventful, but she continued to demonstrate moon faces and experience amenorrhea. Computed tomography demonstrated an adrenal tumor. Laparoscopic adrenalectomy was performed under a diagnosis of Cushing's syndrome caused by an adrenal tumor. Overproduction of cortisol caused by Cushing's syndrome may be related to the development of cerebral

163

aneurysm. (Department of Neurosurgery, Gifu Prefectural General Medical Center, Gifu, Japan. masayasu.kato@nifty. ne.jp)

According to another article in the *Journal of American Physician*, Nieman and Iilias discuss the evaluation and treatment of Cushing's syndrome as follows:

"In rare cases, an abnormality of the adrenal glands, most often an adrenal tumor causes Cushing's Syndrome. Adrenal tumors are four to five times more common in women than men, and the average age of onset is about 40. Most of these cases involve noncancerous tumors of adrenal tissue called adrenal adenomas, which release excess cortisol into the blood. ([1]Nieman LK, Ilias I. Evaluation and treatment of Cushing's syndrome. *The Journal of American Physician*, 118(12):1340–1346.)

I felt like I would leave no rock unturned until I exhausted any legal remedies to bring justice to me and my family for the losses we sustained. These losses were directly due to a catastrophic stroke that in my opinion were caused by the failures of medical doctors that I respected and trusted.

In the meantime, I still have a husband who loves and supports me. I have two daughters to get through high school, and a family that will do anything to help me. I do not intend to ignore the price my family and I paid for the mistakes of my doctors. However, my life goes on and I don't want to miss being present in today or causing my family additional distress. They have suffered so much already.

Missed Diagnosis for Cousin Cindi

Remember, my father died of adrenal gland cancer, and my first cousin had an autoimmune disease. In the middle of 2012, another cousin wrote to me about her personal battle with an endocrine system disorder. It was eight years before she received an accurate diagnosis. She writes:

> Linda,
> I read through your email carefully – and read your medical documents very closely. I have so many thoughts and I'll share some of them with you. First, I agree with your opinion that

164

your stroke probably could have been avoided had you had
proper diagnosis in a timely manner. It's hard to say that with
absolute certainty, but the facts just tend to indicate that. So
naturally that is very upsetting. I did wonder, however, about
the "hemorrhagic disorder" and how that is related since that
is a risk factor for stroke, too, I think.
My first thought is that you are a "miracle." It is a miracle
for you to still be alive and to be functioning as well as you
do. I think you are amazing and you are an inspiration to me
and many others. I also consider myself a miracle. I know how
close I came to death because of lack of proper diagnosis.
Although I have been very angry over the years because of all I
have lost, I never discount the miracle of still being here.
Like you, I have wanted to help others. I don't want others
to go through what I went through. And I have found that by
helping others, it has helped me get rid of anger and has also
turned a bad thing into a good thing. So I totally understand
you wanting to be a "spokeswoman" and to help others who
have suffered. And I understand you wanting to fight for getting
those laws changed!
I looked some at the South Carolina medical malpractice
laws. I think they are ridiculous. I know in my own case that
when you are finally diagnosed and get treatment you have
a recovery period. It took a while before I even realized that
other doctors had so misdiagnosed me. And then I started
requesting medical records from many doctors who had treated
me. And that took time. Then when I got those records, I had
to read them and interpret them and all of that takes a while.
That short statute of limitations is heavily weighted against the
harmed patient.
But I have also learned over the years that the law is biased
in favor of the medical profession. It is very hard to prove
"medical negligence." I've seen that doctors often cover for
one another. And I have especially seen that doctors rarely will
admit any wrong doing. All this can be very frustrating.
Over the years, I've seen many similar cases of people going
years without the proper diagnosis. Autoimmune disease (like
my thyroid disease and others) is said to take an average of

165

6-8 years to get diagnosed. That's just unacceptable. I think part of the problem is that doctors go so much by lab tests and often don't seem to "see" their patient. You obviously had overt symptoms of Cushing's. The doctor should have recognized that and pursued it. Just like with me, everything I ever reported to a doctor or was treated for—was due to the undiagnosed thyroid issue. They should have known that and not relied on one lab test.

You and I are both very blessed to have good husbands who love us so dearly. So many women I've found do not have that support. I think having a supportive husband really helps in recovery and healing.

I appreciate you sharing more of your story with me. One night when I was feeling very frustrated, I wrote out my story. It's long but you might like to read some of it sometime. http:// thyroid.about.com/od/gettestedanddiagnosed/a/deardoctor.htm

Love you too, Cindi

What Life is Like Now?

From the outside looking in at me, the casual observer would see a well-functioning woman who is a stay-at-home mom. She walks, talks, takes care of the house, and takes her daughters to school. She works out at the local gym and is physically fit. She takes pride in her appearance. She maintains her household and enjoys her family and her friends. She takes art lessons and shows her work at local art fairs. She takes road trips to visit her sisters in North Carolina.

A closer look reveals the loss of brain function. Although I feel that I have recovered a great deal, my deficits are too great to return to the classroom or work in a meaningful career. I still have aphasia and memory loss. I still have difficulty learning, imprinting, and retrieving information. I cannot engage in spontaneous discourse with friends and colleagues. I continue to struggle to understand the nuances of conversation. Subtle hints and jokes go right over my head. I struggle to comprehend what I am reading—despite the assistance of a dictionary. I cannot put words and definitions into context.

When Jeff or my girls explain complex thoughts or ideas to me, I still have to ask them to repeat the information two or three times before I grasp their meaning. They are patient and never seem to mind but it is tiresome for me to be a drag on their time. Despite the limitations, I continue to work hard to retrain my brain and I do not give up in despair. No one said this would be easy—and it isn't! But I function well enough to take care of myself and I am surrounded by love.

Art Classes

I have been an active member of the Art Guild in Myrtle Beach for many years. I want to continue improving my artistic expression and techniques. I believe in life-long learning. I have experienced firsthand the crushing blow of memory loss. While I could not remember facts or retrieve stored memory, I could sketch from the moment I could sit up and hold a pencil. It is amazing that my artistic expression was intact. I could draw and paint throughout my recovery. Initially, my scope of vision limited the "size" of my work. I performed better on smaller works that did not require a full visual field. I could see in the center of my eyes only—making larger scale work impossible because the artist's perspective was lost.

I expect and desire constructive criticism about my paintings. Lay persons do not usually recognize defects in my work. My family and friends rave about my paintings but I crave professional evaluations, too. I cannot improve or learn without critical examination. In the early 1980s, I had a wonderful instructor named Tom Moore in North Carolina. He was analytical and taught me numerous techniques and stylistic applications to improve my finished pieces. Today, I have a wonderful "master" named Jim Horton who works with me and seven other local artists. He candidly critiques our techniques and will stop us and say, "Stop right there because you are doing it wrong." Then he demonstrates the correct way to achieve the desired effect. We meet for class and instruction every Monday from 10:00 a.m. until 2:00 p.m. When new people who do not know my story join our group, they think I am "not quite right in the mind." They are right!

I have good friends who are fellow artists who also help me greatly. Many of them have helped me with their friendship and art critique. One in particular, Deb Austin, is one of those lifelong friends who has helped me become a better artist. Together, Deb and I took classes from Kate Lagaly, a very accomplished artist. Many of the techniques I had once known were taught to me again by Kate, for which I will always be grateful. I speak to Deb weekly even though she has moved out of the Myrtle Beach area and treasure my relationship with her. Deb accepted my deficits and provided unwavering support as I worked to constantly improve my speech and art abilities.

The weekly learning sessions reinforce what I am struggling to relearn about colors and applications that I had lost. I had forgotten so much that it makes me cry with joy that I can do this again. *"Oh, yes. I remember that!"* I am so grateful to have an instructor who expects the same from me that he does of the other artists. We chose a great instructor, Jim Horton. At age seventy he does not need money and does not care if he hurts our feelings. He knows we could not improve without his constant, "All right, just stop ... and let me show you again how to do this." His ability to critique and his accuracy on perspective is priceless training for me. Some say he is rather eccentric—I saw him as a godsend. Unfortunately he passed away recently, but the artists in his group still paint together. We like to think that in a small way his legacy lives on through us at the *Flying Fish Restaurant.*

The continuity of working with my fellow artists has helped me regain confidence in my abilities. I am indebted to them for their patience to try and understand my aphasic speech patterns. We have enjoyed learning together and doing art shows together. My son, Larry Bond, arranged for all of us to show our work at the *Flying Fish Restaurant* in Myrtle Beach. It is an uplifting experience to display your art work and see the appreciation that people have for paintings that we create.

In July, I wrote to the editor of the *The Sun News*. He wrote a story about an 18-year-old girl who was sitting at a stop light in New Jersey when another driver ran into her car and killed her. Her mother said she was an angel and said several things that reminded me of my precious daughter, Carmelita. I wrote him and told him I am not as good as I used to be but I would love to try to paint a "Cynthia Ayala" portrait for her mother (for free, of course). When I write something like this I am very aware of my slow and inadequate ability to deal with people and express what I would like to say. It does not bother me and I do not feel sorry for myself. I know I am fortunate to be alive and functioning as well as I do.

Service to Others

I now realize there are better things that God wants me to do. God does not tell me exactly what He wants but I know when an opportunity presents itself to be of service. I think I am an inspiration or symbol of hope to some of the people in my stroke support group. I hope they can regain some cognitive and physical abilities, too. Every stroke victim is different in terms of progress and recovery. A great deal depends on whether they suffer from a vascular, aortal, or cerebral aneurysm associated with a stroke. For that reason, we should not compare ourselves with other victims. In my opinion, we should each strive to do our very best to recover the losses we covet the most. I am motivated to improve my speech and memory by my love of art and teaching. Remember, the first thing I did when they set me upright in a wheelchair was to sketch a picture of another stroke victim. I did it with my left hand, too, as my right was still useless from the stroke.

I am aware of other opportunities I am given to be of service. A runaway black Labrador retriever almost drowned in our pool but I was nearby to show her how to get out of the pool. There was only one section where she could exit the pool on her own. I was able to guide her out before she drowned from exhaustion. I was so happy I could "teach" this dog.

Recently, I received a letter from the Waccamaw Animal Rescue Mission thanking me for my service to help them save abandoned animals. I sketched numerous pastels of dogs and cats which were framed and displayed to raise money for the mission. Their Adoption Day Fundraiser featured the drawings and they earned all of the proceeds.

My mother-in-law, Peggy, has been an angel of generosity like this for all her life and I just really "woke up" after my stroke. It

169

seemed like I was always too busy raising kids, working, and using my spare time to do what "I wanted to do." Part of my psychological recovery has been the realization that God stopped me and made me slow down. He took the "wall" away that I hid behind since childhood and freed me to think more about others. I can still do everything that he wants me to do but he had to "mold me" gently and prove His existence to me.

When I see someone who has the obvious physical characteristics of Cushing's Syndrome, I share my experience with them. My daughters are so embarrassed when I do this and accuse me of intruding in the lives of others. I sincerely hope I am not insulting these individuals. I wish someone would have stopped me in the mall to say, "You know, I have Cushing's Syndrome......" It is hard to approach a stranger but I do it anyway because I just might save one person from a fatal stroke. I can only try. I work to be an advocate for Cushing's Syndrome, stroke recovery, stroke dyslexia and the importance of art therapy.

Living by Example

"Do not be weary in well-doing, for in due
season you shall reap, if you do not lose heart."
Galatians 6:9

My sister, Roxie, shared her wisdom with me... "You are different now ... you think about what you say before you say it." She was right and I am aware that I need to think before I speak. I need to listen and pay attention to what my loved ones are actually saying to me without reacting. I did not do that before my stroke. I have excellent role models to become a better person. Peggy has helped her friends, families, students, and acquaintances all her life! I see her as being a perfect grandmother, wife, mother, mother-in-law, sister, daughter, family, and the best person I know. Her faith and kindnesses are rare. Jeff and I both realize that she loves us and we are better people just trying to live by her example. I fall short below in comparison to my mother and Peggy. I strive to be more like them. I hope our children will pick up some of the "core heart and soul" that seems to come naturally to them. I know Jeff is definitely a better person from the unconditional love and support of his parents. He knows that. We both realize and talk about them as role models. Jeff is a perfect husband and father because of his parents and the way he was raised.

Peggy has taught me that humility is not a weakness—it is my strength. She has shown me that I can be kind and tolerant without being a doormat. Despite all that kindness, concern, and consideration for others—she is no milk toast! I have seen her level the playing field when she sees prejudice and cruelty. I want to be strong without being aggressive and hostile. I want to think before I speak. I want to be a child of God and raise my children to have good character and a moral compass to steer their ships through troubled waters. If I can do these things to be a better person—I will be a winner.

A Typical Day in 2012-2013

The deficits that I had after the aneurysm/stroke every year improve with each passing year. My blessings are many. I spend much of my time researching my disease, thinking about legal remedies, and writing for my book. Due to my aphasia, my writing requires a lot of editing. Peggy knew that, but still encouraged me to write as much as I could. With her wisdom and conversations with Jeff, I realize my progress was considerably fast in comparison to most "stroke" victims. I am less easily frustrated today. I can pause, regain my composure, and try again if I don't do it correctly the first time. Peggy did not tell me what to write, but she gave me suggestions and she organizes and corrects my work. I am sure you would not have enjoyed reading my book without her help.

The aphasia is my biggest challenge because it effects my communication with the rest of the world. The spontaneity of conversation is hampered. In her book "My Stroke of Insight" Dr. Jill Taylor, Brain Scientist, writes: "People who have damage in their left hemisphere often cannot create or understand speech because the cells in their language centers have been injured. However, they are often genius at being able to determine if someone is telling the truth, thanks to the cells in their right hemisphere."

Studying the role of each hemisphere of my brain helps me understand why my former learning strategies are not effective now. My best learning tools were reading, memorization, and drilling with flash cards. These are learning tools controlled in the left hemisphere. Stroke victims should never give up. Personally, I understood that the medication was slowing my ability down to think clearly. To be honest, had I continued the volume of medications I was taking after my stroke, I would not enjoy the improvements I gained after weaning myself from so many medications. However, I am not suggesting people change their medicines without careful consultation with the treating physician. It is also important for me to carry medical information with me in case of accident or injury. I also try to make sure every single doctor I see has a complete and current list of my medications. Both over-the-counter and prescription drugs have potentiating outcomes.

As a teacher, it is my nature to measure progress in my learning. My best yardstick for measuring improvements is in six-month intervals. It is hard to see improvement day to day. I see significant improvements in my writing and composition with time. I get up each morning with a goal and do not go to bed until midnight. I am usually exhausted mentally. I get up and do the best I can each day. It doesn't matter whether I am cleaning the toilet or learning new words. I cannot prove what happened and why I was a survivor. I cannot explain why I am able to do things that the doctors said I could not do. My MUSC doctors are more amazed each time I return for the annual evaluation. Each time I have improved cognition and speech.

After the first two years, my goal was to improve enough that I could return to my classroom. I was even more determined after my trip to Italy. I was inspired by the art and excited all over again. They checked my brain again and I got very excited. I knew I had progressed and I was eager to hear my test results. The neurologist said, "I have great news … your brain is still at the same level … no more damage." I hoped for more. There is a poem written by my former co-worker, Terry Edge, which describes my thoughts and aspirations for improvement.

"Understand
You cannot Know
You may feel
And contemplate
And reason,
But you may never know.
Contemplate
Is to live within your limits
Without being less
Than your destiny demands.

Terry Edge

"**W**arhol shows us our idols,
Segal shows us ourselves."

Phyllis Tuchman

4
LESSONS LEARNED

It is a fact that medical science cannot explain my survival. I have lost count of the dumbfounded reaction of doctors who read through my medical records. As Peggy said, "I kissed the face of God, and came back to tell the tale." Maybe that is the major lesson learned here. "All things are possible under God." It is abundantly clear to me that God had other plans for me. However, I am not yet clear on exactly what His plans are.

In his book *A Purpose Driven Life*, Rick Warren writes that at the end of the day when our time on earth is over the only thing that matters to us is love of family. We don't ask for our diplomas, bank books, or material possessions on our deathbeds—we ask for those we love. He also writes that our sole purpose on this earth is to be of service to God—to carry out His mission for us. That is all we have to do every day—ask His will for us then do our best to do it! Perhaps in the final analysis, this is why my life was spared.

It is difficult to summarize and condense the "meaning" of my own catastrophic medical experience. I am humbled by the fact that I am still alive. I believe that it is only by the grace of God that so many physical and cognitive deficits were restored over the past five years. I realize that many other variables influenced the quality of life I enjoy today. In my case, I believe in divine intervention—it was not my time to go. I believe that my character traits of perseverance and courage gave me the "never say die" attitude that kept me fighting for survival. In truth, my ego probably had a great deal to do with my determination to overcome apparent and embarrassing deficits. I was embarrassed for people to think of me as "less than." I also believe that I am a product of my environment—especially as it related to my childhood which was filled with domestic abuse and poverty. I honed my instincts for survival throughout those years.

I believe that the love and support and patience of family and friends transcended the barriers of physical and cognitive impairments. My loved ones were trying with all their hearts and souls to be there for me throughout the coma. They were all trying so hard to reach me. Yet I was angry at them because I could not comprehend incoming information and I could not communicate outgoing information. I believe mother's love kept me comforted with ethereal affirmations. I felt her calming presence all around me. I remember hearing myself say, "My girls are too young to be without their mother." I had to survive for them.

My lifelong habits of exercise and diet are another large factor in the increased odds for my survival. Twenty years of physical fitness provided me with the endurance and physical stamina to overcome so many physical deficits. Interestingly, I had experienced a lifetime with undiagnosed learning disorders. Thus, I was accustomed to the struggles of reading, comprehension, and memorization. I was definitely not a stranger to dictionaries, drilling, and flash cards. These tools served me well in overcoming aphasia as well as I did. My lifestyle_also played a role. I never smoked, only drank wine socially, and maintained a healthy weight all of my life. My life with Jeff was too wonderful to lose.

Lessons to Share with Others

I have given a lot of thought to the question—*what were my lessons learned?* Generally speaking, the important lessons learned are not earth-shattering, but my thoughts might be helpful for other victims and their families. My mother-in-law Peggy has helped me put together some of my family's lessons learned.

More than One Victim: A catastrophic illness does not happen

176

to just one person. Individuals who love the victim are also victims. They suffer emotional pain, fear, worry, and powerlessness. There is no "rule book" for them to follow on how to interact with a brain-impaired person. They are engaged in a battle to control their own fears and emotions while striving to "be there" for the victim. Their hearts cry out—*please don't die!* While voices sing out—*hang on, you're going to be alright!* After the immediate crisis is over, the family members continue to feel the after burn.

Caregiving: There is no roadmap for caregiving to someone with a traumatic brain injury. Despite a caregiver's best efforts, the impaired person may be angry, difficult, and resentful. The length of the road to recovery is unknown and family members bear the burden of care. No matter how much we love the injured person, caregiving is a heavy responsibility. Like my son, some individuals must relocate and/or quit their jobs to help provide care. In my case, the need for daily care at home was only a few months. We were fortunate. But there are individuals in my stroke group who have been highly dependent for a decade. The demands on caregivers take a heavy toll.

Long-term caregivers need as much support as the impaired person. There is a distinct difference in caring for a person with dementia or brain injury compared to caring for a person with other physical issues, for example. Those with severe brain injuries suffer communication disorders, often have personality changes, lack judgment and problem-solving skills, and deteriorate over a long period of time. Caregiver support groups are an outstanding benefit to families who take on these tasks for the long haul. Basically, attending to the support and health of the primary caregiver is as important as the care provided to the impaired person. Caregiver support groups, respite care, and encouragement are the tools of those who are on the outside looking in.

Extended caregiving at home victimizes the family again. Psychological and physical ailments are common among caregivers. Primarily women, caregivers suffer increased depression, anxiety, and fatigue. They perceive themselves as "weak" if they ask for help or need respite. Abusing medications and alcohol are not uncommon for caregivers. Extended family members and friends would do well to pay as much attention to the caregivers as to the victims. Watching for these signs might signal the need for intervention.

It takes a village: I was so proud to learn how my entire family circled the wagons to protect my children. In a long-term catastrophic illness it takes the entire village to pave the road to recovery. My children were shattered, our finances devastated, my career ended, insurance terminated, relocation to another house, and other dramas were playing out while I remained incapacitated. No role is too small to play in sharing care and concern. Every kindness counts. Prayer chains make a difference.

I was so touched that Elena's teacher took her aside at school the morning after my stroke to find out what was wrong with her. The teacher could see that Elena was pale, worried, and unusually quiet. On hearing her story, the teacher took her under her wing, washed her face, dried her tears, and gave her extra support. I know how good that felt to Elena and as a teacher I know how good it felt to the teacher to give that support to my little girl.

My sisters dropped their responsibilities at home to rush to the aid of my children three hours away. My husband lived in that hospital along with me, constantly trying to reassure the kids that everything would eventually be okay. My sons are my heroes—in very different ways—and they shouldered more than their share of responsibility. Co-workers gave me so much joy with visits and cards. It was an opportunity to keep some small connection with my "professional self." Like other precious commodities, every drop of kindness counts and buoys the spirit of the victims and the families.

Don't Go It Alone: It is okay to ask for help. It is okay to accept help when it is offered. It is not a sign of weakness to allow others to be part of the recovery process. Most people are kind and happy to provide assistance—especially in the beginning of the illness. Over time, when the initial crisis has run its course, help is more and more scarce. It is important to have a support team—don't just go it alone.

As the victim, I was non-compliant! This was probably due to fear of dependency and the unknown. I acted out with obscene language and refusing assistive devices. I created more fear and more work on my family because I wanted to "go it alone" and do it my way. This is definitely one of my important lessons learned. Ultimately, I forced myself to attend speech therapy and support groups. I despised being there. I allowed my son to take me to the bathroom and cussed him every step of the way. I allowed my little girls to be Brain 1 and Brain 2. They answered questions that I could not respond to. They were "interpreters" for me and it was embarrassing. I realize now that it made them feel good and important to be helping me recover.

Most importantly for me, I am stubborn to a fault. I had to learn the hard way to at least listen and consider the opinions of others. Today, I actually ask for the opinions of people I respect and listen to what they say before I make a final decision. You might say that since I lost one third of my brain I need to use the brains of others to fill the void!

Spiritual Fitness: I have been actively engaged in physical fitness all of my adult life. I have also been active in intellectual fitness through education, reading, research, and teaching. But I had neglected my efforts to maintain spiritual fitness. Perhaps more than anything else learned from this experience I have renewed my spiritual connection with God. It was always there, but not in the forefront. With each passing day and by writing this book, I have a new appreciation for the meaning of "God's Grace." I am alive by a miracle, as there is no medical explanation for surviving a stroke of this magnitude. Yes, I am still angry and still grieve the losses in my life but there are moments of infinite calm that I know are gifts from God. I hear that "small, still, quiet voice within." I know that I will be okay even if everything is not okay. I am not alone. I can do this. I am grateful for this new spiritual awareness.

Reflections on Family

With the passage of time and my restoration to relatively good health, I find myself examining my relationships with the people I care about. I wonder whether I have given enough praise to my children. I thought I did but as I write this I wish I had taken the time to praise their work rather than critique it. I know that I cannot possibly bestow the loving memories on the hearts of my children that my mother left me. I can look at myself objectively

179

and understand ways I failed them. My expectations of them were unfair. Especially related to art, I should not have expected them to have the passion for art that I did. Academically, I struggled to get to school and through school. Learning was difficult for me as a child and as an adult in college. Imprinting, retaining, and recalling factual information required exhaustive study, drilling, and memorization. These skills come easily to my husband and to my children. Thus, I have great expectations on them. Because they are brighter and more intellectual, I constantly push them to excel and expect more effort. It is one thing to push myself to study, relearn, and restore my memory, but it is unfair to push them at the same relentless pace.

My own fears of failure are projected onto them. I am constantly fighting for the survival of my executive functioning; they are bright and intelligent. I have never felt incompetent until after the aneurysm. Before the stroke, I could study, learn, and retain data—now I cannot tell someone my home address without handing them my driver's license. I cannot remember my phone number and often get lost driving from home to my supermarket.

I accept that I am powerless to create and accomplish my lifetime dreams of a career in art. I was just getting started. After only eighteen months of teaching, that massive stroke and aneurysm robbed my mind. Some days I don't think about the losses but other days, like today, my deficits are very much on my mind. My youngest daughter started high school today. The principal at Carolina Forest High School in Myrtle Beach is an awesome young woman. She is an enthusiastic educator. Her passion for learning is infectious among these young students. She is personable, witty, and energetic. High school students respond beautifully to her. Her communication skills are outstanding. I am so glad that my daughters are going to school in her district. I envy her future and believe she will go far in her career.

I would love to have her job. For the first time in my life, I cannot say "I can do that job! I would make a great principal and invigorate students to love learning, grow self-esteem and develop good character." Then I remember—*no I cannot do that, I know I cannot.* I no longer have the mental capacity for spontaneous interaction. The brain damage has changed my personality. At times, I am impatient and easily frustrated. Even when I am concentrating as hard as I can, there are long pauses in my response time. Some days I write and speak beautifully … almost! Other days my intellectual function is probably at a seventh-grade level, or lower. I have a long way to go to get back my "self."

Acceptance

Acceptance is an important part of recovery. Yet it is the lesson hardest for me to learn. I thought *acceptance* meant failure. If I accepted myself as I was—there would be no incentive to get better or to work harder at regaining my "self." The truth is that *acceptance* means that I must make peace with the past. When I stop fighting the past and the wrongs of others, I regain inner peace. Acceptance allows me to make an honest appraisal of where I am—where I want to go—and how I plan to get there. If I am constantly looking back—I will miss my road to the future. It is easier said than done—but it is worth the effort.

I am reminded by Peggy that acceptance doesn't mean that I have to *like* it—it means I must learn to live with it and make new plans. If I continue to battle the world, I will lose the inner peace that makes my life worthwhile. I lose the inner peace that allows me to really see and hear my beautiful children and all the blessings in my life.

Yes, I can accept what has happened and live life accordingly. It does not mean that I should give up on my efforts to improve, or seek legal remedy, or to abandon my hope to educate others. It just means I cannot leave the bodies of my family all over the playing field while I do battle against the system.

Gratitude

Jeff's father, Dick, always says that "gratitude is the cornerstone" of happiness. He says that we should go to bed and get out of bed with an "attitude of gratitude." He is right. It is hard to be full of fear or resentment if I am thinking about what is good in my life. I make a big effort to think about the good things in my life and to count my blessings. That doesn't mean I am giving up on my mission—it just means I don't have to be so angry about pursuing a difficult path. I am most grateful for my relative good health in the face of all that has happened to me. I am grateful that God spared my life, and I am grateful that all of my family members stood by me and carried me back to wellness. Now it is my turn.

This poem describes how I think about the valuable lessons of my life.

Van Gogh's Prayer

A battle lost in the cornfields
And in the sky a victory.
Birds, the sun and birds again.
By night, what will be left of me?
By night, only a row of lamps
A wall of yellow clay that shines,
And down the garden, through the trees,
Like candles in a row, the planes;
There I dwell once and dwell no longer-
I can't live where I once lived, though
The roof there used to cover me
Lord, you covered me long ago.

By Janos Pilinsky

Lessons Learned about My Sons

I believe babies are chosen by God to be born at a special time. If children are not born at that time, and that child's time was missed, another child cannot make up for that missed opportunity. There was that special time reserved for my sons, Larry and Nathan. I did not recognize this fully at the time. I believe the children we have are not accidents. God has a purpose for every human.

Larry, my son, is amazing and special in many ways. I will not be able to acknowledge all of his gifts or accomplishments, but I know what they are. His gifts were truly revealed to me and to others the moment he learned about my stroke. My stroke and aneurysm led to a coma—and all the days following that event—showcased all the goodness a mother can hope for in a son. There are many things my son will accomplish and he will fulfill the reasons God has ordained for him.

My son Nathan is an artist, both in ability and in his way of thinking. His gifts as a craftsman in his field of work are an expression of his art abilities. Nathan's gentle, loving soul brightens the world of those around him.

Lessons Learned About My Husband

There are wonderful people on this earth that can get it straight. My husband is one of them. He gets up very early in the morning seven days a week. He is one of those veterans who would be right there to fight again if America needed him. Today we are happy and safe in our own home because of him. Our young girls respect their dad but not to the extent I know they will when they are older. Jeff is one of the smartest people I have ever met and he lives by ethical principles. Is he perfect? No. What he does is keep our home comfortable, happy, and safe.

I have a huge appreciation for men and women in service to our country. I respect and admire the families who sacrifice their time with their loved one due to the long absences of military service. My father and brothers are good examples of this. As for me—I did not want to be a wife living, working, and raising children alone. I did not want to be married to someone in the service.

I believe in the commandment to "Honor thy father and thy mother." My sons have so much respect for Jeff and they use Jeff's advice. I hope all three of the girls find someone as fair and committed to their marriage as we are. The secret is to understand life is not perfect and both of partners have to make it happen. Not one, both. If you are living in a relatively serene home, living a life of good character, happy and safe most of the time—life is worthwhile. If you are miserable in the marriage—then changes need to be made. An unhappy home is no place to raise children. Domestic violence, alcoholism, adultery, and other character deficits are treatable if the individuals want to be better. A father or mother who drinks excessively sets a poor example for children and creates desperation in the spouse living with it. Alcoholism is treatable and people with a problem know it.

When either of the partners are unwilling to communicate, compromise, or seek counseling, then there is really no hope for a successful marriage. Life is too short for me to accept less. I will not expose myself or my children to domestic violence whether verbal or physical. I will not live with an alcoholic or addict who refuses to acknowledge the problem and seek help. I will never live in conflict in my home and I have a husband who agrees.

My life is too precious to waste. I do not know how much time I have left, but whatever time I do have I intend to be happy and to be of service to God and others.

Lessons Learned from Others

Many years ago an employee shared these words of wisdom from his unpublished book of poetry. His words are prophetic and exemplify important guideposts for living a life of character. Given to me as a gift, I share them here with you:

A free life
Is such a precious gift
That even though we cannot conceive of God,
We have need to bow down
And thank Something
For this opportunity
To Be.

Have guts.
Do what is right,
Especially when it hurts,
For that is when it most crucially concerns others.
It does not come off itself.
Use your mind.
It takes conscious,
Concerted effort
To be moral.

Terry Edge, Fayetteville, North Carolina

You alone decide who you will be.
In small steps your character
is formed every day."

Anne Dotson

5

THE FUTURE

This is what I want to share as the final chapter in this book about my current life. It represents where I am today—and where I hope to go. Jeff left at four o'clock this morning and I could not sleep. He will be in the heat outside working with his employees. I am at home safe with my girls and my faithful German Shepherd, Mauser. I know no one is coming into our home past Mauser! Today we also have Diesel, a giant Alaskan Malamute that was a gift from another brain injury survivor. There are so many things I want to say to encourage others and to share what I have learned since awakening at Waccamaw Hospital in rehab. I can talk and understand better now.

I need to say one other thing. I was reading part of my art graduate studies work that I had written for credit. One article was about classroom action—a research project that described how I would teach in a classroom. As I now read the content, it is more difficult than what I remembered. A few activities that are "foggy" (I do not remember how to do them today): student achievements; engage the rational research; aesthetics; speech; and writing about art and activities.

The parts of earlier "Childhood Classrooms Communications," media oral and written language, cognitive/symbols expression in the learning process, design, implementer exemplary content, and reflection to name a few. *(I am writing this as I am reading it, but at this point I do not understand what it means).* I had to excel in grades one through twelve to earn my degree. But I no longer comprehend the meaning of these phrases. If someone showed me each step or demonstrated the correct approach, I could probably do it.

The reading that I had written about my interpretation and thinking was not just for a "grade" or to understand the extent, I had written and still recognize it was the actual real way I taught before my stroke. It was not just to get my master's degree, I taught that quite seriously.

How long will it take to understand a curriculum and again to do this, learn, understand, and comprehend? I do not know. It does not matter. Every time I study I am an inch closer than where I would have been before or would have given up. I never gave up, that is for sure!

In 2009 after Peggy took me to Italy ... I could not read. Words on paper all looked like a foreign language to me. I was still learning words, then sentences that seemed like it took me forever to read. I still cannot easily comprehend scholarly work. Now, I can work my way through the "Reader's Digest." At the time we went to Italy, I could barely read "Dick and Jane!" I was barely able to read at a first-grade level. That is the level I continued to practice. Every sentence took forever.

I went to my doctor's office and I was embarrassed that I could not fill out a form or answer new questions. But the willingness to start at the bottom was essential. I was like a child in terms of reading and comprehension. I had to start at my own starting point. Nothing would happen unless I tried to over and over. I had to go back to Dick, Jane, Look, Help, and Thank you ... over and over. I am not sure what elementary school teachers use now, but I used the approach that my teachers used in grammar school. It worked for me and I became an excellent speller thanks to phonics.

In 2014, I can read and I am starting to understand the materials. It is so important that I fully engaged myself in learning and took it seriously on a daily basis. I study, practice, read, and write at least six hours every day. My speech and communications disorders are still significant. The speech therapist was helpful in getting me started. The real work is the responsibility of the "learner." You are responsible for your reaching out to your greatest possibility. I believe everyone will start at different levels and pace but the effort expended is the key. Looking back at my writing, no one could read my book or understand what I had written in 2009. I could not understand myself!

188

The words made sense when I put them on paper, but everything I wrote in those first two years is disjointed. Realizing how difficult it was to write an entire paragraph that made sense, I made notes and put them on cards. Sometimes it was so offbeat that when I looked at it the next day I did not remember what I meant. My spelling was terrible. I would draw what I thought I was writing.

Drawing to communicate reminds me of cuneiform writing in ancient history. Drawing is a legitimate way to communicate. How did the Votive statues of that time (made of the limestone, alabaster, and gypsum) of large figures communicate with others? Scale of the body might have been small in comparison to a human yet the eyes scaled excessively large. You do not have to say or read anything, you automatically recognize the message! I didn't remember that explanation well enough to write it; I had to look in my history book to explain it correctly.

I remember what I see in my mind but I did not remember the sculptures I had studied and was tested on. Right now I am not able to tell anyone about a specific work of art unless I read it and have it in front of me while I am speaking. Even with those teaching aides, my spoken words may not match my brain's intent. The point is that we have to start somewhere or we might as well forget getting better. I was awful in 2008 and I was embarrassed and humiliated to read "Dick and Jane" in front of my children. They had to help me read it. If I had not started my quest for recovery in 2008, I would be a failure to myself. We do not get better by doing nothing. It takes work, willpower, and willingness.

If you are a husband, wife, caregiver … spend time daily with the basics. Don't necessarily start with words, try to start with form, a line with their side of the hand that they eat with. Do not give up on them even when they give up … keep trying every day! I was miserable because I could not remember my eyes, nose, and mouth, I knew I had them but *why didn't I know where they were … what happened?* Today I know that where the body begins and ends is knowledge provided by the left hemisphere of the brain. I lost one third of my left brain. I know stroke victims are all at different places in their abilities. My goal is to share my experience with others to provide a roadmap and some hope.

How can I help others … set an example? I can only share what

I did and what was successful for me. I can also share what did not work for me. I cannot tell you all those biological parts of the brain. The neurologists use those terms with our families and caregivers. But I do not need to know or be able to recite them at this point in my recovery. I just need to get into action to get better. Like a small child, I had to relearn the ABC's, reading, writing, and arithmetic. I do know that the brain mass I lost in 2007 is still lost. But I am able to compensate and open new pathways in my brain to grow my knowledge and memory a little bit every day. The best way I can explain my progress is that I repeatedly study a word or concept until "I get it!" I do it over and over until I get it. Starting with the applied arts concepts of the line, the form, the value, the shapes, and space works for me. I think we underestimate the value of art interpretations with a stroke victim trying to make those connections in the brain! I believe talking, reading, and comprehension are critical to become productive human beings and to help stroke victims attain their highest potential. Again, there are big differences in functioning based on which half of the brain was damaged. That is, deficits caused by a right brain stroke are different compared to left brain damage.

My goal and desire now is to work with other stroke survivors to share my successes and see if they can benefit. Sometimes I dream of an academy for relearning and opening new pathways in the brain. Ideally, this might be achieved through peer support, meaning one stroke victim helping another with all the understanding both individuals have of the devastating effects of a stroke. I remember speaking to a lady older than I am when I went to Coastal Carolina. She said she wanted to paint and teach art to imprisoned people. I am embarrassed to share how negative I was about her goal. My first thought was "what a waste of time!" God was obviously not finished with me yet. I am definitely a work in progress. Look how long that took me to figure out.

I want to expand beyond art for my personal growth and pleasure using the example of hieroglyphics—communication can be created through art. As mentioned earlier, I could not write out my thoughts for inclusion in the book. I knew what I wanted to say in my mind but it was impossible to put on paper. I had to draw pictures of what I wanted to say. As my ability to express my thoughts on paper increased I went back to those pictures in my files. A year later I was able to translate the pictures into words. How wonderful is that? It was a tangible measure of my improvements and gave me a needed boost in morale. Others telling me I am better is so nice to hear. But seeing my progress in measurable outcomes is awesome!

God took care of my brain, I am sure ... I feel it. I believe it is God's plan that I learn tolerance and acceptance for all of His children. My ethereal experience in the trauma center comes to mind. I was seeing my mother in heaven with her beautiful smile near a fence with Helen. She did not have to say anything. I just felt her presence and the warmth of her smile. I knew everything was okay and I started on my own journey wherever I was led to be. I did not know the doctors were opening up my brain, draining fluid, barely keeping me alive. I was on the fence enjoying my mother and my sister who I had never met. Somehow the words came out of my mouth, "Can I paint in Heaven?" Mom smiled and I said "I don't want to go to Heaven, I have too much I want to paint." My heart smiles when I think of her and I know I will paint her picture when I get to heaven.

Art is beyond "fun." It is the core of my being. God created my passion for art and my desire to create in a medium that transcends "speech." Perhaps my dream of returning to the classroom is foolish and unrealistic. But I cannot fail by trying. I only fail by doing nothing. You might say that I am on the fence again for my life. I am at a fork in the road and I need to find a way to do both of my passions. If I cannot teach high school students, I want to teach art to adults, maybe even to stroke victims. I want to work with others any way I can. I realize I am not at the level I was when I earned my degree. I would want to be as good as I was at teaching. I recognize that I do not have the patience for working with children. Students deserve and parents expect the kind of art education I provided my high school students. God has changed my life and He has other plans for me. (I wish He would hurry up and tell me exactly what those plans are because I am excited and ready!) I know I am His servant and I am okay with that. I will not be contented or complacent with His needs and I know that He is right there to guide me.

I no longer "grieve" my lost ability and broken dreams as I used to do. God has a larger desire that I cannot comprehend ... I do not need to know ... I will continue getting up and trying every day to improve as much as I can. I have better days and then some days I become disappointed that I am moving slower than I think I should. When I am feeling low, one trip to my stroke group leaves me feeling grateful and better. I always get the feeling that I am making a difference. That is a good start on being of service.

I think about those special people the entire time I am with them. We identify with each other. "What caused my stroke ... what caused theirs? It has been at least ten years since most of them suffered a stroke, why aren't they better by now? What can I do to improve myself? What can I do to help them with their depression and loss of hope? Do they think I am just lucky because I function so well? Do they realize how hard I work every single day to get a little bit better than yesterday? If they worked at it hard enough, couldn't they get better, too? Or are their losses permanent? I think about them all the time and wonder about their futures. I believe all we can do is try, try, and try some more. Stroke survivors and their families need emotional and educational support.

The other side of the coin that does haunt me is the fact that my stroke was preventable. I do not know how I can be effective in sharing my circumstances with other potential victims. There are only a few national associations that specifically advocate for stroke survivors who had aneurysms due to Cushing's disease. My goal is to become acquainted with the resources available for people like me. For example, the mission of the Cushing's Support and Research Foundation is to support families and survivors. Two are listed here for anyone interested in finding information about diagnosis, treatment and support, as described on its webpage:

Cushing's Support and Research Foundation

"While the most common cause of Cushing's is exposure to corticosteroid medications such as prednisone and others used in injections and creams, a small percentage of the population develop Cushing's due to a tumor on the pituitary gland, the adrenal gland, or elsewhere in the body. Because Cushing's caused by tumors is a relatively rare disorder and some of the symptoms are common in the population, many patients with Cushing's

are not __tested__ for the disorder and continue to go undiagnosed.

The Cushing's Support and Research Foundation is a 501 (c) 3 non-profit organization dedicated to supporting patients with Cushing's and their families. Since 1995, the CSRF has provided information for patients on the medical aspects of Cushing's, put patients in contact with other patients and worked to increase awareness in the general population and the medical community. We are supported primarily by membership and individual donations and would greatly appreciate __your support!__ __http://csrf.net/__ "

Aneurysm and AVM Foundation

"A brain AVM (arteriovenous malformation) is an abnormal connection between arteries and veins. An AVM is typically congenital, meaning it dates to birth. An AVM can develop anywhere in your body but occurs most often in the brain or spine. A brain AVM, which appears as a tangle of abnormal arteries and veins, can occur in any part of your brain. The cause isn't clear.
You may not know you have a brain AVM until you experience symptoms, such as headaches or a seizure. In serious cases, the blood vessels rupture, causing bleeding in the brain (hemorrhage). Once diagnosed, a brain AVM can often be treated successfully."
www.taafonline.org

My aneurysm occurred in a vein—rather than an artery.

I urge the relatives, friends, teachers, artists, and others to become aware of Cushing's Syndrome/Disease and the associated risks. Survivors are often unable implement an awareness campaign. Please help us. Perhaps the greatest focus of advocacy and education efforts should be directed at the medical community. Neurologists are well versed in this disease. Because it is relatively rare in humans, most other specialists are unaware of the urgency for early detection and treatment.

Stroke survivors—particularly brain stroke victims—need a personal ombudsman to attend medical appointments, take notes, and explain what has been said. Sometimes we are so embarrassed by our

193

language skills, we sit in silence even when we do not understand. Survivors are powerless, especially in the first year. Comprehension, speech, and memory deficits preclude understanding what has happened to us. An ombudsman plays a vital role in taking notes, keeping records, and requesting copies of medical reports. Survivors need time and quiet at home to concentrate and absorb information. At six months post-stroke, I was not capable of understanding the meaning of incoming information. Someone needs to ask questions about medications, side effects, and purpose. When in doubt—trust your instincts. It is difficult to tell your primary doctor that you would like to take your records for a second opinion. A good doctor is not offended by second opinions. Your life may depend on the courage to "trust but verify." Do not assume the doctor did everything he was supposed to do if you suspicion otherwise.

Every state has a statute of limitations for redress of medical neglect or malpractice. Time is of the essence when a medical failure occurs. Something caused that incident. If you are not a medically savvy person and most rely solely on your doctor—second opinions and specialists are imperative. When you know a doctor missed the diagnosis and failed to take proper steps, there is nothing wrong with asking an attorney qualified in malpractice to evaluate your questions. Most do not charge for an initial consultation. The legal system is driven by profit. Rightly so! Be prepared with your records, evidence, and timelines. Again, a personal advocate or ombudsman is essential in making your case for legal remedy.

I was horrified when my doctor used his Blackberry to answer my questions. Some people are impressed by the doctor's ability to access electronic medical resources with handheld devices during an office visit. But I was shocked to think he didn't have the answers without looking online. The PDR is at their fingertips and the physician's drug reference data are easily accessed. The information age and digital age make it possible for doctors to have instant access to diagnostics and symptom checkers. My doctor used a Blackberry to answer my questions. As I said, that was a red flag for me.

However, the information age is an available resource for the general public, too. I was not Internet savvy at that time. It would never occur to me then that I might "google" my symptoms! The thought of that never occurred to me. Today, I urge individuals suffering medical mysteries to undertake the quest for answers. Whether you rely on second opinions, the Internet, or medical journals—just do it because your life may depend on it.

I have not yet recovered enough to educate and answer questions that others have. I can share what has happened to me. I am not yet recovered enough to write a forum myself. But I can urge the medical community to carry the message. Public health educators, national associations, and consumer webinars are excellent tools but I cannot yet navigate the technology by myself.

As to the artistic part of the brain, I am blessed by a miracle. I remember parts of a lecture given by Professor Susan Slavik at Coastal Carolina University. I remember reading her book about learning strategies for sixth-grade students. She drilled our lessons into our brains; perhaps that is why I can still recall the meaning but not the exact content of her message. She was brilliant and I wish I could repeat exactly what she said because she was a master at dealing with children and art teachers. Art is a critical necessity for students to make achieve a full, well-rounded education. It is not a frivolous elective! It is critical knowledge and merges with math, science, history, and English. Visual learners depend on imagery to comprehend their studies.

After listening to stroke group survivors and guest speakers I have a better understanding why I never considered giving up or slowing down. I am not paralyzed; thirty percent of my left brain is erased. But I know that I can learn, open new pathways in my brain, and accept that my efforts are painstakingly slow. I am beyond slow—I move at a snail's pace! For example, my doctor said that the visual optic nerve damage was irreversible. Somehow, my sensory abilities are improving. I could not accept the dependency created by being transportation dependent! I did not accept the disposition … I had daughters who wanted to go places instead of taking care of me. I did not drive because I knew I could not see one third of a car when Jeff drove. He said, "You cannot drive." I said, "I know but I will get better" and I believed it. Positive self-talk is a vital component of recovery. Without hope, courage, and positive thinking, stroke survivors would give up trying to improve. If one learning strategy does not lead to improvement in a few months, try another strategy! Don't give up—no matter what!

About sixty days post-stroke, I studied pictures Larry cut out of magazines to learn to the difference between an apple and an orange. He pasted colorful pictures into a scrapbook for me study basic food items. I still have aphasia and get caught on the simplest words. Stroke educators tell us that the first months are critical to your intellectual capacities. I believe that painting was a significant factor in my progress. My brain seemed to flourish with increased cognition that I cannot explain. My brain was remolded—in artistic terms—to imprint new information. This was an important "reconnection" with the world for me. I began to feel worthwhile and capable of doing something intellectually creative. That was a meaningful breakthrough that reduced the stigma of being a stroke survivor.

Painting was a learning tool for me, as well as a creative outlet. I could not remember the colors of the paint but I instinctively knew to use another object, or picture from a magazine, or from an art book. I do not remember how long I had to "copy" the works of others before I could "create" from my own brain. I attempted to create an exact replica over and over. Did it matter that I had a natural ability and years of training to draw or paint? I do not think so. I drew with my left hand because my right side was useless at the time. I realized the effort to create art is more important than the final output. It is the effort, the effect, the desire that feels so good. Those tiny rewards kept me from giving up. This was a meaningful revelation and turning point in my recovery.

Strokes occur in both sides of the brain—left or right. I started with what I learned about art. We start with a line, it is the key to creating concepts for me. Line is the first lesson to be learned. I believe those lines will eventually become space. Your brain will "connect" through new pathways. The connecting lines create space that opens pathways for synapses to occur. Synapses create new messages within the brain—like a computer that is "back online." As the pathways and synapses increase, brain function improves. Keep hope alive and never give up.

I believe I am approaching the future a little wiser and more boldly. Over the years I have cherished the unpublished poetry of my former co-worker, Terry Edge. Having more time to read and study, I reviewed two volumes of his poetry again. These are treasures that I hope he will publish one day. I find them prophetic and thoughtful.

The simplicity of his writing allows me to more easily comprehend the poems. I hope others will enjoy them, too.

There is no joy
Such as exists in the quiet.
Do not see it out
For it cannot be found.
Simply allow this to be happen
And catch hold of the moments
Of feeling
And thought
And life.
You will find
It is all you really are.

Terry Edge

I know that I have the courage and optimism to view the future realistically. There are many hopes and dreams for my future. My wishes are so simple but will not be easy. Of course, I would love to return to the classroom and teach art history. Perhaps I can return to my field in another capacity in the instruction of applied arts. I hope to travel to Italy again and see the very same sights and works of art. But this time I would give anything to go there with my husband. He knows the history of the Roman Empire, and the battles fought where so many American soldiers fell on foreign soil. We never really had a true honeymoon. *They say love in Rome is unparalleled, Jeff.*

I want to pursue my goals for improved speech and cognition. I know people do not understand what I am saying and that makes me feel like I can only have half of a conversation. I realize that I do not always understand what I hear, read, or study. I struggle every day not to feel like a loser. Finally, I want to be ready to listen and hear God's will for me. The best thing I could do is to be of service to Him.

Currently in 2014 I help run a stroke survivors' meeting and also utilize my art education training in a free Art Therapy class for stroke survivors. I also am a strong advocate for stroke dyslexia and the amazing potential in the use of Art Therapy as a way to help stroke victims. I have been a speaker at various organizations on these subject and also Cushing's Syndrome.

The rest of my time is spent with my family and in art related groups, painting pastel animal portraits for donations, and working on various murals and sculptures.

Be courageous enough
To be curious.
Let not the ignorance of weak people
Effect you in such a way
You do not see to know
And understand.
It is important in your being
That you strive toward those things which see
higher
Than yourself.
Bear in mind
You will never reach the entire depth of your soul,
Therefore, always search for more.
Be careful not to waste
What little precious time
You have at your disposal.
Be wise.
Be.

Terry Edge

"Do not let yesterday use up
too much of today."

Old Cherokee Proverb

6
My Personal Story

Many people say that my ability to survive this tragic experience was due largely to the strengths I developed trying to survive my childhood. When I started writing this, I had very little recent or short-term memory. It was easier to remember my childhood, which made me angry. While I had a loving mother and grandmother, most of my childhood was filled with domestic violence. Those memories came easily to me but the names of my husband and children or where I had lunch yesterday were so difficult to retrieve. It was suggested that I simply start with what I remembered, which was growing up until my marriage to Jeff and the beginning of my teaching career. Memories of my recent past are still impossible to recover without notes and calendars to refer back to.

Peggy gave me an outline to follow of what we should include. My goal was to help other victims and their families understand the inner world of a stroke victim as I experienced it. It was suggested I focus on what life used to be like, what happened, what life is like today, the lessons learned, and my hopes for the future. I also wanted to share the impact on the family and friends in a potentially fatal health crisis and, more importantly, their role in recovery. My personal life story is primarily of interest to me and my closest friends and family. Thus I have included it at the end of my book.

This is the part that took me the longest to write. The rewards to me have been profound. Sharing my story has helped me put my life in perspective. Reliving the bitter past helped me realize the strength

199

I gained from all those hard knocks are the very strengths which probably saved my life. I believe my story is an important legacy for my children. They will know who I am and where I came from. Events may transpire in the future that will impede my memory again and I did not want to lose all my memories at one time.

Birth and Early Childhood

I don't really know if my instincts for survival are any stronger than anyone else's are. But if the saying "adversity builds character" is true, I had all the survival training I ever needed in childhood. These were the most challenging years of my life. I feel guilty saying this because my mom's life was much worse than mine.

My mom had two husbands who were unable to provide the love and support she had every right to expect. Her first husband was an adulterer and the second husband was a violent alcoholic. Working full-time, paying the rent, buying food, and trying to hang on to her sanity, she raised four daughters virtually alone. Although she had love and support from her mother and sisters, the men in her life were physically or emotionally absent from the home. Mom also suffered for many years with undiagnosed bipolar disorder. The primary symptom I witnessed as a child was bouts of depression. I don't remember seeing her agitated or manic until many years later as the disorder worsened. (She was eventually diagnosed in 1990 at age 52, when I was 32 years old.) She never complained about anything. I always felt her love and devotion no matter what happened in our house. Being the oldest daughter and the most outspoken, I suffered the brunt of a very sad childhood at the hands of a violent step-father. Yet I never doubted my mother's love for me and I always took comfort in that—and I still do.

My Aunt Jean dated (the future) Uncle Tommy Cornwell and mom dated my future dad Kenneth Baumann on double-dates. My dad was a soldier and worked at Fort Bragg. Uncle Tommy was very good-looking and was compared a lot to Elvis Presley when he was young. Uncle Tommy had his own car. My cousin Lynn always said they were Italian instead of Indian because of the stigma they perceived about having Indian blood. Mom looked like Pocahontas, but prettier! Mom had Indian heritage on her father's side of the family. I think her third great-grandfather was Indian. People usually asked me if I was Indian. I had dark skin, black hair, brown eyes, and high cheekbones. Aunt Jean and my grandma knew we had Indian heritage, but for some reason they were ashamed of the background. Mom was five years old when her dad died. He was killed by a truck. Mom's siblings, Uncle Leslie and Aunt Jean, always told the best jokes and would keep everyone laughing. It bothers me that they all denied Indian ancestry.

I have a friend who has been working on my genealogy for several years. She is trying to trace the ethnicity of my roots, but has not yet identified the Indian connections that I know are there. I consistently asked Grandma but she would not admit we were Indians until she told me that on the Buck side of the family, there was Indian background. The census showed them as "white" and there were no Indian names in their family bibles. Most of them, I suspect, were not willing to accept the truth. My mom was the only one who would be proud of an Indian heritage. She would tell me the truth, without hesitation, if she knew it. I can feel Indian ancestry in my soul. When I hear Indian music, visit a powwow, or hear Indian prayers, I am viscerally affected in a way that I know these are my roots. I feel the Indian oneness with the universe and feel calm in the presence of the Great Spirit. (In 2013 I met Larry and Mary Broome, American Indian Ancestry Experts. They were able to identify my Indian ancestors for me on my Grandma's side. I had no idea I was Tuscarora Indian!)

My pre-school childhood from birth to age four was seemingly safe and normal. My parents met when my father, a young U.S. Army paratrooper, was stationed at Fort Bragg, North Carolina, in the mid 1950's. My mother lived in Fayetteville, the town adjacent to Fort Bragg. Although dating GIs was frowned upon in our family (my grandparents feared their children falling in love and moving far away), my mom met my dad and was smitten, and nothing anyone else could say made a difference.

Their first child was a little girl, Helen. By all descriptions Helen was a special child and was the light of my Mom's eyes. When she was about 11 months old, Helen woke up one night swollen and screaming. Mom and Dad rushed her to the hospital, but the doctors were unable to save her. They were told that Helen had died of spinal meningitis, possibly from a cat scratch. After Helen's death my Mom got pregnant with me. My Dad was then restationed to Korea.

Mom was absolutely devastated and grieved throughout the rest of her life for the loss of her first little girl. I was the next child born, in 1958; I will always believe that Mom and I shared an especially close bond because as a baby my mom was able to get through some of her grief by taking care of me. A few years later we moved to and Army base in Kentucky and my sister Roxanne was born.

Life was pretty good until I was about four years old. We had plenty of food, nice clothes, a stable place to live, and medical and dental care. Then my father met an older woman and began an affair. Over time, my mom discovered the affair and decided to move back home to Fayetteville. I still remember vividly that Dad's new girlfriend Katie came over to the house and asked my mom to leave her two little girls (me and Roxanne) with them. Dad and Katie would be able to raise them better, she said. Outraged, my soft-spoken, petite mother beat and kicked Katie to the door and watched her crawl away. This is one of my most vivid memories.

Mom didn't have a car or even a driver's license, so she bundled up our clothes and some photos in a couple of suitcases and we took a train back to Fayetteville. When we arrived we stayed with my grandmother. My mom didn't explain any details of why she had left my dad, just that she could no longer stay there in Kentucky. Grandma had come to like my dad and to appreciate the security of the military benefits, and she could not understand why my mom had left him. She constantly told my mom that she had made a mistake in leaving my dad, etc. I never heard my mom respond about my dad when Grandma criticized her. My Aunt Louise lived next door to Grandma and we spent a lot of time there, too. Aunt Louise was wonderful to us and helped us a lot over the years.

Freshly divorced, Mom got waitressing jobs easily. She was friendly and pretty and a hard worker. Without a driver's license, she walked everywhere. At first, Mom got a job at a downtown café and she would often take me to walk to the cemetery where Helen was buried. Fayetteville was a tough town in the 1960s and we lived right down town and pretty much just walked everywhere. Mom could have started over and met someone nice and possibly gotten remarried. That was not to be.

It wasn't long before there were some men trying to get Mom's attention, one in particular named Felton, a young man Mom had known in school. As soon as he heard she was back in town, he started stalking her. Mom tried to discourage him but Felton was very persistent and had a very violent streak to him. He would hang around her work and cause her problems with her bosses. I can remember clearly when she came walking home one night bruised and disheveled, with her clothes torn. Her eyes were red from crying. Felton had waylaid her on the walk home, pulled her into a corner and had his way with her; then left her to find her way back.

I remember another nightmarish incident. Mom was trying hard to get Felton to leave her alone and would refuse to go anywhere with him. One day Mom and I were walking together along the banks of Cape Fear River. Felton just appeared out of nowhere, grabbed Mom, and dragged her down to the river. In a flash, he hit her in the face with a brick. Mom's teeth were all broken out in the front and her lips and gums were mashed. She had very little income, no insurance, and no money for dental care. She did not smile much after that and felt like she was not as attractive. All of her pretty teeth were gone, she was ashamed and demoralized, and well on her way to an emotional breakdown.

Felton was actually arrogant about that incident. He told her that if he couldn't have her then no one else would. I am not sure what my mom told the rest of the family about the blackened eyes and broken teeth, but they all despised Felton. At the young age of 25, Mom was increasingly depressed and defeated. She continued to take me to the cemetery every Sunday. She told me the cute things that Helen did as a toddler. She repeated each week that "Helen was an angel with pretty black hair and blue eyes." People would always came up and tell her how beautiful Helen was.

I loathed Felton so much and still wish I could have done more to prevent what continued to happen. It was unrealistic for me to feel guilty through those years, but like many abused and neglected kids I felt responsible. Police, landlords, and the courts all had the same response. This was her responsibility, they said, but they didn't believe my mother was trying to work and take care of her kids while a stalker was beating and abusing her. After being threatened by the custodial loss of her children, she never complained or explained again. I was increasingly angry and bitter inside and Roxanne just hid a lot. I recognized that my attitude toward Mom was wrong, too. Even I was mad at her that she did not kill him in self-defense! I feel bad about that now—if I was mad at her, too, she had absolutely no one on her side.

We lived in a neighborhood with prostitution, drugs, and whatever else came along. Mom did not socialize with the neighbors and told us not to. She told us to stay away from their houses and to never get in a car with them. She was desperate for childcare but never allowed them to watch us. Some had offered but she never did. (*That song "Luka" by Suzanne Vega is playing in my head..."I live on the seventh floor. Don't ask me awhile, if you hear something...*)

I realized even then that the bad neighborhood was the best we could afford. I assumed the role of parent and feared for her safety. I still tried to protect her. I felt like a failure because I could not spare her the pain of Felton. Through the thin apartment walls we heard way too many things and saw men who left as women and came home as men. I remembering thinking as a child, *what is wrong with this picture?* It was confusing to me.

Mom became pregnant and was physically and emotionally sick. She went to talk with my grandmother and told grandma about it right in front of me. Grandma was religious and must have thought I was too young to understand her or she forgot I was in the room. She was very upset with my mom. Grandma told her to have an abortion and that we could *not* move back home with her. Grandma couldn't believe that mom would have a baby from Felton. She was cruel when she told Mom, "Christine, you can't even take care of the two children you already have." Grandma suspected that Felton had beaten her up many times. (These were terrible, hurtful things for her to say to my mom. I held it against my grandma and have never forgotten or forgiven the way she talked to my mom. Perhaps that anger and resentment is why I could not cry at her funeral. Deep inside, I was still offended by her insistence of an abortion and for not allowing us to escape to her house).

When we moved out of my grandmother's house before my other two sisters were born and before she married Felton our life was calmer even if we didn't have enough money to make ends meet.

Mom did well enough to keep us safe and hide where we lived so Felton wouldn't find us. Eventually, he always found us and broke into our house. Mom would pay the rent because she wanted to have her own apartment with me and Roxie. There were other people who took care of us when she had to work. My cousin Marie came to take care of us one night but Felton found our apartment, broke the lock, and scared Marie so badly she never came back to our house again.

After that break in, the owner evicted us because we could not pay rent on time and it cost him more to repair the door and locks. It still did not stop Felton—he always found our house and broke the locks to get in. She tried so many times to prevent him from breaking in. He didn't care about anything. After a while she seemed defeated and hopeless. I was aware but did not know what to do, either. Roxie was about three years old and I was about five. We were never left by ourselves at that time.

Mom rented trailers, rooms, or apartments after that. Most of the time these apartments were in large old houses in downtown Fayetteville that had been converted to have a few apartments in each house. These were rough areas to live. Without much in the way of furniture, most of the time we all slept in the same bed. Felton would get drunk and show up at the apartment late at night. He would break into the house through the flimsy door locks and sexually assault Mom right next to me in the bed. He had convinced Mom that if we screamed or caused trouble he would hurt us. It wasn't long before we were evicted because Mom couldn't fix the locks and the landlord didn't want the trouble.

Mom pretty much gave up and Felton soon ended up living with us and eventually married Mom. Over time Mom had two daughters with Felton, my sisters Gail and Carol. I hated him for the way he treated us all and as I got older and approached my teen years I was never shy about telling him what I thought of him.

As I said, during that time Mom almost never complained and was usually upbeat. (Many years later, she was diagnosed with bipolar disorder and suffered manic behavior and occasional suicidal thoughts throughout her life. She was almost fifty years old when we finally managed to get a good diagnosis and began medications to stabilize her moods and manage her disease.)

Due to circumstances that followed, I don't remember having a

205

childhood of playing, picnicking, or family gatherings. Why didn't I play with dolls and do things with friends who asked me to come out and play? My mother tried to encourage me to go out or visit friends but I was afraid to leave her alone. She seemed fragile to me. My mother was my hero. She suffered in silence, did her best, put one foot in front of the other, and kept moving forward as best she could. She never quit on us, she never gave up in despair, she loved us unconditionally, and stayed alive for us. I don't think she ever fully understood that she had a mental disorder that caused her so much despair and anguish in life. She never understood that it wasn't her fault. She had a serious medical condition that required medical intervention. In short, betrayed by a philandering husband and living with a violent angry second husband, her life was pure hell.

Growing up, I wish I had known she had a mental condition and was not responsible for her behavior and decisions. I must have sensed it because I tried to become her self-appointed protector. It was my mission in life to look out for her and keep her safe. She must have felt cornered and helpless. I suffered witnessing her pain and I was full of anger and rage throughout my life.

Acknowledging the abuse in our house and our helplessness just made me scream—like the subject in the painting, "The Scream" by Edvard Munch.

This painting expresses exactly how I felt. When I tested for my degree, Munch was one of the artists I studied. Just looking at the subject I did not want to delve into the technique or the meaning of his work. Even at first glance the viewer is instantly in the grip of the tragic circumstances unfolding on the canvas. As a grown woman it immediately took my heart and soul right back to my mother's condition. I could see the torture the artist conveyed. Edvard Munch also suffered a tumultuous childhood, losing several of his family members. When I look at "The Scream" and see the main subject holding his head walking down a dark road, I immediately sensed that my mom must have felt that way inside although she did her best to conceal her condition. The emotional trauma is captured by the artist's colors and shapes, too. Ironically, her favorite color was orange, the same dominant color depicted in "The Scream."

This painting would not leave me alone no matter how many times I refused to learn anything about it. Even before my studies in art history, I saw prints of that painting for sale at malls, museums, and in the libraries. I was reminded every time of how many years I witnessed the abuse in our home. How could she possibly act normal with her torn clothes, bruised and swollen face, and limping walk? Yet she usually acted as if nothing had happened! She did not appear to respond emotionally to the abuse, but I did! I wanted to scream like the painting.

Mom only ate crackers and Pepsi on her job and smoked cigarettes. She did not have much money. I would cough a lot, and still do at night. I'm sure the smoke or the asthma had something to do with it. When we lived in a two-room apartment, my coughing would enrage my stepfather. He would yell at me to stop coughing. I tried but he would come over and hit me hard. That would make mom tell him not to hit me because "she can't control her coughing." In retaliation for speaking out against him, he would hit her and say, "That half breed knows what to do, she pretends so I can't get my sleep." The girls wouldn't say anything, especially Roxie, because she was so quiet. I don't know if my sisters were mad at me for coughing. They still had not started to school. They did not know about asthma. (After my coma my asthma abated. I stopped coughing for about two years. Now I have a very mild asthma unless I am near smoke or a smoker.)

I know my sisters wished I would stop coughing and just go to sleep. They were always afraid I would start something to rile Felton up even more. On those days when I didn't cough, he would say "I told you there is nothing wrong with her!" He had several names he liked to call me but I just ignored them.

When Gail and Carol were older, Felton was less abusive but he did verbally abuse Gail and Carol; they also suffered low self-esteem when they were young. Today, they are both happy with two children each and good husbands. Gail is very strong and I think is the most responsible person I know. She has made a career in special education with children. I am so proud of all three of sisters in many different ways. I have wished often that I would be more like them; they are the epitomes of sisters, mothers, teachers, friends, and community givers. Gail has been married to her husband since high school. She has a wonderful husband (also named Jeff) and he dotes on her.

Carol has a wonderful husband, Eddie Guyton, and they are doing well. She works with autistic children in an elementary school and both she and Gail are held in high regard by the parents and administrators of their respective schools.

In August 2011, Roxie divorced her husband and decided to move to South Carolina. She stayed with us until she got back on her feet and got a beautiful little place of her own in North Myrtle Beach. She is a trained dental assistant and is also attending college full time and wants to work in Gerontology.

It was fine with Felton if Mom was working in the Holt Williams Mill. As long as she paid the bills, Felton didn't want to beat her up too much because she would miss work. We still moved often because there wasn't enough money to feed the family and pay bills on her salary. I have to say when Gail and Carol were little girls, Felton's two sisters and their mother gave us many nights of shelter and food. Even before Gail and Carol were born, their family let us stay with them and eat when we had no food and no place to go. Roxie was so beautiful with green eyes and the sweetest personality; everyone liked her. Today, Roxie stays in contact with some of their family. Gail and Carol had little to do with their side of the family. I remember one of the cousins who was married and had her own house let us stay with her many times. She made us some strawberries and cool whip one time. Roxie and I had never eaten that before. She took us to the store to get it. We stayed with them often and they never seemed to mind sharing their food. If I saw them today, I would express my gratitude.

Roxie stayed mostly with Mom, Gail, and Carol. I stayed mostly with Grandma and for the first time, I was allowed to visit friends and walk around freely on three different streets nearby. It was a luxury to have a safe place to walk in a three-block radius. Maybe things went better for my mom and my sisters when I was not around. I was outspoken about what I thought was right or wrong. I stood up to Felton and he did not like anyone to oppose him. (I asked Roxie later and she said that Felton was still violent about other things even when I wasn't there).

My friends on these streets near Grandma's house were an important part of my good memory reserve. I don't remember their names, but they made a significant impression on me. There wasn't any violence in their homes like there was at mine. They were not rich but had normal lives and we confided in each other. I think their parents probably knew I was poorer than they were. They were tolerant people. In the early years before I lived with my grandmother we had ended up on their porches or back yards in early morning hours. Whenever Felton became too violent, Mom took us to spend the night in the woods, or to those neighbors' yards. That happened more times than I can count—it was an exodus in the night.

One of those special friends was like a sister from first grade until today, Ms. Sheila Gray Segura. We have stayed in contact over the years and know each other pretty well. She has had a lot of hard things that happened in her life, too. In childhood and today she is strong and always tries to do the right things. I could count on her over the years no matter what. We had another friend named Rutha. We spent all our time together in third and fourth grade. Her mother was so beautiful and ended up with cancer. She had three brothers and a good dad. She always had beautiful dresses and her blond hair was always in a different style. She had the prettiest things to wear I guess because she was the only girl. I was so happy for her. I do not even remember asking for or wearing any of her things. I never thought about that.

Rutha's house was comfortable and there was no yelling. We always watched "Batman" together. I felt like others thought I was a poor little dirty girl compared to Rutha. The most significant incident I remember was a school play in the third grade, *Cinderella*! Our teacher asked me to be Cinderella. We were all surprised because Rutha was the only blond and the perfect Cinderella. She was upset and told the teacher, "I should be Cinderella instead of her." Our teacher said "Linda is the only one that can remember all the lines." I said "That is okay, I don't mind being an ugly sister; I will help her if she forgets." The teacher said, "I hope you kids understand how unselfish she is. Many of you could benefit from her example." That compliment stuck in my mind forever. These examples of small achievements have run in my mind over the years. I did not mind being an ugly sister.

In second grade, I was in a play to read the entire *Bedtime Story*. I was supposed to sit on a bed and read the story out loud. I was told to wear some pajamas. I never had the appropriate kind at home. At home, I slept in the clothes I wore the day before. For the play, I had to borrow a pair from a friend down the street. I remember where she lives but cannot remember her name. I am sure I took good care of the pajamas, but she gave them to me afterward. Felton made sure that I did not have them long. I was so happy my mother came to the play. She was so proud of me. She went on and on bragging about me to anyone she saw for the longest time. She always gave us lots of praise. I think she did more for me because she sensed I needed more self-esteem. I think she felt that she could not give me anything else but her love. That was all I needed like a flower to bloom. Our play was very good. Afterward, I saw the silhouettes of our cast on the billboard in front of the principal. I remembering telling Mom, "I can paint people like that." She said "I know you can, you can do anything you want to do!" I was convinced of that because I wanted to please her. I never thought about how a mother's devotion and unconditional love contribute to a child's self-esteem. If she had been the only person in the audience I would have done the best job I could to get her approval.

Another special friend was Betty. Her childhood was a lot like mine, except her dad was in jail of most of their childhood. Betty's grandmother raised her son's children. For some reason, Betty's mother lived in another state. I did not remember every meeting her. I used to go by Betty's house to walk with her to school. It was dangerous walking alone on some of the streets, so most of us stayed together going to and from school. When I went over to see Betty, it reminded me of life with my grandmother. Her grandmother made them sit down and listen to her read passages from the Bible. Then they had to close their eyes and pray. I think Betty had at least two other brothers and a grandfather. Her grandmother did not seem to mind if I walked to school with Betty. I remember that Betty had a Collie and I had a German shepherd that someone had given me. Betty and I agreed on everything except boys and breeds of dogs. Of course her dog was Lassie and she would say my dog was mean. We argued all the time about which one was smarter and meaner. Of course, I didn't have a dog, but would show a neighbor's dog and pretend it was mine.

I escaped some of the madness of my home life through prolific reading. As soon as I learned to read, I devoured whatever I could find or borrow. A friend of mine who did not like to read would sell her parents' old copies of *Reader's Digest* to me for five cents. Of course, there were other paperback books and magazines that were missing the covers (usually sexually explicit stories) that I also read. It seemed like we moved every time the rent was due, at least several times a year. People who lived in a place before we moved in would leave old and used books in the drawers or trash. When I found a book I hadn't read I felt like I had won a lottery! However, some of those books I read were inappropriate for my age group, such as *Rosemarie's Baby* and *Valley of Dolls*. Most of the books with the front cover torn off were definitely not age-appropriate for a pre-teenaged girl. Those were the types of people we lived around my entire childhood. Like some of the trashy novels, the lives of the people around us were pretty trashy, too. I developed contempt for men because of the way I saw most of the men around us act. I vowed I would never get married because I thought all men were worthless, abusive womanizers like the men in my mom's life.

My mom had to move us again, and it was farther from Betty's house. During that time, Betty's grandmother died. Her father had served his time in jail, and Betty and her brothers began living with him. Betty often dreamed that her mother and father would get back together. When I could go see her, we danced and listened to Elvis Presley on the radio. She could dance very well, but I couldn't.

Betty was full of sexual questions. I don't think her grandmother had told her anything. I did not want to share what I knew, which I had read in those sexually explicit books and magazines with the covers torn off. Betty kept asking me questions and I finally suggested that she ask the lady who took care of us when my mother was at work. "You should ask her, she will tell you what you need to know." I figured the lady was older and experienced and I had only read about sex in those books. She was about the same age of my mother but not as attractive. She did a good job telling Betty the facts without explaining the anatomically correct terminology. Betty was shocked that people had intercourse and her face turned red. I was speechless because she described it in a way that sounded uncomfortable rather than a pleasure. She said it was something men want to do and women want to avoid unless you have to. I understood that she evidently had not experienced "making love" the way it was described in the books. Based on the novels I read, I determined that she was probably "frigid!" Betty was a little upset by the discussion. I decided the best thing to do was be quiet and I didn't want to talk about it when we were so young. Betty grew into a lovely woman, wife, and was a good mother the last time I saw her.

Betty was friends with another blond girl who played piano and sang like an angel. She lived in the biggest, prettiest house in town and they owned cars! I remember that they could afford three dogs! That was amazing to me. During the summer months when mom was working, I got to spend a lot of time there.

There were other kids on my stepfather's side of the family. Their family thought that hearing their kids cursing was "cute." Mom would not let us curse nor comment about their kids. Felton's older brother had a wife with three boys and one girl from a prior marriage. Felton's brother and his wife had a little boy. Marilyn and her brother were from her previous marriage. In between evictions, we stayed at their house for a while. Both of them died within a year after we left. They were both alcoholic and drunk all day. There was a lot of that in Felton's family.

Their daughter, Marilyn, had beautiful blond hair and was smart. My skin was so dark next to hers. I tried to wash my dark skin away but it did not get any lighter. She and I talked a lot about how much we hated our stepfathers. She was a year older than I was. She and I went to the same school for a long time. She talked a lot about boys, which I hated hearing about, and we played cards because they had poker games at their house every Saturday night.

There was one major thing that I remember seeing her do at school. We were crossing guards for the school and had to stand watch at the end of our day. One day, after our duty, we walked down by one of her classes to get her books and things. I watched her as she went by several desks and took the pencils out of the other students' desks and took them home. I said, "Marilyn, what are you doing?" She told me what I thought was a lie, "They always take mine so I'm just taking them back, and I will give you one." I told her no and that I did not steal! I was mad at her for stealing when she didn't have to for survival.

We would eat mostly with Felton's family when there was no money left to buy food. I think his family felt sorry for us because Felton beat my mom pretty bad. After grandma died, Mom slid into an even deeper level of depression. Grandma had prayed for Felton all the time and Mom knew she could always go to my grandma's house if we needed food; now her safety net was gone.

Felton started to encourage my mom to drink because she would get intoxicated on two beers. Sometimes I think it made her feel better— she could escape the reality of our lives. She was self-medicating her disease. I immediately recognized when she had been drinking. At that time, no one had ever heard of bipolar disorder and neither did I until her formal diagnosis in 1990. Back then, we just thought it was depression. Doctors were only used if you broke an arm or leg. Despite her undiagnosed mental illness and spousal abuse, she still managed to work, clean house, and love her girls. She was always kind to us even in the worst of times.

I found ways to call the police several times when Felton would not stop beating Mom. Eventually the judge finally threatened Mom with removing her children if he saw her in the courtroom again. After the courtroom incident, she was increasingly complacent; it seems she had just given up. We still ended up losing our rented rooms several times a year, then had to move and stayed hungry. Several people in Felton's family would feed us fairly often, especially after our grandmother died. All of his family liked my mom. I do not remember any of Felton's sisters ever working outside the home except for one sister, and all of their husbands had jobs and supported their families.

Their food was good, their house was clean, and they never seemed to mind us being there for supper. Mom always went to work, but did not eat anything at work except soda crackers and drank a Pepsi. Mom couldn't keep waitressing jobs because Felton would ruin her clothes, but was able to get a job in a factory. It was very hard work in the factory, but she had a lot of pride and did not mind to work.

Mom's sister Aunt Jean had a hard time keeping up with where we lived, but she did. Aunt Jean saw me reading those old books with no covers and she scolded me, "Don't believe everything you read … that is trash … you should not read that garbage!" It was ironic that she was concerned about what I was reading. Little did she know that the thin walls to our rented room left little to the imagination about what was going on in the bedroom next door. I do not remember if Mom looked at the books or not or if she thought I shouldn't be reading them. I never remembered seeing Mom read a book. When she was working she came home and cleaned up the house and started cooking. She never just sat down and rested or read.

I was one year late starting school for the first grade. I had an outbreak of impetigo. There were yellow crusty sores on my legs that were contagious. The principal could not allow me start school until I was cured. I was allergic to fleas and scratched the bites and it made the condition worse. I loved dogs and their fleas would jump off of them and get on me! The fleas caused the itching and the scratching caused the infection. My mother was as upset as I was that I had to wait a year and start school when I was six years old.

By the time I started first grade a year later, I could already read. I practiced by reading all the books at my aunt's house. Those were appropriate books. Aunt Jean always let me read and watch television at her house. My cousin, Wayne, is the same age as my sister, Roxanne. He did not like me because Aunt Jean would let me stay at their house and sleep in Wayne's bed. My sores would ooze onto those clean, white sheets. We never had clean white sheets at our house. I tried not to scratch and I liked being there because it was the only place I felt safe enough to sleep. I would sleep so soundly that my sores would stick to the sheets. There was not any money for medicine, but I remember a teacher telling Mom to use a yellow salve. I don't blame Wayne for not wanting me to stay at his house but Aunt Jean asked him not to complain because she could wash the sheets. His sister Lynn is a year older than I am. She never made me feel inferior but they never went to our house because our neighborhood was not safe.

Grandma kept all four of us when we were young while Mom was working. I do not remember many toys. We played next to the railroad tracks. When a train was coming by, we put pennies on the track to see if the train could smash them flat. Grandma had a vegetable garden but we had to be careful around it. If we trampled any of her vines, she would make us get a switch to keep us in control. Wayne got along great with Roxie and I got along great with Lynn. We still see each other as much as we can. Thinking about it now, Lynn and I never argued. She never said anything bad to me because that was not her personality. She was very easy going. I would not cry if someone said something bad to me. I just told them off and used words I should not say from those books I read.

My grandmother made biscuits every day. For breakfast, she let us have day-old biscuits in a coffee cup, with coffee and sugar. That was our cereal; I am sure a few kids still have to eat like that today. I remember it being delicious. Roxie and I would eat one egg each. But Lynn and Wayne ate as many as they wanted, like six whole eggs! Roxie and I were too thin and Lynn and Wayne were a little too chunky.

Aunt Louise was always sick and had four daughters at home. The oldest was Dottie, then Barbara, Marie, and Ann. They were teenagers and she had her hands full. Although Grandma read the Bible to Aunt Louise all the time she still ran the house with a "big stick." She married Barney Bradley after her husband died. He was about 20 years older than she was. He rode a bicycle everywhere he went. We tried to ride it as kids but it was too big and heavy for us. He was already retired and "whittled" all day. I remember thinking *that is the most ridiculous thing I have ever seen somebody do with their time.* I would never waste my life like that! I do not remember seeing him much at the house, but I was glad because I did not like men except the ones who were teachers. I was convinced that given the chance men would try to do something to me that they should not do. I was totally on guard around men.

I was thirteen years old when I went to live with my grandma for a year. She died a year after that. Living with her was peaceful but she ruled the house with the fear of God and lots of rules! Going to school without the drama of life with my violent stepdad gave me a chance to focus on doing well in the classroom. My mom made sure that she saw me every day before or after school. I was lucky I had a year to stay with Grandma that year before she died. Going to school without the drama and seeing my mom daily gave me a chance to focus on doing well; school was a refuge for me. I stayed after school to learn anything I could from my teachers.

My favorite school teacher became Ms. Alma Weathers. Even after I passed to the next grade, I was still going to Ms. Weather's house for art lessons once a week. She knew the safest place I could be was at her house. She never asked questions like "Why do I have to take you to a different house every other time I take you home?" She recognized I had way too much "street smarts" and I could easily take the wrong road in life. She was a safe haven after school, and taught me to mind my manners and focus on my art lessons. She was observant—but never minded my family business, although I'm sure she would have stepped in if she ever saw any signs of abuse on me physically. She was black and she could connect with the lowest self-esteem students and make them shine. I am not black but she treated me the same way. I think it was because she wanted to show the poor people where she lived. The murals, her art students saw how we could live better. Most of her students lived in worn down apartments or projects. I believe I would have been that kind of teacher had I been able to continue teaching after the stroke.

I was grateful for male teachers who were excellent role models. I thought my sixth-grade teacher was the smartest man in the world. He was a black teacher named Dr. Hill. Desperate for a male figure in my life, I tried to write down everything he said as if he was Socrates. I got into trouble for talking and/or fighting. Two of the fights I had at school, he assigned me to clean up the trash inside the school yard. The other punishment was that I had to hold up a book for a long time. I'm sure he felt sorry for my skinny arms. I did not get mad at him. I recognized I had broken the rules. He helped me to be a better student and a better person by fair and even-handed discipline. By the end of the year I was voted the sixth-grade student body president! Dr. Hill taught me how to respect him as an authority figure, that there were consequences for bad behavior, and that there are men who treat you fairly.

I was a teenager when Grandma died. It was not the best time in life to go back to the harsh world of life with my stepfather. My absence had not improved the temper or attitude of my stepfather. Making matters worse, my grandmother's death pushed my mother further into depression. For Mom's sake, I tried to argue less and keep my peace when I could, but I couldn't always do it. I became the de-facto 'mother' in the home and tried to make things normal to the best of my abilities. Each night I would walk down to the Mill where my mom worked and walk her home. I felt like I had to be my mom's protector (as if I could have protected her as a scrawny, skinny teen). I remember once that my three sisters were asleep and it was time for me to walk down to the Mill at 11:40 p.m. to walk my mom home. I saw that my stepfather was passed out drunk on the floor and I took the heavy door mat and hit him over the head with it until my arms got too tired to hold it. He either figured it out or one of my sisters told him, but he became aware that I was the one who made his face all swollen and sore. No one would believe that this skinny girl could be guilty of such a thing! My mother somehow knew that I did it but she never spoke about it. Like many nights, I prayed that night as hard as my grandma prayed that he would be gone when I woke up the next morning.

My stepfather seemed to be proud of the trauma he caused in my mother's life. After Grandma died, I felt that I was the only one left who could protect her from the abuse. I suffered with soul sickness believing that the only way for my mom to survive was for Felton to die before he killed her. These are the twisted thoughts of a young school girl who was traumatized by family violence. I was that young girl who was loved by her mother and grandmother but who had to shoulder too much emotional responsibility in the home.

Life inside our house was difficult and life outside wasn't any better. There were all kinds of debris throughout the yards and alleys where we walked, and we could sometimes recognize a condom among the rest of the trash. I walked Roxie to school in the mornings. On the way, we always found stashed supplies of alcohol and cigarettes hidden in the trees. It was a rough and poor neighborhood. That was our life. Whenever she could, Mom would walk with us to school. However, most of the time my baby sisters, Gail and Carol, could not be left alone. Mom never owned a baby stroller, and couldn't carry both of them on her way back home.

Many horrible things happened in this part of town. The police never found the man who raped and murdered a first-grader who lived down the street. At her autopsy, the coroner found her own little teeth had been knocked out and were lodged in her stomach. Some people may ask, "That was a long time ago, how could you remember that?" I just shake my head without saying anything. I have not forgotten the things that I saw as a child. I have not forgotten the face of that little girl nor will I forget the abused face of my own dear mother.

Mom always tried to tell us that "tomorrow is a better day." As kids, we responded to the hostile environment internally; we had to keep our emotions under control because we were so vulnerable. Sadly, my heart hardened with time and I was so filled with rage. I would have done anything to get that man away from my mother and out of our lives. To be honest, my whole childhood was spent trying to figure out how I could get rid of my stepfather and live to tell the tale. I was too young to understand why Mom made the choices she did, but I intuitively knew that God wanted me to protect her. And I did that to the best of my ability until she died many years later.

Times were so different then. The terms *spousal* and *child abuse* were unheard of in the 1960s. It took many deaths and tragedies in so many families before these issues reached public awareness and eventually became criminal activity. In my childhood the system usually blamed the victims—especially women and children—for dysfunctional family life. As I mentioned earlier about our courtroom experience, the authorities at the time told Mom to stop calling them for help. They indicated that if she couldn't take care of her situation and her children they would take her children away to social services. I was there many times when the police came. She was easily intimidated and submissive. Because of her disorder, she could not explain her circumstances adequately. The police just didn't want to be bothered by domestic arguments.

Several times a year, I went next door to call the police when Felton beat her up, because of course we never had a telephone. It was usually when she got paid and he wanted to take her wages and go to the bars. When he became violent, I thought calling the police would save us and it was the only thing I knew to do. I probably did not weigh fifty pounds. My stepdad was very good at lying and twisting the truth when the police came. Because I was a skinny little child they did not listen to me when I tried to tell the truth. I cannot tell you how much hurt and rage those men caused me to feel! After I had spoken up and told the truth the police left me behind with the perpetrator. I had to run like hell and hide when the police left. I knew what would happen in the wake of his fury.

Sometimes the police would take him to jail, but they would hear the same old story from Felton—that the problems and violence were caused by my mom and me. That I had no respect for him and he knew it. I would tell him exactly what I thought then run and hide.

After one particularly bad beating of my mom, the police took him in. I was very young when I went with Mom to court for a hearing. We were both afraid. My mother did not like the courtroom at all and it was overwhelming for her. We had been to the courthouse before appearing in front of hearing officers but never appeared in front of a judge. When she tried to speak to the hearing officers, she was stricken with so much anxiety that she opened her mouth and no words would come out. This time—in front of a judge—she was almost paralyzed with fear. The consequences were horrifying. If the judge didn't like her—he might let Felton go or even worse take her children to protective services. I was in fourth grade and so hopeful that the judge would send Felton away for good. We had suffered his violence for years and we finally had our day in court. It was devastating! We were defeated before mom could speak a word. The judge asked no questions and simply said, "Madam, if you call the police one more time we will take your children from you and place them in the custodial care of the State of North Carolina." It was a cruel blow and one more time, the abuser was safe. Worse, he was in the courtroom and heard the admonishment of the judge. After that, he used the judge's words to keep my mother "in line."

After that day in court, Felton was also gloating because my mother basically gave up. She did not want to lose her kids and did not know how to prevent it. All my prayers for him to go to hell and leave us in peace went unanswered. My grandmother took me to church often and she was so proud of me for praying but she would not approve of what I was praying for!

I believe that because of my mother's bipolar disorder, God gave her a daughter with a strong, stubborn, and driven personality to protect her. I am afraid of many things, but I will not let fear control me in ANY way because I've always felt that I've already seen the worst side of people. I often wonder if I helped or hurt her with the strong personality I seem to have been born with. It often seemed like I was the adult and she was the child. I lost my childhood in order to ensure her survival and that of my sisters. This stubborn, defiant attitude came to me instinctively. Was it a curse or a gift?

My mother was the strongest person I ever knew but domestic abuse and mental illness exceeded her capacities. This was the life God gave me to live and I have no regrets. My mother was an angel. Even my husband Jeff, a former Army Ranger, said after watching her fight cancer later in life that she was stronger than any of his soldiers when he was in the military. We all realize she did the best she could under the circumstances. Even all these years later, reflecting on the abusive traumas of childhood, my blood boils and the hairs on the back of my neck go up when I think about it—like a dog's tail, back, and neck when he feels threatened.

To my shame, there were things I had to do that were against the principles I believed in. It was embarrassing to beg for food, ask for handouts, take charity, and go through trash for possible "treasures." I hated being sent to a neighbor's to borrow food items that I knew and they knew would not be repaid. My younger sisters were barely old enough to walk. My stepfather did not keep a regular job and rarely provided any money to the household. None of my family ever received a welfare check. Mom was proud but I do not think she ever understood that public assistance was available. Mom worked every hour she could and did whatever work was available.

My real Dad never sent us anything for holidays or birthdays, no cards or presents nor acknowledgement of any kind of our existence. We just lived on a small $50.00 monthly military child support check, mom's wages, and tips. Felton would not work consistently and my mother was typically the only breadwinner.

Although our food was always just the staples required to get by, when that military money arrived and we went to the grocery store we felt like we were rich! There were no extras and hardly ever did we get a treat. We couldn't get fruit because they were so expensive. I tasted one grape when we were at the grocery store—it was my favorite. From the time I began to work until this day, fruit is in constant supply in my home.

I thought the food at school was delicious. I loved school so much that I cried if I had to stay home. I recognized that education was fun and it was my way out, to do well. We had so many luxuries at school like peanut butter sandwiches, soup, chicken, fruit, apples, and desserts. These were things we never had at home. I still smile when I remember those wonderful cookies served in the cafeteria—they were delicious called Peanut Butter Delights. We would get to eat breakfast at school and had a snack sometimes. Most of the time, it was orange juice and a cookie. The snacks were in the classroom in elementary school. There were other poor students who loved the food as much as I did. I can't remember ever having orange juice at home, what an incredible luxury!

My kids are so spoiled about their food. Both Jeff and I are disappointed at times. We try to limit the junk food and insist on nutritious evening meals where we sit down and eat at the table together. I do not take having a full refrigerator and full pantry for granted. Fresh fruit and multiple cookies are always available. When we are at the store and ask them what they want for breakfast or lunch, they know to have some suggestions. Jeff and I grin and shake our heads when any of our kids comment *"We have no food!"* They have never had an empty refrigerator or pantry.

The same concept applies to having enough clothes to wear—and the right clothes to keep us warm enough. Our kids have nice clothes, shoes, and clean beds to sleep in. Yet they will stand in front of their closets and lament, "I don't have anything to wear to school!" When I was in the sixth grade my wardrobe was pretty simple. We received our clothing from the Salvation Army, teachers, and churches. At the beginning of school or Easter Aunt Jean would take us to get a few things and a pair of shoes. I never thought about the sacrifice she made to do this for us. Compared to the way we lived—Aunt Jean seemed to be rich. She and Uncle Tommy worked very hard, saved, and remained married until his recent death. I know Aunt Jean also gave my mom money when she had little to spare. Mom did the same nice things for her nieces when she worked as a teenager. Ann, Marie, Barbara, and Dottie (my cousins from my Aunt Louise) told me that before mom was married she worked part time at a restaurant. They told me mom would come and take them to the store for a "moon pie and Dr. Pepper" but Mom just liked Pepsi and peanuts.

Mom wasn't able to figure a budget, one of the common problems among people with bipolar disorder is the inability to manage money. We never had enough money to get by more than a week or two and military checks came only once a month. The last two weeks of every month was a struggle to keep food on the table.

One thing I remember specifically and will never forget. This particular week, Mom bought a small jar of chili powder. It was almost as expensive as some of the meat we ate, but Mom could make a delicious spaghetti sauce with it. Typically about mid-week I knew what was coming. Mom would choose something left over from the grocery purchase the week prior and tell me to take it to the store and return it for money. There was only one lady who would accept my return and give me a cash refund. I'm not sure how many times I did this, but this time it ruined our dinner. Mom had added salt to the chili powder and mixed it up in order to return it so that it appeared full. We used the money from the chili powder to buy some bread; we had often had bread and butter sandwiches for our meals (butter, not peanut butter). That is what we ate that night. The next week, no money again, so she sent me back to the store. I returned something and picked up a chili powder. That night we had our favorite food—Mom's spaghetti. Her sauce was our favorite. We sat down to eat and we looked at each other in anguish with the first bite. After one bite we all spit it out and drank some water. I had picked up the same chili powder we had returned, and it was about half salt! This was one of the few times she showed her devastation. Remembering what happened is sad and embarrassing. Again, we had butter and bread for dinner and mom did not eat anything. From then on I looked carefully at those mid-week purchases to make sure I wasn't getting our 'special' returned items. Afterward, I remember that I was secretly glad that we didn't ruin someone else's dinner!

When I was in middle school, I remember Grandma made pickles. We had pickles everywhere! When Roxie grew up and married she made pickles every year. We were so proud of her when she won the 1st Prize at the North Carolina State Fair!

My grandparents had a dog similar to a black and tan mixed chihuahua, but she was old and fat! I loved dogs but I did not like Poochey I think because she had health problems that made her smell bad. Grandma did not believe in doctors or veterinarians. She believed in God and had all kinds of White Square prayer pieces from Mr. Barber at church. The White Square pieces were prayed on at church then taken wherever you went that needed a prayerful touch. Poochey had one, too. I found those White Squares all the time when I lived at Grandma's. I wonder if she was trying to keep the devil from taking over my heart! When my grandma and I were living there alone, we had the chance to talk about more grown-up things. There were so many things I wanted to know. Mainly, my grandma was a devout Christian. I wanted to understand, "Why did God allow such a piece of worthless man like Felton to ruin our life?" "Why did my mother tolerate years of abuse?" I had many more questions that cannot be explained to the satisfaction of an angry teenager. Grandma gave me many quotes from the bible—but none of them soothed my angry heart.

When Grandma died and I had to go back to the real world, my absence away from home had not improved the temperament of my stepfather. Perhaps those childhood experiences honed my instinctive fight-or-flight response. Perhaps that instinct for self-preservation kicked in when I wanted to defend myself against anyone who came near me after I awoke from my coma. It had to be a fight for my survival. (I am not sure what happened to cause the terror, cursing and fear after the coma. Was it typical for someone who had a stroke or is it the result of things that I had been exposed to as a child? Is that the result of surviving the "catastrophic aneurysm and stroke," or God's work to save us?)

Many times I witnessed children being abused and heard their personal stories of molestation. Someone attempted to molest me but I was able to fight my way out of the situation. One of my friends lived with her grandma. She was big but her grandma was real short, tiny, and had polio as a child. She invited me to join the Salvation Army, which I did for two years. Her grandma lived on Russell Street in downtown Fayetteville. There was a single male about forty years old who lived next door. My friend was about twelve years old. The man next door had never been married. Her grandma went on and on about how nice the man was. I think they had lived there two years before I started going there after school. She let my friend go a lot of places with him alone. I listened about how nice he was, how he wasn't interested in dating, and how much he loved kids. All the stories I heard from them about this man raised a lot of red flags. I knew that if he had not molested her yet, he would. I shared my fears with them. Even at my age, I realized how naïve she and her grandmother were.

We were in middle school and I went home with her after school. Immediately the hairs on the back of my neck were raised up! She had a lot of material things from him, another red flag! How can anyone be so naïve about the risks of a grown man giving gifts and trips to a pre-teen girl? She went to the drive-in movies with him, and took out-of-town trips with him when he played guitar. She asked me if I could go with them. I didn't even ask mom because she would probably say *yes*. I thought afterward, maybe I should be brave enough to go with her a few times to see for myself. I was ready to pounce on him if I saw anything with my friend or if he tried anything on me! Did he sense that? I don't know. (Looking at that now, it was a very poor decision and I feel lucky that my friend and I did not end up buried in the woods somewhere!) I felt sorry for her and later talked to her about it. "Does he treat you like a date or girlfriend?" She had strabismus in her eyes so I couldn't really tell if she was embarrassed or lied. I told her that if he did treat her that way, it was wrong and she needed to tell her grandma right away.

I wanted her to know what I thought and to warn her because I thought she was vulnerable. She knew that I didn't own any jewelry or pretty things—in fact, I had next to nothing except used clothes from charity places. Oddly, she mentioned this lack of material things and said she thought I should "be friendlier to him and he would buy you anything!" I said, "No thank you, I do not like him and you better be careful." I said, "I will come to see you but I do not like him and I will not go to his house." After that, she was not as close to me.

Still worried, I decided to talk to her grandmother about what I suspected. I thought well "what if he kills her or her grandmother, like my friend, Becky, who was murdered?" I told her grandma the things I was seeing and what I was afraid of. Apparently, whatever he was doing to her granddaughter did not bother her and she said I was too nosy. There was so much going on at my home I just stopped going over there after that. She and some of my friends who I visited asked me if they could go to my house. I was honest and said, "You wouldn't like the way things are at my house. You wouldn't like my stepfather and you shouldn't trust him." Some days he was okay to be around and other days I didn't like the way he looked at me and I left home as soon as possible because of it.

There were days we only had the clothes we were wearing because Felton threw our clothes away or ripped them up in his drunkenness. When we grew up, we were so ashamed when we obtained copies of our school records. The teachers had written comments about our dirty hair and clothes. It was documented that we were given clothes from the Salvation Army because ours were dirty or torn. We were heartbroken when we found out what the teachers had written about us. After that, we were more aware of our appearance and tried to maintain our hygiene, hair, and teeth better.

One hurtful memory was that Felton destroyed almost all of our family photographs from Kentucky. Mom brought many pictures with her to North Carolina on the train from Kentucky. Grandma and Aunt Jean had some of them, too. One day when Felton was in a hostile mood, he saw those pictures and ripped them up. Mom managed to salvage one picture. It is a crumpled and torn picture of me when I was four years old. I found it in her things and saved it. It is on the cover of this book. Mom could never afford to buy any of our school pictures growing up and these pictures my dad had taken were very precious to her.

As the oldest, I assumed the role of parent to my mom and to my sisters. That was a lot of responsibility and I didn't have the emotional maturity to cope with all of it. I just did my best. I was not focused on myself other than going to school. I was focused on my mom and I did not talk or listen to my little sisters about their problems and lives while we were growing up. They have grown up as wonderful women. I have often wished I could be as carefree as they were. I knew what kind of life I did *not* want when I grew up and I always had goals to get a job, support myself, help my mother, and get an education. That was all I wanted. I'm glad my sisters still love me. I look back and feel like I cheated them by my single focus on our mother. There was no room left in my emotional reserve to be a good sister, too. It is a shame that we lived a life of poverty and domestic violence. I hope by writing about this part of my life—the truth will set me free. I am sad with myself that I can remember every detail of the darkest years of my life and I cannot always remember the names of my own precious children today.

I am comforted that my mother loved us, and did the very best she possibly could for us. We loved her for it until the day she died in our arms battling cancer. It is also a comfort that our children all loved and worshipped her—she was warm and loving to them. She told them how much she loved them every single time she talked with them in person or on the phone.

Mom was a magnet and drew her grandchildren into her heart. I have always known that I have a strong personality and tend to say what I think. As a result, I am not always well-liked. I do have some special friends who love me unconditionally. They have seen the best of me and the worst of me and still love me. I cannot ask for more than that and they will be my friends for a lifetime. I do not think I am special or rare and believe there are a lot of people out there who were raised just like I was. Please write a book, it is good therapy.

225

Just don't lie to yourself. I am embarrassed about what I was thinking … sometimes … but I want to know myself better and recognize the good and the bad. Someone once said, "The unexamined life is not worth living."

Writing about this and thinking about my mother is heartbreaking. Here was a good person trying to work and take care of her children. She was beautiful and upbeat when we were all three together. She had been devastated after losing her baby girl and caught her husband cheating on her during the whole time she was pregnant with Roxie. As I said, Mom divorced my dad because he would not stop cheating. Mom kept her torment to herself for twenty years.

She was on the brink of a nervous breakdown and talked less and less. She looked so sad sitting on the bed, just staring at the floor. Sometimes I would just sit beside her and hold her hand without saying anything. It was all I knew to do to make her life easier. She would eventually look deep into my eyes with such emptiness in her eyes and then she would smile at me. After that, on those blue days, she would say, "I'm so sorry, Linda. I wish I could make it better and I could but I'm too selfish to let you go and give you to someone better, it will get better, I don't know how or when." I could see fear and desperation in her eyes. If the doctor told her she will die if she had a baby she would die because it is not in her heart to abort a child.

Someday, I will paint her. Paint all the triumph in her eyes— she deserves that. Despite the terrors of our lives, her dream was to keep her girls as safe as she could and to keep us all together. She succeeded against all odds. In the end, she won. No money, food, job, or place to go but we were all kept together. And by her teachings we are all together and close today.

Grandma was critical of her and constantly told her everything she did was wrong and that she should have gone back to her husband in Kentucky. Mom never explained why she didn't. Would Grandma even have listened to her? There was so much I didn't know and yet I knew too much. I did not want to know all that stuff or even try to understand it all. I just wanted help. Despite Grandma's willingness to take me in, I still wonder and feel a personal concern about my emotions at the time of her death. Why didn't I cry or hug my grandma when she died? Why didn't I cry at her funeral? Other people commented about my lack of emotion, too. I was not affectionate with people. I hugged Grandma sometimes. She smelled like pretty rose scented powder, especially when I wrapped my arms around her and put my face against her neck. At her funeral, I remember mom and my aunts and cousins were crying but I could not feel anything. As I'm remembering that now I suspect I had watched my mother struggle so much that my feelings were numb.

My mother-in-law, Peggy, read my first draft about my childhood years. She talked to me about my feelings and resentments. Afterward, she said, "Linda, I want you to do something for me. You carry too much wreckage from your past. I want you to go to the beach by your house. Take these painful memories with you. Walk along the beach that you love and let the sun shine on your pretty face. Get on your knees and lift these agonies up to God. Just like you would release a helium balloon into the sky, release this burden. Let go and let God. He has been waiting for you. Do not tether yourself to the past, dear."

I cannot bring myself to do that. I told her I will never forgive Felton—ever. She said, "Then you will never be free. He still has a grip on your heart and is taking up space you could use for happiness. It is time to run and play, Linda. Forty years is long enough—let go."

The old memories keep crowding into my mind. Mom would tell people that the reason she left her husband and came back to Fayetteville was because, "I missed my mom in North Carolina and Ken was always gone in the military." My grandma visited Mom and Dad in Kentucky many times after Helen died. Grandma remembered the casket and we still have the pictures. My cousins will tell you today about how nice my dad was to them. He showed them how to brush their teeth and brought them whole milk—which they seldom had at home. My grandmother worshipped my dad and had all of these nice stories and memories about him. Mom just kept the story of his infidelities to herself. I wonder if the truth would have made any difference to my grandma.

Grandma tried to call Dad and talk to him about reconciliation with my mom, but she said she never reached him. My dad had an education; my mom quit high school in her junior year to marry Dad. She knew intuitively to protect her children from knowing bad things about their father. There are studies that show children gain self-esteem from having a positive view of their parents. Mom never wanted us to think bad things about our dad because it would make us feel bad about ourselves. Some divorced parents turn their children into their private battlefield and the kids get caught in the crossfire. I am grateful my mom didn't do that to us.

I like to believe that my dad realized many years later that he was not a good father to Roxie and me. I think my two brothers (his sons with Katie) and Roxie forgave him. I made it clear to Dad when I saw him again, in my mid-twenties that my mother had been my father *and* mother. I told him that she raised me as best she could and that I am a loving mom and responsible adult because of her. I told him as honestly as I could how I felt about the past and his abandonment of Roxie and me. However, I knew he wanted to be a grandfather to my children and that I was willing to start over with a clean slate to have a relationship. It was the right thing to do—especially for my children. They did not need to grow up with a closet full of skeletons. Sometimes what children imagine is far worse than the facts.

I am grateful he rarely said anything negative to me about my mother. He did not know that I knew about his affair. When I asked him questions about their separation he avoided answering. I guess his silence was understandable. There is no defense for cheating on a woman who had lost a baby girl and had two young girls, one still in diapers. I wonder if he would have paid any of the $50 monthly child support if the military had not deducted it from his pay.

As young adults, we learned another sad truth. Roxie and I were deeply hurt that our dad told all of his family not to let our twin brothers know that he had two daughters by a prior marriage. To him, we did not exist! How could he defend that decision? Obviously, he could not. He tried to avoid answering our questions by telling us something different and changing the subject. He said that he did not know where we moved after we left Kentucky, and he did not know where we lived when we were little. He married his girlfriend who was well-off while my mother was suffering from depression, trying to support two little girls, and barely making ends meet on $50 child support a month.

One of the worst days of my entire childhood was when I came home from school and noticed my mom was unusually despondent. I already knew she was on the brink of an emotional breakdown. She was pretty beaten up that day—she may have had some alcohol, too. That evening she climbed up a power pole and I panicked. I knew she would get electrocuted by the wires. I was only ten years old and immediately started climbing up the pole after her. I was saying everything I could think of to get her to come back down. Finally, I just screamed, "Do you want me to go up there with you so we can get electrocuted together? Felton is not worth it!" Who is going to take care of Roxie?" I finally had her attention and she paused a while then came back down the pole. I was terrified when I had to leave for school the next morning. I was afraid of what she would do while I was gone and I had so many things to tell her. She had never done anything like that before! When I got home I told her if I can finish high school, I would get a job and take care of her. I'm so glad she didn't hurt herself again because I had no idea what to do.

Somehow, she gradually started fighting back. She was five feet and four inches tall and probably weighed ninety pounds. I remembered her being tiny, like Roxie, but shorter. She survived, she kept her family together, and she was still my hero.

When this book is finished, if it helps only one person I will feel successful again. One good outcome is that writing down all my memories has been therapeutic for me. I can see some of the good things now. I feel proud that my husband and I were able to bring my mother to our home and take care of her the last six years of her life. She was in a safe, peaceful home where everyone in the household adored her.

My husband never complained about bringing my mother to live with us. He accepted her mental illness. My husband took the best care of her when I went back to school and was her primary caretaker when I began my first year of teaching. He was by my side when she was diagnosed with cancer. We all took care of her until she died. My sons and daughters loved her, laughed with her, fussed over her, too. Those memories make me smile. My sisters Gail, Carol and Roxanne went to many of Mom's medical appointments in Myrtle Beach. Their children came to visit mom often in Myrtle Beach during her last years, and most of mom's family were there when she passed away.

I compare Mom's victory in life to this parable about crabs. Several crabs in a bucket would try to climb out, but each time on crab reached the top, the other crabs would pull it back down. Eventually they all died, but they could have all made it out if they helped each other. She was the crab that managed to climb out of a bucket! She raised four strong daughters who grew up to marry, raise families, get good jobs, and who continue to love each other through thick and thin. A case in point—all three of my sisters stepping in to take care of my home and family while I was in a coma for 28 days. They also helped me constantly through that first year of recovery.

It is gratifying that all of her grandchildren loved her very much. They still remember her as a loving grandma. My mother's crowning glory is that she had four daughters and many grandchildren who loved her. She was the mother and father of those four daughters and overcame so many obstacles with courage and determination. She loved her children above all else. These are my memories of our lives growing up. My sisters may have memories that are different from mine but I am compelled to write my own truth. This is my effort to seek justice for Mom and to honor her strength through so much adversity.

Later in my life, especially when I taught high school, students commented about their childhood. They often used bad circumstances at home as an excuse for being late, not turning in homework, or missing tests. These excuses fall in the category of "woe is me," and do not capture my empathy. Poverty, broken homes, illness, and domestic strife are part of living. As a survivor and as a teacher, it was paramount to me that these students understood they are personally responsible for their actions and the outcomes. I couldn't let them use the failures of their parents to become failures themselves. I could not let them give up. Their situations will probably not improve at home and they need to learn survival skills. Privately I would meet with certain students that were full of "street pride" and talk with them about expectations and consequences. I used techniques that were used by my teachers—firm but fair. They had my empathy— not sympathy. I had been there and I wanted to make a difference. Sometimes the only role model that a child looks up to is a teacher.

"It is better to be a lion
Than a sheep all your life."

Sister Elizabeth Renney

High School Years

Some of my most asinine decisions in my life were made in these years. The first crisis was the derailment of my plan to finish high school and enter college. I was blindsided by my high school advisor and by my step-father. I always held my teachers and advisors in the highest esteem. I thought most school officials had the wisdom of Solomon. But I was victimized by the prevalent stereotypes about "poor white trash." My high school advisor looked at me and sized up my potential by my appearance and long list of street addresses. He was adamant that I get a job and go to work rather than pursue my then-dream of becoming a veterinarian. How could I take the path of vocational classes and getting a job rather than focusing on a curriculum that would prepare me for college? Why did I cave in and agree with him so easily? In retrospect, I wonder what would have happened if I had waited and solicited the advice of my favorite teachers, or school counselors, or our minister.

I was doing so well in high school and getting excellent grades. I loved school, the order and organization, the food, the knowledge that was available, the library. I wanted to get a good education in a professional field that would provide a better life for me and my future children. I loved animals and that was my dream career for as long as I could remember. When I met with my high school advisor, he was quite blunt. I had been living with Grandma until she died, and after a couple of horrible years around Felton I was now staying with Aunt Louise. He told me I was too young to go to school by myself. He said, "Linda, you have to go back home, get adopted, or get married. You need to get a job and support yourself." In addition, the advisor's records were erroneous. He had been told that by Felton, my stepfather, that I was a runaway and caused problems at home.

There was a lot of prejudice against poor kids from the wrong side of the tracks, then and now. I tried to explain but he would not consider my side of the story. He had to approve my study plan and now I felt cornered and angry. One more time I was a loser.

The parents of my friends and most teachers were eager to help students finish high school and get good jobs or an advanced education. I was in the opposite situation. My stepfather actively blocked my efforts to stay in school and now my advisor was doing the same thing. My only choice was to go along. It was a hard blow.

In Fayetteville most jobs were related to the military base at Fort Bragg, the Holt- Williamson Cotton Mill, or the Kelly Springfield Tire Factory. These were the major employers of the community. The lower income people worked in service jobs and most young people started out as restaurant help. I decided to get a job as a waitress. My mom had waitressed but she was friendly, outgoing, and fun to be around. I was serious, angry, and suspicious of others.

My first job was at the Waffle House, which was within walking distance of Highway 301. Having never worked for pay I felt rich when payday rolled around! My tips were not very good because I was not friendly enough to the customers. I worked after school. The manager decided to change my work schedule to the third shift which was usually midnight until 6 A.M. I needed the job and I took the shift change.

During that shift the local male customers came in drunk and the long-haul truckers flirted with me or propositioned me. I was definitely ready to find another job after a few weeks of third shift. It was still dark and dreary when I got off work in the wee hours of the morning. Whenever she could, my friend Linda Bond would try to pick me up on her ancient motorcycle. It was so old she could not get parts for it. Sometimes she had been out partying all night but I still hopped on the back of her motorcycle and rode home. Like most teenagers safety never entered my mind. Yet I was wary of the men.

One good memory of the Waffle House was visiting and talking with a tiny little man who was so gentlemanly to me. His name was Willie Shoemaker, the famous horse jockey. He was very polite to me and left me a very good tip. He even gave me his autograph! The married and drunken men that flirted with me and tried to get me to go out with them were disgusting. My attitude was showing at work.

I finally had to quit my job before I was fired.

My next job was at the Holt-Williamson Cotton Mill—one of the oldest cotton mills in the United States. It opened in Fayetteville in 1898. I was the third generation of the Buck family to work at the mill. It was originally a white yarn mill. Colored yarns and knits were added later. These products were sold to manufacturers to make the cloth.

Life was getting a little better for me the more I stayed away from the house where Felton lived. I started dating a boy from school named Larry Bond, my friend Linda's (the one with the motorcycle) brother. I was living with Aunt Louise when I started working at the Mill and was glad I got to see Mom every day after work. Mom worked one of the hardest jobs in the factory. The mill was steamy hot inside, and thick cotton balls and fibers clung to her clothing and her long black hair. Mom was an amazing worker. She worked all day on her feet, no goggles or masks to protect her eyes or lungs and no rubber mats for leg and back support. Yet she broke into a huge smile when she saw me waiting for her at the gate. Despite blisters on her feet and holes in her shoes she always took overtime if it was offered. As a child I told myself *I am going to go to college so I don't have to work this hard physically to make a living.*

During my freshman year, Mom was the only one who told me I was smart and could do anything I wanted in life. When I told her I wanted to go to college and get a job to take care of her, she said, "I know you will because you are so smart." She was always positive and made me feel good. Her special face just made me want to take care of her but I was so helpless. I would often ask her, "How come you are the one to work hard and Felton sleeps all day and doesn't have a job?" She would look at me with such distant eyes. It was a far-away stare that was not in this world. When she had that look you almost lost her and she didn't even hear anything else you said. When she came back to the present she would always smile, as if I just appeared in front of her.

I didn't mind working at the Mill. It was a tiring job but it was a company town that hired employees for life and successive generations came to work at the mill. Observing the people walking out after each shift, I could tell by their physical shapes which jobs they were doing because they had worked on the same equipment all their lives—the men developed a lower shoulder on their right sides, for example.

There was a very nice German boy who went to the same high school I did. His mother had a heavy German accent and she worked at the mill, too. He was tall, smart, blond, and had the prettiest blue eyes. We talked every day. We both wanted to go to college. He had two older sisters in college and both of them wanted to become lawyers. He was so interesting to talk to. He knew I was dating another boy named Larry and I had no romantic interest in dating him. I guess the right chemistry just wasn't there. But I enjoyed him and wanted to be friends. One day I was walking to Larry's house and the boy drove by and offered me a ride. He knew that I was dating Larry a lot. After we drove a little distance he shocked me by telling me his feelings toward me. He said that he loved me and was a better man and would be a better husband than my boyfriend would be! Then he surprised me by kissing the top of my head! "Linda, if you just give me a chance you would see how much more of a man I am than he is. Larry is not very bright—and you are. You need someone like me, Linda." I was speechless and have no idea how I responded! Needless to say, we were not close friends after that.

During the summer I worked as much as I could and saved some money. Larry Bond and I were dating more often. He had a severe injury to his neck and was in the hospital a while. I lived near Larry's family and knew his mother, Johanna. My mom really liked Larry because he had been working at various jobs since he was thirteen years old. He obviously had a strong work ethic. Larry liked me and his younger brother liked Roxie. I was so surprised when Larry sent me a card and some money for my birthday in May. No one had ever done that for me before. We dated and worked all summer. On the weekend we would go to the drive-in theater. We were both so tired from working we could not hold our eyes open through the second movie. When Larry graduated high school I still had my junior and senior year to complete. He knew all my goals and I knew his.

I lived with my Aunt Louise and she let me use her car. I took her to the store, out to lunch, and to church. My biggest concern was that I needed a car for school and a job. I was wary of asking to use their car because I feared her husband would expect "favors" in return. He had already been to prison for nearly cutting a man's head off in a fight. I did not feel safe around him and made certain I was never alone with him. My cousin Ann used the car to help her mother, Aunt Louise. Ann had graduated, had a good job, and was smart enough to get out of the state and away from Aunt Louise's husband Henry as soon as she could.

When high school started that fall, I was still working third shift. I could barely stay awake in my first period class. Larry let me use his car as much as possible because he was worried about Henry doing something to me, too. When Aunt Louise went into the hospital for surgery I knew I could not stay alone in the house with Henry. It was another turning point in my life. Knowing the circumstances, Larry's mother, Johanna, invited me to live with her. She liked me and I liked her a lot. I didn't own many things anyway so it was easy to move to Johanna's house and I was grateful for a safe haven. The downside was that Larry's three sisters did not like me living with their mom and brothers at first. But they got used to it and gradually accepted me.

As I mentioned earlier, it was then one more time Felton hurled a roadblock in my path. He tried to get me kicked out of that high school because of the residency requirements and he succeeded! Although I was a good student, attended classes regularly, paid for my own lunches, and caused no problems in the classroom, Felton's interference was costing me the chance to remain at the same high school. He told a lot of lies and half-truths to pull this off. This was the first time I remembered becoming emotional and mad on my own behalf. I was devastated. In order to be admitted to Central Carolina Technical College in Sanford as a vet technician I had to complete specific courses in high school. Due to Felton's interference the time delay would cause me to lose my slot for entrance at CCTC that year. This was the only school available on the east coast at that time for a veterinary technician degree. I already felt like a failure and one more time I felt like a total loser. My long-range goal was to become a veterinarian—*a doctor not a technician*! I finally realized that six to eight years of college was unattainable without support but I knew I could somehow manage enough money to finish the technical college courses and get my license.

At that time, Larry Bond never told me he loved me and I did not love him. We had a good time together, had very similar goals, and were both workaholics. After the incident about my legal enrollment at school, Larry hatched a plan. One morning I dropped Larry off at his job at Kelly Springfield Tire Factory. Suddenly, he took both of my hands in his, looked into my eyes, and starting talking about a future together. I do not remember everything he said, but I was shocked. He told me his dad was about to lose their family home on Rockfish Road. He said we cold both use our tax returns to save the house from foreclosure. His dad said he would sign the house over to us when we got married. He said I could finish school and we could split the proceeds from the house if I decided to do something different. It felt like it was a business plan, not a proposal of marriage. My mind was whirling. He said "just think about it and don't say anything until you pick me up tonight."

I was stunned. I knew we didn't love each other but the friendship was great. Getting married for these reasons? I had to think about it all day long. My first thought was, "What about his mother?" She raised her five children in that house. I knew she was not happily married because her husband was an ass and everyone else thought so, too.

I had never had a home before. My first priority in life was to get an education and become a vet, not get married and buy a home. This "proposal" was unexpected and overwhelming to a 17-year-old girl. *Who can I talk to? Who can I trust to give me accurate advice? What am I worried about?* I was not afraid of divorce, but he has enough money to get the house without me. *What is he thinking? I've never had anyone make a decision and drop it on me like this and give me eight hours to think about by answer! He is not desperate or an old man, he is one year older than I am. We are friends. He is the only one I dated. What does this mean?*

Later, his sisters told me that Larry *loved* me. I said "He is not saying those words and those are powerful words." They countered with, "He is just afraid of love. It will work out." I thought about what his sisters said and their comment that they thought we were "in heat!" Well, I was smart enough to take birth control. I really wasn't interested in a relationship. I had never given any thought to marriage to anyone. School was the most important goal I had. We both enjoyed the physical satisfaction we got from each other. My street-savvy experiences from the past immediately kicked in. I would be adamant about a monogamous marriage—but doubted that he would feel the same way. We were too young. *Are we crazy?*

By that evening, I had a lot of questions to discuss with Larry. My main objective was to finish school in Sanford to get my vet tech degree. He said, "Save your money now, because you won't have time to work and go to school full time. I know that's what you want to do." He seemed to have all the "right answers," but love was never part of our discussions. Friends and family thought it was a great idea for us to marry. Mom and Johanna went with us to South Carolina to get married. I do not remember the rings or circumstances. It seemed surreal at the time and my memories of that trip and the ceremony are dim at best! I just thought, "Here we go!"

Life with Larry
The Happy Years

We married and did not have any problems blending our lives. We were busy working and studying. In the summer, he started working on the house making all kinds of repairs. I started gardening and planting. For fun, we went out to clubs after second shift—about midnight. There was a bar in downtown Fayetteville where Larry's mother, Johanna, worked. We hung out there at nights and played pool. I always dressed nicely and looked my best. Larry loved the extra attention from the guys of having a beautiful wife. He never drank and I usually had a couple of drinks. There was a club near Kelly Springfield where everyone knew him. Larry was a great pool player and almost always won money shooting pool. We also loved to dance at the nightspots. We loved the Michael Jackson songs from the late 1970s. We had so much fun dancing—we actually went to a studio and took lessons. We were usually the best dancers on the floor. These were the first really fun times of my life!

Through the end of high school, everything was great. Larry began noticing my drawings and the posters I designed for the senior prom. He constantly encouraged me to paint and bragged about my artistic ability. I was very happy. It was an especially happy day when I was accepted as one of only eight new students for the new semester at Central Carolina Tech in Sanford for their Veterinarian Technician program! I graduated high school in June 1977 and entered college in August. I was so excited. I was also happy because my mother and sisters seemed to be doing fine and things were better at home without me living there.

Finally, everything in my life was coming up roses! The relationship with Larry was good and solid. He was proud of me and showed it. I graduated high school after all those years of abuse and struggle. I felt triumphant at last! Now I was accepted to an outstanding college for veterinarian technicians. And most importantly, my mother and sisters were doing better at home without me being there. I was so happy with my life.

This was definitely the best time of my life thus far. Starting school at Central Carolina Technical College was wonderful. The classes were harder because they were intensive. I enjoyed studying animals except for the rats! Lab work was the favorite part of my schooling. There were so many interesting aspects to it. I also enjoyed surgery, X-ray, delivery, and biopsy. Remembering this information reminds me of people who have extensive sports knowledge. They have memory banks filled with facts. They know about all of the plays, statistics on every athlete, and the details of games played in the past decade. People can memorize when they played, how well they did, how much each weighed, and countless details of sports long past. Memorization was not a problem for me—it was easy. Math was the greatest challenge and technicians needed to be proficient at it. Calculations, weights, proportions, formulas—all were critical skills needed. This was a big challenge for me. The most difficult part of a technician's job emotionally and intellectually is to calculate the exact amount of medication required to euthanize an animal based on breed, weight, and other factors. I loved learning and was excited about my future.

On the home front, things were beginning to change. I loved that Larry and I had lots of friends and they came to our house for picnics and barbecues on the weekends. Larry got involved in water skiing and that gave me time to study. He always wanted me to ski with them but I had to have study time. He began to get annoyed with me and said I always "had my head in a book." He continued skiing and

I studied. I had no desire to be on the boat when I needed to study. I would fail school if I didn't stay focused and disciplined. Learning was difficult for me. The more I studied, the more our relationship seemed to change. After a year together, everything was going well. I decided that I loved him and told him so. I also told him that I was going to stop birth control for a while. I knew it would take a while to get pregnant.

I had a nagging feeling that Larry was slowly drifting away and I thought it was because I was so occupied with school. I made more effort to spend time with him and go places that he enjoyed. I wanted him to be happy. Recently I had also noticed there were a lot of female friends hanging out at his boat. I never cared about that previously, but now I did. I started dropping by where he was playing pool. It seemed like things were okay again. The more time I spent with him the happier he seemed to be. He paid all the bills and paid for my tuition and books. He bought a small Renault car for me to drive to school. I had never had life so good.

Despite my renewed efforts to spend quality time with him, I noticed again that he was gradually changing his attitude toward me. When I suspected that something was wrong I tried to talk to him about it. I told him how much I loved him and wanted him to be happy. At the time, I decided he resented me being in school. Because my education was part of our plan from the beginning, I was baffled by his change of heart. He was perfect in every way except telling me he loved me.

The happiness was short-lived. He started lying about things and his personality and attitude toward me was different. He was aloof and distant. I could feel the discontent but he would not discuss it with me. His moodiness and lack of communication was driving me crazy. I knew he was hurting, but I didn't know why. I felt like a Cinderella suddenly turned back into a street urchin. *What was going on? What could I do about it? Yell at me—scream at me—but please don't just ignore me!*

The following week I had an appointment with my gynecologist. I did not have a clue that I might be pregnant yet—but I was! We had been married a year and I was just beginning at school in Sanford. I was so stunned I thought the doctor had made a mistake. I was immediately euphoric! As it was sinking in I felt like I was walking on air. I was so excited I thought my heart would explode. This news made me even happier than my acceptance at Sanford! My second thought was how thrilled Larry would be! We would be having a baby together! On the way home I was planning how I would tell him. I knew it would be perfect to go down to Hope Mills Lake where we had always discussed the major issues in our lives.

I was so excited to tell my mother and sisters. The first thing my mother said was, "It's going to be a boy!" Mom grinned from ear to ear. I walked on clouds the entire day. This baby was the most exciting thing in my life. I decided I would walk down and meet Larry that night and tell him. I had gone to my favorite fast food place that afternoon—Taco Bell and I had an epiphany! Was it safe to feed this baby Taco Bell? *Even as I write this story now I am so excited ... and hungry! This is one of my sweetest memories.* That night I asked him to meet me down at the Hope Mills Lake beach.

I had graduated from high school in June. Larry and I had been married a year when I became pregnant. Little Larry was born December 21, 1977. The marriage was becoming rocky for reasons I did not grasp or understand. Larry became more and more distant after I became pregnant. We seemed to be in a constant state of conflict. I started my training to be a licensed veterinarian technician in August, 1977. I was still size 8 in my uniform and my size didn't change much during pregnancy. My belly grew—but the rest of my body remained pretty much the same.

Except for the frequent conflicts with Larry, I was so happy again! I was going to college for the career of my dreams! I was married to a good man, had a secure home, and I enjoyed the experiences of having my first baby. Still, I was a bit cautious about my husband Larry. It was important to me to see whether Larry was going to follow through with our original commitment about my educational goals.

We shared similar views. I thought the things Larry said were as important as the things I said. We listened to each other. He said the reason he did not want children was because he knew the world was a hard place today to raise kids. We discussed that before we got married because he did not like being raised by his father and mother growing up. They argued all the time and had an unhappy marriage.

I told him I knew exactly how he felt. He knew my childhood

was so much worse than his. I felt our relationship was different than our parents. We were stable, we loved each other, and we had a good future ahead of us. We listened and respected each other. I was disappointed that he was not excited about our pregnancy—but I was sure he would understand the situation. I told him I took birth control and told him when I stopped taking it and if he was so adamant against having a child he should have helped prevent it. I did not agree with him having a vasectomy even if he did not want any more children. I reminded him that I had just started to college and I was not planning a pregnancy. I told him it was not my total responsibility. We did not plan this but it happened, this is our child, and we should just be happy. No matter how many times I reminded him that it was *our* responsibility, I could tell he did not accept it.

Practically speaking, I told him that having a baby would not change our life that much. I was still going to finish my schooling and we each had three sisters that would help with babysitting. They would all love to have extra money while I go to school. He thought I should quit school and it felt like he was punishing me with his insistence. I told him it would be too hard to get back in this school. "I know I can do both." In exasperation, I said "you are saying one thing but you are not telling me exactly what the problem is! Please tell me how you feel now." His only explanation is that he did not want children. I said, "Larry, we are going to have a baby so we just have to be happy and continue our plans as much as we can. Yes this did happen a little sooner than I wanted but I was very happy that it did."

It broke my heart that Larry changed almost immediately after learning of our pregnancy. It seemed like I had heard and read, *"Don't get pregnant because you will be stuck and the father does whatever he wants and you have to do everything by yourself."* I did not feel used. I knew that he was not so upset that he wanted to end our marriage right away or that he even mentioned abortion.

I loved him and wanted for him to be as happy as I was. I did not mind finishing school pregnant or having to do everything at home. I was very content living in the first house I had ever lived in. Larry was gone a lot and told me he was working longer hours to make up extra money for the pregnancy. Trusting him was becoming increasingly more difficult. He was emotionally unavailable. I felt my insecurity growing and I had seen a lot of cheating men and women in my life. It was important to trust him but there was still the gnawing doubt because he no longer treated me the way he used to. His behavior was not tolerable. He was a good provider, did not get overly angry or swear, and he never physically hurt me. I knew I could tolerate almost anything except lying and cheating on me. I had zero tolerance for adultery. But our happy little life had changed forever.

I continued to attend classes and study, but I stopped studying and talked to him when he came home. I had no reason to suspect that he was not honest because we had long discussions about lying and commitment long before the marriage or pregnancy. We agreed if one of us wants to end the marriage we would make that happen, but we would not engage in the battles we had witnessed in our homes.

Larry had a lot of friends—both married and unmarried. He always wanted to socialize with couples. I knew that was important to him, so I went as much as possible. I knew his motives were related to his business and status. These couples were wealthy business owners and successful in life. His personality and character were different in these social situations. His conduct was embarrassing to me; he had an arrogance and false pride about him. He inflated his financial situation and exaggerated about his material possessions. No matter how much I wanted to excuse and justify his behavior, it was indefensible. I had never known him to be deceitful except when he was around the wealthy friends. It was sad to see a good man in his own right turn into a "wannabe." On the other hand, I was pretty much the same person regardless of the company I was in. I am pragmatic and direct.

His real motive was to be someone that he wasn't. In retrospect, I think he had such a low self-esteem that he tried to be someone that people would be impressed with based on illusions of wealth and material things. It was increasingly obvious to me and I knew his "friends" thought so, too. Gradually, he began to embellish even the most minor things. It hurt me to see him do that to himself. He was better than that.

His behavior was getting so phony. It drove me crazy because he was wonderful the way he was. I tried to discuss the matter with him without anger, one on one. I never wanted to humiliate him in front of others. He tried to justify his lying. He was convinced he needed to do so in order to achieve his goals. Finally, I gave up with the velvet glove approach and told him he was making an ass out of himself and losing my respect. Lying was just poor character parading around as success. I did not like a lot of his friends and decided I was wasting my time. He sulked like a child whenever I brought it to his attention. We would probably get along better if I stayed away from his dream world.

For years after this failure, I analyzed over and over again the ways I could have responded differently to make our marriage work. Perhaps I could have kept my "know it all" ideas to myself. Was I as immature as he was? Was I expecting more from our "arranged marriage" than he bargained for? At the end of the day, I knew that I loved Larry and I lost him at some unknown point along the way. I grieved that loss for a long time.

There were friends who called me or stopped by to go places with me after they found out I was pregnant. They were happy and excited for me. Larry and I had increasingly different friends. He was so much more social than I had ever been or needed to be. Although the wives of his friends were friendly to me, I had little in common with them. When they made comments about things my husband and done or said, I was matter-of-fact. I would say "Really, Larry said that?" It was ludicrous because most of the things they shared with me were untrue.

Larry's friends came down or called me to go out, but I did not accept very often. There was not enough time to read and paint and grow a baby. How did I ever work and do the things I wanted to do? One of the wives was more special to me and I enjoyed her. I never shared my problems but I listened and responded to her in a positive way. I had made up my mind that I would not give her advice unless she asked me. I would answer most questions that she asked me except questions about my childhood. Most of the decisions I had made were not exactly the right decisions and I felt unqualified to give anyone advice. She had told me her husband did not want any children because he had a daughter from a previous marriage. He did not want any more children with her. Normally I do not say much but we had spent enough time together alone that I shared my thoughts with her. Personally I thought she was making a mistake regarding a permanent decision to have tubal ligation. People change and you should not let someone else convince you to make a decision that cannot be reversed in the future. I asked her, "Well what about you? Do you want to spend the rest of your life without a child?" She said that it was fine with her. I told her I thought that he was kind of selfish to deny her from having any children and convincing her to have a surgical procedure that was irreversible. I told her that things change, and your marriage may not work out.

Although the choices Larry and I each made ultimately ended our marriage, I will never be sorry about my pregnancy. I believe babies are chosen by God to be born at a special time. I believe there was a special time reserved for my son, Larry. I did not recognize this fully at the time. I believe the children we have are not accidents. God has a purpose for every human. Larry James, my son, is amazing and special in many ways. I will not be able to acknowledge all of his gifts or accomplishments, but I know what they are. His gifts were truly revealed to me and to others the moment he learned about my stroke. An aneurysm in my brain—and all the days following that event—showcased all the goodness a mother can hope for in a son. There are many things my son will accomplish and he will fulfill the life God has ordained for him.

The conversations that my husband and I had were leading to constant conflicts. I felt he was deliberately punishing me for getting pregnant. He actions were calculated and pushing me into a corner, forcing me to agree to with him. He was leading up to the ultimatum—I must choose marriage or choose school. I refused to do that. It was a no-win proposition. He couched his words in a hundred phrases to trap me into a decision. He did not have the ability to be direct and honest with his ultimatum. Conversely I refused to be trapped into submission to his manipulations. We reached a painful impasse.

I had experienced and witnessed more than any young girl should endure. I knew that I would not be forced to make a choice. I was married, I was a mother, and I was a student. There was no other choice. I think he wanted a divorce but he was too afraid of losing material things, all those toys we purchased together and all the things we bought for our house. Looking back, and looking at his conduct in the years since then, I think that material possessions and status were more important to him than relationships. Things and image-making were integral to his future goals. He was disenchanted and frustrated that I did not conform to the things he valued. We had different values about how to lead a successful life. Ultimately, the pregnancy changed our relationship and changed me. I was a different woman now. Our basic character would not permit either of us to compromise at the crossroads.

The war of words continued. With a new baby coming, I knew I would have to schedule my return to school immediately after childbirth to meet enrollment deadlines. Again, Larry used my registration date and fees to box me into a corner. We needed to arrange childcare for the next semester but he refused and insisted that I would have to stay home and take care of the baby.

Despite our previous agreements, he was not budging to support my educational commitments. We could afford childcare. There was an excellent childcare center that our friends used. Despite any solution I proposed, Larry persisted with his arguments, "You shouldn't go to school for this—you know veterinarian techs don't make any money when they graduate. People work with veterinarians as volunteers for free!" I told him that my goal was to become a veterinarian and that unless I went to school I would feel like a loser. I already achieved part of my dream becoming a technician, but I sacrificed my dream of becoming a veterinarian doctor.

When logic failed, he resorted to ridicule. Maybe because I was pregnant and my hormones were crazy I was more emotional than usual. I was furious with his assertion that finances and childbirth should end my education and career goals. I recognized it as another manipulation and I refused to give it up. Being true to my core self was at stake—my integrity was not negotiable!

My baby was due on December 25th and my doctor agreed to induce labor on the 21st. It all worked out and I was able to return to class on time. We placed Little Larry in KinderCare and I shared rides with three other students or rode the bus. I just used the extra travel time to study.

Larry tried another approach. He had friends who owned a gorgeous pet store. She was a veterinarian and paid people to work in the store. His friends travelled all over the world and the owner worked only when she wanted to. Larry thought managing or working in the store should satisfy me. I reminded him again being a clerk or

store manager was not my goal. The discussion ended predictably—
he left to go to the mountains to ski with his friends.

I could see the handwriting on the wall. I was heartsick at what
was happening but practical by nature. I had to be in survival mode
most of my life—and now I had to do the same for myself and my
son. *What can I do to accomplish my goals and take care of my son?*
He continued pushing for the outcome he wanted.

The more Larry pushed me into a corner, the more I hated the
dilemma I was in. Now he refused to help the way he promised. I
only needed two years to complete my goal—I could not see a way to
accomplish this without Larry's help. Looking at it more accurately
I realize my part in this. I used to think I should have stayed on birth
control until I finished school. I thought it would probably take six
months to get pregnant. But today, I know the reasons. There was
something special about my son, Larry. Had I not had him then, there
was never going to be another opportunity to be born. All children
are precious and God had made my decision for me. Larry has been
born to accomplish his destiny. It was Larry—and all of my other
children—who helped Jeff keep me alive when I had that aneurysm.

My Service in the United States Air Force

I finally realized that I needed to have a new plan to survive and
take care of Little Larry. I could not afford childcare and tuition
without an income. I had to put my dream on hold. I also had to
face the realities of my marriage. I had lost respect for my husband.
We had both changed. The rules of engagement changed, and our
priorities in life changed. Neither of us was willing to compromise. I
knew I had to start over. *How? Where? What next?*

Having lived in a military town all of my life, my next thought
was to see a military recruiter. My father had been successful in the
military. My decision was to go into the military with a guaranteed
job in a hospital at the end of my tour. I saw all of the videos that told
about the benefits and the child care on the hospital grounds for my
son. When I learned that after completing my military tour of duty,
a veteran's benefit is paid-for education, I was convinced. I could
actually go to school and get paid for it! I was so naïve and didn't

know anyone locally in the military. I hoped I was making a good decision—and I hoped Larry might reconsider his position.

I was so desperate to make sure I would not be a loser. Now Larry was faced with the ultimatum. All Larry had to say was, "Don't leave, you can finish school." I would have stayed with him and kept my family together. But he didn't say that. I told him that he gave me no other choice and I enlisted in the Air Force.

Basic training would start in April and last six weeks. I arranged for several sitters to take care of my son until I finished basic training. Larry was only four months old and it was an agonizing decision to leave him. After basic training I knew I could take Larry with me to my next assignment. I was convinced that everything was going to be perfect after basic training, but I knew it would not be easy. What I didn't know was that this was really the perfect opportunity to end the marriage. Larry said he would not take care of me. How could I make such a mess of my life and marriage trying to be successful in my own right? I was shocked that Larry did not attempt to get me to change my mind.

Larry told everyone that I had abandoned my family and he had to make arrangements for family members to take care of Little Larry. Still stunned by the turn of events in our marriage I was prepared for a divorce when I completed basic training. Now it was Larry's turn to be shocked when I told him I didn't want anything from him except my son, Larry. Was I crazy?

When I received my "guaranteed" job, I also realized that the "Air Force needs came first." I was stationed at Valdosta, Georgia, as a supply specialist, not as a medical tech. *What in hell did I do?* This was becoming more complicated than I anticipated. I needed to talk to someone who could guide me. I was making adult decisions as a 20-year-old single parent and raw recruit. I could not trust Larry enough to just call and talk with him about it. He said he wanted to see other women. I told him that I hope he enjoyed it and I would leave him alone.

When it was time to finally leave for my first duty station, Larry seemed to be glad to drive his wife and son to another state. I was glad he offered and I accepted the ride. I met a lady who had been in the military six years. She was married and had two children—ages two and three. She helped me by answering my questions and telling me where to live. Across the street from the military base there were several trailers for rent. I rented one for us to live in. Child care was available for twenty-four hours a day—seven days a week, if needed. How convenient. The only negative thing I could see immediately was a long road and a thirty-minute to drive the nearest McDonald's! In Georgia, there was a church on every corner and nothing else I could see near the base. My new friend said that she goes down to Dayton, Florida, once a month for a weekend. She invited me to go along too and arranged a sitter for her children and mine. She was good with the kids.

Larry came down and decided to help me buy a new car. It's a shame he didn't volunteer that when I wanted to continue school! We had a good time together before he left. It was bittersweet for me. He was happy for his freedom and I was still trying to figure out how to add school to my hectic life. I was told about a college twenty miles away and started thinking more strategically. Although vet tech was my first love—I realized that a guaranteed hospital job was a promising option. Registered nurses made three times the salary of vet technicians. My job on base was from 7:00 P.M. to 3:00 A.M. I made a new plan. I enrolled in nursing school, worked all night, and attended classes until lunch time. I had afternoon time to study, spend time with Little Larry and report to work for my shift. Little Larry was such a good toddler. He would play beside me in his playpen as I stood there and studied. I was not excited about my situation. I was making the best decisions I could under the circumstances. It seemed there was no time to waste.

I missed my mother and went go back to Fayetteville whenever I could afford it. I went over to Larry's at night and stayed there with Little Larry. I'm sure he was enjoying the situation. I hated it, but he was not interested in commitments. I told him I was not interested in my job on base but would make the best of it. I had already signed the papers over to Larry to give him the house and the bulk of our furniture.

Larry was different toward me after our divorce. He seemed concerned and said, "Do you need anything for the baby?" He had seen someone visiting where I lived in Valdosta and asked why I did not say anything about dating a man. The last few times I visited my family, I told them I was dating, but nothing special. I told them

Larry now had exactly what he wanted—his freedom.

Larry had not dated very much before we were married. In fact, I had not dated much in high school, either. We enjoyed learning what you were supposed to do sexually and got good at it. It depends on who you talk to—but many people say the only time you should make love is with someone you love. Wrong. Maybe I read too many books. I know some friends of mine told me they did not enjoy sex, but I disagreed with them. Sex is a normal and healthy part of an adult's life. At any rate, Larry was dating now and seemed to be enjoying his new freedom.

I was struggling making a new life for us but defiant about asking or letting anyone help me. By now, Little Larry was walking and was so cute. The single mom thing was a challenge. Larry did not ask to keep the baby or play with him. Larry did not ask to visit. I dated, went to work, and went on with my life. But I soon noticed that Larry had parked his car down the street and watched the house. There were several men in the military who asked me to lunch, dinner, the beach, and wanted to take me and my son to Orlando.

Friends told me that Larry was dating and it was a lot worse on me than I wanted to admit. This situation was still hard but I did not intend to turn into a nun. I was not interested in romance but I enjoyed dating. There was only one person I saw frequently. He had a beautiful voice and played guitar. He sang a lot of James Taylor and he was very good. He had friends next door and introduced himself when I was sunbathing. He and I played cards several times. Several married men were the biggest turn-offs. Here is exactly how and what I was thinking. With the exception of my son being taken care of, I was only concerned with my career goals and school.

I'm not sure why Larry watched me at my house but I continued to enjoy dating. For the first time in a long time, I was having a good time in life. *Well how did you leave him if you loved him? I did love him, but I recognized that life is too short to settle for someone who won't support you in your own dreams and goals.*

One night Larry came to my trailer when my date left. He saw the other guy's guitar, some playing cards. Little Larry was up, fed, and dressed. His dad did not pick him up and hold him, he just said, "Hi, Buddy." Little Larry smiled at his dad—just like he would do when anyone says hi. Larry invited us to go out to eat. He seemed to know exactly where he was going and where everything was located in town.

He started driving down to see us more frequently. He was definitely showing interest in me again. There were several things I wanted to ask him, but I was reluctant. I said, "Larry, are you going to lose your job driving here from Fayetteville so often?" He said, "I thought you wanted to stop working?" I had already told him that Air Force needs come first. I started nursing classes at the college about twenty minutes away. He said, "I thought you have a job guaranteed at the hospital, why are you still going to school?"

Once more, I said "You still don't get it! I am still trying to accomplish my goal of becoming a vet!" Without playing games or hiding anything I told him I was not interested in his car or his money.

Larry had driven down in a brand new car and tried to start all over again as if nothing had ever happened. I was actually very happy and eager to hear what he had to say. Sadly, he still would not communicate openly and he would not say that he loved me. Larry acted like I had hurt his feelings. But he still refused to tell me how he felt about me. I wanted to hear him say he loved me. I was through with the cat-and-mouse pursuit. He asked me to listen to a song and words about a necklace and a cross. It was tender and romantic!

I cussed him out so bad for a lot of different reasons. He started to talk to me—but never did. I begged him to talk to me. Even if he had lied and told me about his feelings—I could have dealt with it. After waiting for shared communication so many times—I just got tired of him controlling me with silence on the most pressing issues in a marriage. I told him that now it was too late because I had to stay at Valdosta and "you started the divorce, Larry. The military made it clear that 'Air Force needs came first,' I am committed and it will be three more years. I don't know what you expect?"

The next few months Larry came down and "dated" me often. It seemed like too little, too late but he was trying. That was the first time he was around his son and wanted to buy things without my suggestion. I let him buy Little Larry toys and clothes. He could buy dinner for me, but no things for me and that was it. I was concerned about exactly what he was doing. "Larry, you are going to lose your job. How can you leave Fayetteville and come to Valdosta, Georgia, this frequently?" I learned later he was paying someone to work for him on the weekends.

Always in control, now he was talking reconciliation. I was flattered but suspicious and angry. I said "You should have thought about that before I made the commitments and signed contracts! What about all the lies you told? What about lying to me saying you were at work and someone would call and tell me you were actually at the bar? You are making me crazy! Now you can go there anywhere and see anyone you want—yet you are driving down here and we are six hours away!"

I was instantly mad at myself for bringing up the past. I realized I was livid that he wanted me back but refused to say he loved me. I had been waiting for those words since our wedding day. I could not remain silent another minute. "Why did you have to lie to me? We had a perfect life then. Our marriage is over now so find someone else! I have my life in order now, Larry. Don't worry about me and get on with your life."

Undaunted as if I had said nothing, Larry continued on with his new obsession to reconcile. He said he an idea on how we could make it work. He said that we were separated, not divorced. He suggested that he was willing to meet me halfway and we could still have a life together. It might have worked, except for one major thing— I was in the military. I did not tell him that I had previously inquired about getting out of the military. I did that when I learned that I did not have a guaranteed job, after all. I failed to read the fine print in the contract.

Now I was straddling two worlds. I realized that my pride was ruining my life. I spoke to a military lawyer a few weeks prior. Although I was not getting the job promised, the military lawyer said that I could not leave even though they led me to believe that I would have a guaranteed medical job. He showed me what I had signed at the end of the forms "Air Force needs come first."

I explained why I was disappointed to spend four years doing something other than medical in my life. I said that I did my job to the best of my abilities "and I will continue but I am not happy." I was fine with the people I worked with and was not miserable on the job—it was just disappointing that I had made such an egregious error. I was just 20 years old and the youngest person in my unit. I was the only new person who worked in that area. They were very

251

helpful and knew nothing about my background. The sergeant in charge knew a little more but I was very careful and kept my business to myself. I was happy enough but wished I had asked more questions and paid attention to what I had signed.

After that bittersweet incident with Larry, I did not date anyone else but Larry. We tried to go on with life and accept the circumstances we were in. He was finally playing with Little Larry and being a dad. He drove down to see us even more often and I was actually glad to see him. When I went to Fayetteville, I spent time at our old house when I visited him in Hope Mills. I was glad to go "home" again and see the old place and check on my mom. I loved to spend time with her.

I had the weirdest feeling driving out 301 onto Hope Mills. I was passing the place where Larry's mom Johanna lived at Hope Mills Lake. This is where Larry and I fished and had so much fun. We had such good times...*does he remember that?* I did not see him that day. I kept wondering why he would not compromise with me before the separation and military obligation. Why did I have to do something as drastic as going into the military to get his attention? I have seen him more now than I ever did when we were married. Does he miss our son? I had to constantly remind myself to *stop thinking!* "I am in the military now and separated ... well, now we are not legally married. He took care of that." I was really hard on myself after that day and tried to tell him not to come back. I retorted that he could have gotten laid faster and closer in Fayetteville instead of going to Valdosta, Georgia, if that was the reason he was coming around! As usual, he ignored me and he continued to come down to see me every weekend.

I went to see my mom in Fayetteville and I decided to stay Larry's house, our last house together. I did not make myself at home there. Everything was like it was before I left. I had not taken much. School classes were going to start soon and I tried to focus on the future and not the past. I went back to Georgia and the other guy I had dated tried to see me again. I explained that as long as Larry was making a sincere effort to reconcile, I did not want to date anyone else. He was shocked after all of the complaints I had made about Larry.

On his next visit, Larry had *another proposal* for me! This time he thought it would be a great idea for the two of us to go talk to the base colonel about the changes we were going through. He got my attention when he said, "I think if I go with you to the Colonel and explain that we do not want to be apart—and that you were misled by the recruiter's representations that you would have a job guaranteed in the medical field—we might have a chance to get an honorable discharge for you. We will tell the colonel that we are very unhappy with the deception about a job." He wanted me to talk to a military lawyer, too.

He basically said that he wanted me and Little Larry to come home. He said, "You do not have to work. I will buy you everything new in the house! We can start over!" I sat down and took his hands and said, "Larry you do not understand. I do not want any of those things—and I will not be satisfied staying at home. I don't want you to take care of me. I cannot trust you to keep your word. I want a career in the veterinary field. You need to just go home. I cannot go back because you still do not understand or hear me! I still have three years to serve on a four-year tour of duty."

Once Larry had a plan, he would not be deterred. Larry persuaded me to go with him to talk with the Air Force chaplain and the base colonel. He was convinced that he could make the difference. We met with them and the colonel did say he would write a letter on our behalf—but even if I was discharged, I would have to remain on inactive duty for the remaining three years of my service. After this joint effort, we went about our lives and hoped for the best. I did not date anyone else.

Reconciliation

At the end of August 1978, I received a letter from the Air Force in a light brown envelope. I let it lay there until that evening before I opened it. Little Larry was beginning to walk now and he had the sweetest smile—I played with him to avoid what was inside the envelope. I remember thinking that I was not going to sleep no matter what it said. My hands were sweating and trembling when I picked it up. My fate was about to be determined by the contents of that envelope. I had to read it several times to believe the words on the paper. The letter stated that I was to receive an Honorable Discharge from the military and that I would remain on Inactive Status for three years. The Air Force had the right to recall me to duty in the event of war. I was stunned and suddenly I did not know whether to laugh or cry. I was in disbelief about the turn of events. Overwhelmed, I picked up Little Larry and held him to my chest and cried quietly for a long time. For some reason, Little Larry put his head on my chest and remained still the entire time. Maybe we both realized we were starting on a new journey.

Still in shock, I called Larry and told him the news. Was it the talk with the colonel, or the chaplain or the attorney? My head was spinning. I told Larry I would have to stay here with Little Larry and I would find a job and I was babbling about having a car payment. There was silence. He said "why don't you come home and you can find a job here and save some money?" Thinking more clearly, I told him I would be there soon. My next thought was that I was relieved that I had not paid for the August semester classes yet. Although I was relieved and happy—I had a nagging knot in my stomach. The old thoughts haunted me—*I am just a loser and making more bad decisions! Am I?* I do not remember exactly when I moved home with Larry. It was sometime before Thanksgiving.

On my move back to Hope Mills, I started thinking about the changing tides of our marriage. On that long drive home, I retraced the milestones in our marriage. I was a junior in high school living with my Aunt Louise. Larry was a senior and we were attracted to each other right away. We dated and became romantically involved, and I became suddenly homeless when Aunt Louise went into the hospital. Larry's mom, Johanna, opened her home to me until I could finish high school. It was a safe haven. Unexpectedly in the same year, Larry offered me an "arranged marriage." He said we could buy his parent's home out of foreclosure, fix it up, then sell it and go our separate ways after I graduated from vet college—if that was what we both decided. He did not want children and I just wanted to become a licensed vet tech. It seemed to be a logical plan. We married, I started to school for my license, and his business flourished while he continued to work a factory job at Kelly Springfield.

The "business-like" strategy might have worked, but somewhere along the way I fell in love with him and became pregnant. Little did I know that this pregnancy would mark the beginning of the end of our marriage. Because of my pregnancy, he suffered in silence, sulked, and began to play around. I was determined to proceed with my goals and really thought he would come around to my way of thinking—especially after his son was born. We had been so happy and had so much fun I could not imagine that this could end our marriage. By the time I finished my first semester, he drifted away from me. We separated, and I joined the Air Force for four years, raising Little Larry as a single mom. I decide to take nursing assistant classes and enroll at a local community college. Before I finished one semester, Larry decides he is still interested in me and begins to court me back. After a few months he develops a plan for me to obtain an honorable discharge and reconcile our marriage. After a brief separation, here I am driving back home to spend the rest of my life with him. *Why did this happen?*

As I came off of 301 from Valdosta, Georgia, I had to stop for gas. I had everything I owned in my little Chevette. I spoke to the manager there and asked about job opportunities. She said they would be hiring for extra help around the holidays. I took the part-time job. As soon as I could, I went to the local vet's office to see if there were any openings. The technician at the front hospital told me they only hired certified technicians. I told the girl at the desk I wanted to take the application anyway. She reluctantly handed me the application and I smiled broadly. I was hoping that my semester of classes would be enough to get my foot in the door.

On the back of the application I quickly listed all of the kinds of worms animals get. I wrote the biological names and sketched the shape and appearance of each one. (*Amazingly I see the worm shapes in my mind now and it is exciting to discover I have this image in my memory bank!*) Next, I listed the technical terminology for each inoculation used for cats and dogs. The receptionist said she would put my application on file with the others. I told her, "No … I will wait. I would rather you give it to him as soon as he finishes this appointment." She did not know what to say… I still smiled. I think she understood I was not going anywhere.

Dr. Tygh came out in about ten minutes. All I can remember is he said "I am impressed with your knowledge." He interviewed me and asked a series of technical questions. I am good at memorization and I was able to easily recite the answers to all of his questions—and then some. He immediately asked "When can you start?" That girl at the front desk was obviously shocked that her boss had told her not to handle applicants in this manner. I had learned to be proactive in childhood and it was reinforced in the military. I smiled and told the girl thank you, real sweetly. I am glad that I did not have to work with her, but I could have.

I worked about ten miles away in a satellite office in Spring Lake, near Fort Bragg. I did everything a veterinarian technician did and I loved it! Larry was right. The other girl did not make much more money than I did. I learned fast. The doctor was great to work with and became a good friend. I drove my car to the Ambassador Animal Hospital each morning. At the end of the day I loaded the animals to transfer to the main hospital on Ramsey Street.

I lived in Hope Mills, and it was a lot of driving to get to the clinic, then to the hospital and back home. I again enrolled Little Larry in KinderCare. I did that job for a year. There were three veterinarians I worked with in that satellite. Larry was right— I only made enough money to pay KinderCare, my car payment and gas. Larry did not complain. He knew I loved my job. Dr. Tygh invited his doctors and some of his technicians to his home for social gatherings. Larry loved being in the social groups and went with me eagerly. Larry was paying our bills and we seemed happy. I was so content.

One day I was driving through Hope Mills where we lived saw a sign that read "Dr. Hill—Veterinarian." I asked Dr. Tygh for his opinion about Dr. Hill the next time I saw him. He told me a lot of funny stories about Dr. Hill. He basically said "You are too pretty to work for him" and everyone laughed—they knew him well. I said "Well his clinic is right where I live. If I get hired there I will give you two weeks' notice!" They all said he was demanding and hard to work with, but to "Come back if you cannot stand it!" Being the person I am did not deter me from the hard work!

I was hired right away! The girl I worked with told me her impressions and experiences with Dr. Hill. The part that I really cared about was that he works right down the street and I could save a lot of time and gas. He had the reputation of being one of the best veterinarians in Fayetteville. Before he retired, Dr. Hill owned Dr. Tygh's office. He missed working with animals and decided to start another office in Hope Mills. It did not take long for me to realize Dr.

Hill was a brilliant veterinarian. He already looked like Ben Franklin in the 1970's and he still had an office when I visited him in 2010, still working at what he loved most—he could simply not get away from helping animals.

He had a receding hairline, bald pate, and long gray hair. He wore small wire glasses, exactly like Ben Franklin. My family members still living in Fayetteville use his clinic. I cannot believe he and his wife still work there. His wife works at the front and he had another lady from Germany when I worked there in his office in Hope Mills. She was a lot like Larry's mom, Johanna. She told you what she thought and I appreciate someone who does not hide his or her thoughts. We got along great. She told me what his expectations in regard to my job and that is what I did. I was there a year and had watched several certified veterinarian technicians and students who wanted to be veterinarians come and go. They did not last long. Dr. Hill could have avoided the high turnover but he was very hard to deal with. He would hurt their feelings. Not intentionally—he was just abrupt. But if they listened to him they would learn so much about surgeries and treatment.

I enjoyed watching the surgeries and working in the lab. Because I lived nearby he asked me to assist with emergencies in off hours. If I didn't have a sitter, I had to bring Little Larry with me. He sat in the chair and never said a word until we finished. Even as a youngster Larry was fascinated with what we were doing to the sleeping animals. Dr. Hill was the only veterinarian where we lived who helped dogs with hip dysplasia— mostly German shepherds. He would remove a muscle section in the hip over the top of the femur. He also performed numerous cataract surgeries. Dr. Hill would always call me in to help identify the mixed breeds. I was very good at it and had learned all of the AKC breeds and been tested on them at school. I even remembered the appearance, movement, and temperament characteristics of each breed. *(I had forgotten so much of this terminology after the stroke. Writing this, I am excited that some of it is coming back like the art history and painting).*

Dr. Hill worked with the Humane Society and that was the worst part of my job. Thank goodness it was rare. He handled the sick animals and the ones that were not going to survive. It was my job to set up the right amount of phenobarbital for the doctor to euthanize the animals that could not be helped. Most veterinarians I worked with hated that part of their jobs. Under the law, if the owners wanted to put their animal to sleep and signed a receipt the doctors were required to perform euthanasia. *(I remember Dr. Tygh had a really hard time with his emotions when one lady insisted that he put some puppies to sleep. He had tears tolling down his face during the procedure.)* These puppies' parents were brothers and sisters that had been inbred too many times due to owner negligence. Those puppies would have experienced significant mental and physical defects.

The things I remember most about Dr. Hill was his fondness of singing Janis Joplin's "Bobby McGee." He would tell us interesting stories about our favorite songs when he was doing surgery. When I saw Dr. Hill and his wife in 2010 after my stroke, he explained with a tear in his eye that the lady who worked for him all those years after I left his clinic had breast cancer. He said he could not work for about five years after she died. He sold that office and he opened up on 301 in Hope Mills. Dr. Hill's daughter is a lawyer and his sons are both doctors. He looked the same, his mind was still brilliant, but he no longer performs surgeries. He was an important part of my life history and working for him gave me a new level of self-respect and a sense of competency I had never experienced before. I have a lot of fond memories working in these clinics with excellent doctors and technicians. I was also grateful for an opportunity to work in a field that I loved and have enough income of my own to maintain some independence at home.

Meeting My Father

My life was finally going in a positive direction on all fronts! Happy with my job, my marriage, and my family relationships, I began to think about making contact with my father. After all these years, it seemed the right thing to do. I made first contact and it was difficult and awkward. I found my dad by asking the Veteran's Administration to forward a letter to him from me. After a few months of letter-writing and telephone calls, it seemed more comfortable. Initially, my dad came down to Fayetteville to see us after I contacted him.

It was the first time in almost twenty-five years. Roxie was about six months pregnant. It was an approach-avoidance conflict for me. Part of me still resented the hell out of him and part of me said it was time to see if there was anything salvageable for a father-daughter relationship.

Before he came to visit us the first time, I made it clear to my dad that when we met I did not want to hear any explanations or excuses why he did not keep in contact with us when we were growing up. We never heard from him on special occasions, holidays, or birthdays. I told him my mother was our mother and father and that I did not want him to ever say anything negative about her. As a father and daughter—we had to start now and move forward—the past did not exist.

Roxanne and I called and wrote to Dad for several months and he came to visit a couple of times. He did not try to bring anything up about my mom. He sent a lot of pictures of my half-brothers (they were twins) Terry and Perry as they grew up and while he was away in Vietnam, Germany, and Korea. Roxie and I were glad to know that our brothers had a good home and lived so well. After a few visits, letter writing, and telephone conversations, my dad extended an olive branch.

My dad invited Larry and me to drive to Missouri to meet and visit his family. Dad said they were going into the military and it would be a good time to get together. My brothers were very friendly, smart, and nice to spend time with. Larry got along well with them and they all went skating together. It was a nice memory. My brothers were fraternal twins and did not look alike. Their mother Katie had a twin sister, too.

Little Larry was four years old at the time and I was glad he would meet his grandfather. As soon as we arrived the first evening, my dad showed us pictures of my handsome twin brothers growing up. I had just met my dad a couple of times and he showed me what seemed like hundreds of pictures of the cutest twin brothers, depicting them living the best childhood possible. What exactly was Dad's purpose in showing these to the two girls he had abandoned and forgotten? Was he just proud of his sons and wanted to show them off? Didn't he have any idea how rotten our lives were and the hardships my mother faced trying to keep food on the table for us?

What is wrong with this picture? How can a career military man, police chief, college graduate, and father proudly raise two sons with his new wife immediately after abandoning his two baby daughters and his first wife? I promised myself that I would not dredge up the past and ruin the present with angry recriminations. I kept my thoughts to myself—but it was hard to reconcile the discrepancies. He knew how desperate our situation was. Grandma had thought about calling him several times to see about a little help, but in the end, she decided against it. She worried that if he knew, he would have had us removed from our mother. Even if Roxie and I had lived with him and had better economic conditions and some stability, my mother would have been stripped of her self-respect. After mom's breakdown, Grandma also realized that mom needed help emotionally and my dad could not provide that kind of support. On the other hand, I felt relieved that my brothers did not have to live the poor life that we had. There was no jealousy on my part. But I was so disappointed when I thought about what might have been a kinder, gentler lifestyle.

I forgive Dad for his abandonment and his denial of our very existence. It was the worst kind of benign neglect of small children. His own two boys had no idea Dad had other children. Still, I had to go on with my life. Obviously, he was too embarrassed to answer my simple questions about his courtship and marriage to my mother. He would not answer my questions about how they met, where they were married, or what made him fall in love with her. He could not even look me in the eye when I asked for these memories to cherish.

The only thing Dad disclosed that was new to me was his statement that my mom was never the same after Helen died. I already knew that the death of her baby girl and dad's womanizing were too much for her to handle. Her mental state was increasingly fragile. I know my dad married Mom because she was beautiful, social, and fun to be with. She had a warm and loving heart and people felt comfortable in her presence. During her marriage to him, he was overseas in the military. He served in Vietnam and in Korea. My mother loved children and became pregnant each of the three times he returned home. After Dad cheated on her, she would not accept the marriage bed again.

Katie was friendly and I was as cordial as I could possibly be. She was not sure what my mother had told me or what I remembered when I was living with Mom in a trailer near Massey Hill when her marriage to my dad ended. I always believed that my mother's first mental breakdown was due to my dad's extramarital affair with Katie combined with the tragic circumstances of baby Helen's death. Helen was buried in Fayetteville and I was born at Fort Bragg in May 1958. My dad was deployed to Korea right after I was born. My dad's sister brought mom and I to live with her in Ohio during Dad's deployment. Mom needed extra care and attention and she was grateful to my aunt for her help. When she was more recovered, my mom moved back to Fayetteville for the remainder of Dad's deployment. When he returned from Korea, they moved to Kentucky where Roxie was born almost two years later.

According to mom, Dad and Katie were having an affair when mom was pregnant with Roxie. Mom had suspected it for a while but it was confirmed when she saw them together at the mail box. After Roxie was born we took the train and moved back to Fayetteville. When I was about 4 and Roxie was 8 months I remember Katie coming to talk to my mother. I remember my mother being upset. Katie wanted to take us away with her, but my mom refused. I can still visualize that scene of the two women squaring off. My mother had custody and she was not permitting anyone to take us away.

My dad was the chief of police in Missouri near an outstanding veterinarian college. I had told him about my lifelong dream to be a veterinarian. I didn't go into the details of my career being sidelined by marital problems.

Dad never missed a step—he immediately invited us to move there so I could enroll in the college! He offered us a place to live in their downstairs apartment, too. It was a generous and amazing offer. He asked us to think about it and encouraged Larry to consider a career in law enforcement working with him. Dad drove us to see his office and he told Larry he could train him to become a licensed polygraph examiner. (I did not know that Larry had his own ideas about his future which he just did not share with me). Larry took the lead right away—telling my dad that we were very interested and grateful for this opportunity! I could not believe my ears. It was an important visit for a possible new beginning with my dad. We had a really good visit and everyone was on their best behavior, then it was time for us to take the long drive back to North Carolina for Larry to get back to work.

I asked Larry later that night about whether he was serious about moving. "Larry, are you sure you are willing to do this?" One more time he supported my dream and I became so excited about this new possibility to capture the dream! I thought because of what happened during our marriage that Larry realized compromise was not that difficult and he wanted to do the right thing. He told Dad and me that he was all for the plan to relocate to Missouri and launch two new careers. He said he needed a year to make house repairs, sell the house, and get his finances in order. Dad was so excited it made my heart sing.

The visit went so well and the outcome exceeded my expectations. We all began planning the move. Dad would be fixing up the apartment, Katie offered to babysit Little Larry while I was in school, Larry would be getting our financial affairs in order and preparing for the sale of our house, and I would continue working and saving as much money as I could. What else could I possibly ask for?

On the way back to North Carolina I could hardly stop smiling. I could not wait to tell Dr. Hill about the plan. He had said to me a hundred times, "You should have been a veterinarian, Linda." Now I had that chance and I knew inside my gut that I would be a good veterinarian! I was very excited as I told Dr. Hill my plan and he was very happy for me. He thought that this was an extraordinary gesture by my dad. Knowing a little bit about my history with Dad, he warned me that my Dad's wife would not really be happy with this idea. "She may agree—but she will make you miserable." The "other woman" would never be at ease with the daughters of the ex-wife! I started asking myself whether I could accept the situation if I was Katie. I thought Dr. Hill was probably right, but I did not want it to be true.

Dr. Hill was a father figure to me. He was usually direct and honest with me. He shared his thoughts and wisdom with me. I appreciated his forthright manner and words of caution about the role Katie might play in this new chapter of my life. But I wanted this to happen even if she made my life miserable for a while. I was willing again to do whatever it takes to realize my dream. Even Dr. Hill's nurse said, "Katie is not going to like it if she has to take care of your son while you go to school." Somehow I knew they were both right but I did not want to miss this opportunity. I wanted to make it real. I was childlike in my thinking: "Besides he didn't do a damn thing while I was growing up so I want him to make up the lost time!"

Dad was so excited in the months that followed. Katie was always cordial. Larry told my dad he looked forward to learning how to do polygraphs. Dad took me all over the city to meet his friends. He took me to the college. It was snowing and we were trudging to make the rounds. My dad was in pretty good shape at that time and it was fun to be doing something to make new memories in our relationship. We planned the transitions ahead. My husband was supportive and took care of Little Larry so that Dad and I could have time together. Dad went with me to meet the professors at the school. He bought my first semester textbooks and mailed them to me. I wanted to start studying before classes started, especially since I was slow at learning. Dad was generous with his time and money to help me get into college. I will always cherish that memory.

We came back home and returned to our jobs. I had left Dr. Hill's veterinary office to take a much higher paid position at the tire factory. We were so excited about the plan to move to Missouri. I stayed in touch with my dad and I was studying the books he sent me and saving my money. He came down for a visit and I took him to the plant where I worked. Larry, Dad, and I all talked about what it would be like when we moved, our new jobs, our apartment, and where Little Larry would attend school. We both planned to work right up to the last minute before the move. Larry told me not to worry about selling the house, that he had someone who would handle the sale of the house for us. I told him he should go ahead and sell before we moved.

Larry's Second Betrayal

That night when my dad was preparing to leave, everything suddenly changed. Out of left field, Larry dropped a bomb on me. He said, "You and Little Larry can move with your dad. I like my job and I want to make a business here. I do not want to move, but you can." I said, "Larry, why didn't you tell me during this entire last year? It is

263

my dream and I do not want to make another drastic change because you decided to break our agreement!" He said he knew that I would not want to do that, and I should go ahead and leave. There were so many questions and emotions that I did not know what to say or do. I was certainly glad that I had not quit my job yet at Kelly Springfield.

I felt like my whole world tumbled down. What should I do? Who should I talk to? My sisters were so busy with their own lives. They would listen but I am embarrassed. I felt like I had to make a good decision—especially now. I am a private person and always kept my business to myself. I knew it would upset my mother for me to move—but I knew my sisters would take care of her. I could return to Fayetteville when I finished school in Missouri. My sisters did not know the "dark side" of Larry and they would be so surprised. I knew my mom would be disappointed for me to lose my dream. I knew I could come back to Fayetteville and work as a veterinarian. I even had a photo taken of where I wanted to build my animal hospital when I graduated. I had told me cousins in Fayetteville, Michigan, and Massachusetts that they should say I was leaving! How embarrassing this was for me. No one would ever believe anything I said again.

On the other hand, I realized that I did not want to give up my marriage. I did not really want to go by myself. I talked to Larry again and asked why he did not tell me sooner. I would not have planned this change and put my dad through all of the hassle and expense of preparing for us to move. "I thought we were going together!" He had business plans all along that he never discussed with me. I began to see that he was not interested in "us" leaving—he was interested in "me and Little Larry" leaving. I did not want to end my marriage and I realized that I would be so far away from my family and friends. In all honesty—my dad was a new person in my life. I did not know what it would be like living there with Dad and Katie and my little boy. I was going crazy with information overload—and I wanted to make a right decision this time.

The next day I called my dad and told him that Larry had decided not to move and that I did not want to leave without him. Dad tried to talk me out of my decision. He reminded me of all the plans we made, and the long-term benefits of this education. I told dad I had given it careful thought and felt it was not a good idea to leave him again. Later, I told Larry what I had said to my father and he was shocked that I was not leaving. He never told me his real feelings. He never did.

His habit of surprises and betrayals continued through the rest of our marriage. He had betrayed me with his promises of a college education six years ago. Now he was betraying me again. He always took me to the edge of the cliff where I had to jump and take my chances or stay with him. This time I stayed.

He acted like nothing had happened. He told me to buy all new furniture—and I did. He brought home a new gray Camaro for me—which I loved. The payments were $350 a month and I earned more than enough at Kelly Springfield to keep my payments current. I was still reeling from his secret plans to quit his job and open more businesses. Larry was an entrepreneur and I never realized it until that moment. He operated in his own business world and no one else was part of his decision making. He was a one-man show.

I continued to feel terrible about the impact of Larry's sudden change of plans. It was a terrible insult to my dad and I hoped he understood that I was not part of that betrayal of his generous offer of help. I called to talk with him and learned that he and Katie had moved to Fort Meyers, Florida. The unexpected drama with Larry had damaged the relationship I now had with my dad. I really felt embarrassed and ashamed.

I have said many times that I am a very slow learner. But learning my lessons about Larry was almost impossible. I kept doing the same thing while expecting different results. My plans and his promises were broken the first time when Little Larry was born. Why on earth did I think it would be different with the second plan to move to Missouri? What was I thinking?

I did my best to put my disappointment aside and return to my normal life in Fayetteville. I loved my job as a manager and was earning excellent money. I was happy being with my family, taking care of Little Larry, and being a good wife. But Larry's old habits quickly returned. We were back in the "party" spotlight. We lived in a big home, all the amenities, three pool tables, and room for lots of parties and ostentatious living. Larry loved being the center of attention and to be perceived as the big successful businessman. It also seemed that our relationship had matured. We got along great and we each enjoyed the independence of doing the things we loved to do. Life was good.

I told Larry that if we were going to have another baby, we should do it soon because Little Larry was in the first grade. I only wanted two children. I had gotten used to Larry's deceptions and exaggerations but I loved him and was not interested in a divorce. We were happy and contented. It seemed like the next natural progression to finish having our family before we were too old. Larry had not committed one way or the other about having a second child. I was pregnant within two months.

When I told Larry—his behavior toward me immediately changed. He was distant, started staying away from home, and started telling obvious lies. I had no idea he would respond like this a second time! I ignored his response and felt that he would accept the pregnancy when he got used to the idea. I told him I would have a tubal ligation after this pregnancy and it would be our last. I tried to tell him that I was getting older and that he should be happy even though we did not plan it. I was still holding it against him that he had broken his promise to let me finish my schooling. But I did not dwell on it.

He had plenty of money so that was not the issue. One night I sat him down and tried to talk to him about why he was so upset. His response was a repeat of the last pregnancy. "I do not want children, I never wanted children. I told you when we married that I did not want children. Linda, you chose to get pregnant knowing how I felt!" I was still convinced he would change his mind just as he had with Little Larry when he got bigger and started school. I thought it would be the same way again and he would be okay. I was dead wrong.

He had his mind made up and was not about to change it. He gave me an ultimatum: get an abortion or get out. I was stunned into silence. I did not believe in abortion and he was well aware of that fact. Our intimacy and relationship ended that night.

Abortion was not an option. We had not discussed any options but I could not wait to get divorced. I knew that I would be alone with my two children and that I made enough money to take care of us. I did not even have to think twice about it. Our marriage was over. He agreed to put the house up for sale, and I moved into the guest room. Larry engaged in a dozen more tricks and deceptions along the way to a final divorce decree. He proved he could not be trusted to keep his word—why did I think it would be any different now?

I bought a house that was just being built. I loved the house. I sketched out the landscape I wanted and decorated the inside of the house to be a good home for me and my two children. I continued to focus on my job and moving up the career ladder. But I was bitter about the betrayals of a man who I loved so much for so long. I realize his colors were there all the time, I just did not want to acknowledge them. I thought I could change him. I thought if he loved me he would want what I wanted. Perhaps the Ray Steven's song verse is true, "There are none so blind as those who will not see."

Life with Jose
Marriage on the Rebound

I was so busy working long hours that I had very little time to buy groceries or cook meals. I often took Little Larry to a cafeteria style place called K & W. He was a picky eater and he found things that he liked there. Everything with my husband happened so fast that I did not even have time to cry. I was still so upset with the way Larry tried to cheat me. He was really angry because I would not sign the papers for him to sell the house. He moved out and stayed with one of his friends. As a manager, it was important that I kept my personal business to myself at Kelly Springfield. Unfortunately, Larry worked there, too. He apparently told people negative things about me and our marriage. The more I heard from others, the more determined I was to move on and start another life. I am sure he was relieved to be free again. We had tried but he could not seem to muster the character to meet me halfway in repairing the damage in our marriage. I told him I would sign the house if he made the legal arrangements and told me the truth. The house belonged to his parents before we bought it. I contributed half of the improvements and house payments and taxes after we assumed title. It was the principle of the way he handled the transaction with me and his life-long effort to manipulate people to his financial advantage—let ethics be damned!

One of Larry's friends was a body builder named Jose. One evening Jose and his girlfriend stopped by the house. I had seen him with Larry a few times because they were friends and went to the gym. Several of our old friends stopped by this final month of our residency in the house we bought together. Jose and his gorgeous blond girlfriend stopped by most frequently. They said that Larry had told them what had happened. I told them I was fine. I was happy about the baby I was expecting and that I planned to take care of my kids on my own. The new house would be finished in November before the baby was expected in January. If it wasn't ready for occupancy, I planned to stay with my mother. Felton was in jail at the time so I felt comfortable being at Mom's. Gail and Carol had gotten married and lived nearby. I was working all the time and would work as long possible.

My job required focus. I had ten problems when I started in the mornings and ten new problems by the end of the day. I was in a 24-hour continuous observation mode. I loved the job and proving to the men that a woman can manage sixty employees in a twelve-hour shift—and never cry. Although I cussed under my breath a lot, I firmly corrected problems and smiled when the employee learned the procedure. Good Year Corporate insisted that managers be master trainers. I worked in several departments in the plant with the exception of the cleanest part of the plant where the tire was created. Most of the employees stay in their area of expertise. Despite the ups and downs, I was respected and gave respect to the employees.

Most of the people Larry worked with were in the tire build area. They had the only air-conditioning in the plant—the cleanest environment—and I never worked there. I am sure Larry took the simplest job he could take. He was not lazy but did the minimum to get by at the plant. He was industrious in his other ventures to make money. He sold jewelry and a variety of cars, coins, and boats. He always had money to loan with a significant pay back. I never knew Larry to have less than $500 in his pocket. I was so surprised that no one robbed him because everyone knew he carried money. If anyone needed extra cash he loaned them money with hefty interest rates. If you did not repay him on time he would not loan to you again. He would also loan money for gambling debts. He also ran a "lottery" pool based on employees' paycheck numbers. He was also an agent/promoter for musical groups and ran multiple businesses. He was an entrepreneur on multiple fronts.

The next time Jose and his girlfriend came over they asked me to have dinner at Red Lobster that weekend. They came by to check on me several times and invited me to dinner. Jose's girlfriend was a body builder also and a very sweet girl but I could tell they were more friends than lovers. I had known Jose only through Larry and they worked out at the gym together. I agreed to meet Jose and his girlfriend for dinner at the Red Lobster. His girlfriend did not show up because she was sick—or so he said. I was hungry and not interested in him anyway so we had dinner. Ironically, I think Jose was motivated to spend time with me because of Larry's negligence about fatherhood. Jose loved kids and came to the middle schools at the request of teachers to teach children about life and customs in a different country. Jose was from the Dominican Republic and was excelling in competitions as a body builder. Kids loved to look at his muscles and let Jose lift them up using one arm—sometimes two children at a time. You could understand his accent and he was very well spoken. Teachers called him often. He also showed nude at art classes when teachers needed nude models.

At dinner with Jose, I do not remember much about the conversation but he made it clear that he and the girls he dated were not serious relationships. He must have been shocked that I did not respond or get excited just because he was "available." I really was not interested in him in any way. I had already accepted that I was going to be a single mom with a small child at home on one on the way. Maybe it was because I was so contented taking care of myself and my children. I did not respond to his opportunity and I ended my dinner pleasantly and that was it.

The next weekend I took Mom and Larry to a swimming pool we went to every year. While I was there Jose showed up. I did not invite him or think anything about it. I just wanted some sun and to play in the water with Little Larry. It was obvious that I had started to show with Nathan but it did not bother me and I was not embarrassed. He came over and sat down right beside us. Of course, there were so many women of all ages and shapes who pointed at Jose with admiration. He acted like his appearance at the pool was unplanned—but I knew that was too coincidental. He had never been there before. Women were crazy about him.

For whatever reasons, I simply was not attracted to him. He wore the tiniest bathing suit possible. Everyone was speechless. I almost had to laugh! I recognized that he had a great physique, but there was nothing there intellectually that made him an attractive choice as a mate. He was a cook by trade and made a decent living. His Spanish accent was the best thing about his voice. He laughed and told me I should go with him to the Dominican Republic. I said "No, thank you, I do not like flying and I do not want to leave my children." He had every woman at the pool, including my mother, staring at him. His body was just not enough to have gotten my attention. You could tell that Jose was accustomed to being a public spectacle and he enjoyed it. As for me, I continued to let my pregnancy show. Since all of his friends were body builders, you would certainly think that my obvious pregnancy at four months would send him away!

I got ready to leave and he asked me to go to dinner again. I said, "No, thank you, I am going in early and I am eating with my mom. See you, Jose." I am sure he was not used to women turning him down but I was not looking for a relationship of any kind. I was pregnant and I still loved Larry. I was just sick about what Larry said about our baby and sick of men in general. When we left the pool, my Mom went on and on about Jose. I told her I don't like that type. I expected to be alone, divorced with two kids. "That is okay. I am fine." She looked at me quizzically and I'm sure she thought, *what is wrong with my daughter?*

Jose began showing up my gym which he never attended. He only worked out at Gold's Gym. He still knew several people at my gym who greeted him. I continued to work out as if he was not there. He asked me about my dogs. "What are you are going to do with your dogs?" I said "I have to leave them at Larry's house until my house is finished. I have to go sign the escrow papers sometime this week, as Larry sold it." Jose said, "I love dogs. I have a big backyard and I will take care of them until your house is built. " I said, "I think they will be fine over there or I will board them for a while."

Over the next two weeks I went over to take care of the dogs and finally signed the papers for the house. After all expenses, there was only $10,000 and the undeveloped land next to the house. Larry was not so smart trying to be his own lawyer. My lawyer had written the settlement papers stating that I would get $10,000 for my interest in the property and Larry would get the rest, regardless of the sum. Well, by the time he tried to cheat me and sell the house I received the $10,000 but Larry only got the land next door.

As I was leaving Larry said, "I heard you are going out with Jose." I said, "He just shows up sometimes where I am." Larry said, "Yeah right. I wouldn't worry about it because he can see anyone he wants, why would he want you and pregnant?" It took all my restraint to not slap him. I said "Say that again." He repeated it and I said "Okay!" and smiled. I never thought of Larry as being vindictive but I thought he had guts to say that. I could not believe his blatant insult and thought a lot about his whole attitude. Larry must really be sickened by the appearance of the pregnant female form.

My mother was pensive and quiet when we were doing laundry. Finally, she mentioned that she had talked to Larry. I asked what they talked about. (He knew how protective I am of my mother.) Mom said, "I told him if he wants to save his marriage he better do something because that guy is after you." I said, "Mom I am not interested in him. I am pregnant and will get bigger. He is not interested in one woman and I am not going to share a man! I expect to be taking care of me and my kids. He might take care of my dogs, though!" She had the strangest look on her face.

I went over at my usual time to take care of my dogs and Jose pulled up. I said, "Don't you have a job? You keep being in places 'coincidentally." He said he came out there with Larry earlier. I just kept busy cleaning outside and combing their hair. Collies have to be combed or their hair will get thick and tangled. He said, "You should see my yard and you won't have to do this. I will take care of this for you." I said, "Jose, I can take care of myself but thank you." He asked me if he could take the dogs to the park off of Highway 301. I said, "You want to take my dogs to the park?" He said, "Yes that will be fun!" I told him I used to do that with Larry or his sister. He asked, "When will you be off work?" I told him and we made arrangements to meet with the dogs. He said, "Linda, Larry said I could ask you out and he did not care." I asked, "You asked him if he minds if you ask me out?" He said, "Yes and he said your marriage is over. I matter-of-factly replied, "I do not need his permission to do anything." He said,"I know, but because Larry and I were friends and I did not want to look like I was going behind his back." I said, "We are just going to the creek and take the dogs." He said, "You can sit down while I play with the dogs." Reluctantly and annoyed with the discussion, I said "Okay."

The next week Jose pursued me relentlessly. The more I thought about it I decided I would try dating Jose. Larry must think that being pregnant looks gross. You would think when you are creating your husband's child it would create more love and closeness. I was so wrong. I lost so much respect for Larry because he simply did not want children nor appreciate the miracle of birth!

The next two times he called me I was uncomfortable and I told him I was busy. I knew there was definitely a feeling developing between the both of us called lust and I knew he felt the same way. Love was not in the same league. Previously, there was no attraction to him on my part. I was mystified and did not realize that he had skillfully seduced me and I didn't even know it!

I had read about the seductions, rapes, and perverted people. I thought most were fiction and this was the first seduction that I had experienced. *Think about it with your brain, Linda, your brain.*

Jose asked me to go out dancing. It had been a long time since I had been dancing and did not know what it would feel like being six months pregnant on a dance floor. I went upstairs at work to talk to the only other female manager in the plant. She knew who Jose was and she wanted to know everything that was going on. She told me that Larry had told everyone that the baby was not his. I was so mad and told her that Larry was a liar. I was sure by that time things for Larry were not going as well as he thought.

Jose and I had been seen together and I think they assumed because of the timing—that Larry's lies might be true. For that reason I could understand the gossip. It was rare for someone, especially like Jose, to date and take care of the dogs and be in a platonic relationship! I was stunned that Larry would tell a lie that would affect my work. He followed up with another lie, telling everyone my baby could not have been his kid because after Little Larry was born he had a vasectomy! The lies did not seem to bother Jose. He was fine with the rumor mill. It was so soon to be dating and unusual to date a pregnant woman. Larry thought of me as fat and unattractive—he did not want any part of it! I made up my mind to ignore the lies and enjoy my pregnancy.

Jose was very considerate of the pregnancy and spent as much time as possible with me. Rather quickly Larry realized Jose was spending so much time with me, taking me dancing and swimming. He tried to tell me Jose sees several women at one time; I said "Really?" Larry told everyone that Jose was moving from woman to woman because he could. I still worked my regular schedule.

I did not feel very desirable but Jose did not treat me as if I wasn't. He was so very different. He was very careful about his diet and had given me cantaloupes when I went over to see the dogs. On that visit, I had forgotten that I was pregnant and thought *Larry who?*

He made me dinner and asked me to stop going back to work. "They will let you off until six months after you have the baby." I didn't even consider that. He said we should get married before the baby is born and I reminded him that was not possible. Larry and I were not legally divorced and this baby should have the father's name. I simply needed to think and said, "I need to go back to Mom's house because she will be worried." He asked me again to let him take care of me. Miraculously, I did not feel ugly and pregnant anymore.

I was still bothered by all of Larry's lies. Little Larry and I went over to Jose's to check on my dogs. Larry wanted to pick up Little Larry and I told him that I needed to talk to him. I wanted to ask him why he was telling those lies. It did not look good with my management position, especially the lie about vasectomy! He changed the subject without answering me.

The other female manager was the only person at work who I felt I could talk with candidly. We were told not to get close with people you have to manage so I did not. She did not work for me and never would because we had different departments. We shared a lot and I cherished her friendship and still miss her friendship. Are there things I told her and had forgotten? Of course I am not proud of what happened but it is the truth.

Jose took me dancing and he was not embarrassed and did not explain that I did not have his baby. He basically ignored gossip. He was not embarrassed to take me to the gym. All of his friends and many women he had dated were there at the gym, too. We danced often, went to the beach and gym. He was never embarrassed and most of his friends knew I was pregnant when we dated. Jose kept my dogs and some of his stuff at his house until I moved in. My house was finished in November 1983. Jose asked me to marry him again before my baby was born. I told him "No."

Jose did not have children and I did not want any more. I also thought that after he saw the continuous demands of being a parent he would change his mind. I also knew his reputation of having lots of different women on his arm. I never fell in love with Jose like I loved Larry but I was not good enough for Larry. I did not want José's kids. I only wanted two kids. I loved Larry so it was natural that I wanted my sons to be his children.

Women always left notes on Jose's car, even when I was with him! I overheard two girls talking in the bathroom at Chi Chi's Restaurant. They did not see me in there or maybe they did. One girl said, "Can you believe who he is dating? He can do better than that!" I just washed my hands, smiled, and left. Jose continued to ask me to marry him and I told him I would when Nathan was six months old and if he still wanted to. I am sure it was lust that kept me interested and it gave me enough time to focus on my goal of being the first female plant manager in Goodyear! I expected him to be gone and I would be fine without him.

After Nathan was born we went to New York and met all of Jose's family before we were married. Jose went to schools and the Boys Gym. He talked to kids about fitness and body building and described customs in his country. I saw him at Little Larry's school class. I was impressed the way he handled the kids. He was like a hero to them. When Nathan was walking we planned a trip to the Dominican Republic. My sister Gail agreed to take care of the kids while we took the trip. We stayed at the resort and visited his sister on one side of the island and his father and step-mother on the other side. His mother had died when he was born.

I was not prepared for the poverty there. They did not seem to be bothered by the standard of living. The exception was a trip we took driving up a mountain. The people were homeless on the road, beggars. They were begging for anything—food, money, handouts of any kind. Some were developmentally disabled or seriously handicapped. The little children were walking around naked—with no parents in sight. They were dirty and hungry.

Jose chose a buggy and horses to ride in, but I refused. Not because I was too good for a buggy but because those horses were emaciated and had all kinds of flies on them. Almost all the dogs had mange and I could smell disease on them. We slept in a house that had no glass windows, just an open area. We slept with a thin net cover that prevented mosquitoes from biting us. I did not eat anything unless I opened it like a banana! I lost five pounds in one week! Jose was not ashamed of his country; it was the homeland he was born to and lived there until he was a teenager.

His older brother grew up and moved to New York. When he could afford it, he returned to the island and took Jose back to the United States to live with him. I asked Jose why he moved to North Carolina and left his own country. He never told me until after I visited his country. I asked him why he left New York and moved to North Carolina. He said his brother was a drug dealer. He was so disappointed that his brother was into drugs. Jose found out what his brother was doing so he disappeared. He got a job learning to cook at a restaurant owned by a Mexican family. The owner had all daughters about the same age as Jose and was fond of Jose and enjoyed having a male around. The family supported him until he learned enough English and graduated high school. I spoke to those girls many times. They owned the most popular Mexican restaurant in Fayetteville, North Carolina. I had gone there often with Jose to have their salsa and meet the family, his adopted family. They loved him very much and considered him part of their family. I am not sure if they tried to talk him out of a marriage or if they thought I had his child.

After leaving New York, Jose never saw his brother again. I never knew him to curse, steal, or drink but he loved women and they loved him. I think because I did not love him it was a good relationship and one of convenience. Because I loved Larry and he hurt me deeply— it did feel good to me that I could prove him wrong about Jose's affection for me. I am not sure why Jose wanted to marry me with two kids.

I tried to learn Spanish before I went to the Dominican Republic. I am not sure why it was so hard but I did not grasp the language as much as I thought I would. I had heard it was easy. They did not speak English and I could not speak Spanish. I could understand more if they slowed down. The parents who raised him were considered "wealthy" in comparison to everyone else. Jose called them mom and dad. He did not complain but he did say that his parents did not treat his older sister and brother like their "real" kids. Jose and his older siblings were born to a different mother. Thus, they were not allowed the same amount of food, clothes, or material things. They also had to work and their half-brothers and sisters did not have to.

At the resort it was a totally different story. He is the one who scheduled our trips and arranged everything that we did there. I was still a size eight after Nathan was born. It did not take me more than three weeks to get back in shape. We went to the gym there frequently. Jose was very knowledgeable about health and fitness. The environment, music, dancing, and romance was like a dream. He showed me everything he could possibly arrange in the time we had there—including the main zoo. The only comment that his family shared with me was that they expected me to be blond! I asked Jose to explain to them that my ancestors were in America long before the blonde people came. I had already explained how important the Indian blood was to me. His family looked very much like Jose. His stepmother sold cakes and his dad was a photographer and both worked out of their home.

Jose was kind and good with my sons. When Nathan was six months old, Jose took him everywhere to show him off. He treated Nathan and Larry as if they were his own children. I never heard him say in public that these were not his children. He just acted as if they were. I deeply appreciated that. Despite his earlier accusations, Larry knew that Nathan was his son without a doubt. However, Larry was not prepared to take care of an infant by himself. He spent time with Little Larry, but did not take Nathan for visits or spend much time with him. Larry picked up Little Larry sometime when he was in the first and second grades. As he got a little older, Larry spent more time with him. Nathan was too small but Larry did pay child support, $300 a month for his boys.

Jose continued to work as a cook and I still worked at Kelly Springfield. Jose insisted he still wanted to get married and invited several of his family members to come from New York. We were married on the Rose Garden at Fayetteville Technical Community College. I was not in love the way I should have been to remarry. I felt like our marriage was a sham. We got along well and he was good to me and the boys. But there were incidents that I recognized later as his infidelity. My mom had told me that she thought Jose was cheating on me. Later, others also told me that they saw Nathan with Jose visiting a girl at Belk's. I just did not "feel" the way about Jose that I should have.

After hearing the rumors, I told Jose that I would end the marriage immediately if I caught him cheating and that infidelity was the point of no return. We had often gone to Body Building Competitions and Jose was doing very well. I had to understand about how the women acted. After all, he had a magnificent body and excited a lot of women. During the first year of our marriage, Jose treated me with respect and consideration. Maybe I thought ignorance was bliss but I was not interested in "catching him in the act" of cheating. We had a stable marriage for five years. I hired a lady to clean house once a week and Jose took care of the kids at night, cooked for them, and continued his job at the family restaurant.

Jose knew everyone in the family and they all respected me as Jose's wife. I remember the men did not like always him and several of the wives had come to borrow some "sugar" he said. Why did I think that that was ludicrous? I am not naïve. My best friend, Linda Roney, came to a New Year's Eve Party with us. Afterward, she told me that Jose had "kissed her a little too much" and she wanted me to know. With her assistance I decided to bug my telephone to see what was going on when I was not around.

Kelly Springfield started hiring again and I tried to discourage Jose from applying. I told him building tires would affect his "body building" competition. He thought it would make it better. He just did not understand how long and hard the hours were and that it was not the same as lifting weights in an air conditioned gym full of mirrors and admirers. He eventually started working at Kelly Springfield, too. I was fully committed to become the first female plant manager in the Goodyear system. I worked hard and took every opportunity for new assignments and additional work. I moved throughout the plant wherever they needed me. They even sent me to Ohio to qualify for a higher management job.

Jose knew that I did not want any more children. About fifteen months after we were married I had to have cervical surgery that required the removal of most of my cervix. The doctors advised me that I would not be able to carry a child to full term. That was fine with me because I did not want any more children. I was not thinking about him. Again, I was selfish in our marriage as for me it was a convenience instead of love. It had already lasted longer than I thought it would.

Jose had a second job selling cars at a dealership. We had gone to several body building shows where he competed. The shows were in other towns and some required an overnight stay. Our relationship was consistent throughout our marriage. I never noticed a change in his demeanor toward me. He always wanted to make sure I was there when he competed and won. He won "Mr. East Coast" and did very well in competitions until he actually started building tires. I was aware that he was using steroids almost immediately after he started at Kelly Springfield. That was the first time we had a major disagreement. I knew steroids changed your personality, caused liver problems and tumors, and had multiple negative side effects. Jose also read about the dangers of steroid usage and was well aware of the risks involved. He was in denial and insisted it was safe and a good way to buff up. I was not interested in steroids and I did not want to be too muscular. I supported him at his competitions and I was sure he would do well. Although he started taking steroids he did not drink alcohol. I still had a problem accepting his usage of steroids. After about six months, I began to notice a change in his personality—and I did not like what I saw.

I researched and read about side effects that occurred among body builders using steroids. The trade magazines did not discuss the side effects. The more I read about it the more I tried to talk Jose out of it. The tumors and liver problems were scary. The steroids that he took started changing his personality. He started cursing. He developed a short temper. He was easily agitated. He was not willing to stop steroids despite knowing that I hated it.

Larry opened a new convenience store right across the street from my house. Of all the locations he could have chosen, he was opening a new business right next door to my home! Every time I came home or left home—I had to see his business. He had already stopped working at Kelly Springfield and opened up several jewelry and convenience stores in Fayetteville. I thought Larry would be married to a bimbo by now.

One day I received a call to meet a friend of mine who lived nearby. He and his wife had been at several parties with other employees of Kelly Springfield. I thought he needed some advice or had another problem at work. I had told him I would meet there at the Pizza Hut for lunch. He and his wife lived in a trailer right behind the restaurant where Jose worked. They were much younger than I was and had no children. He came to meet me by himself. I used to be his manager and they had been to my house before. He started off with a blast! He said, "Jose is seeing my wife." He said they had been secretly meeting each other since Jose's birthday party. He said, "I think that you and I should have sex." I looked at him and said "Hell no!" He said, "What is the matter, I am not good enough for you?" I was shocked and started laughing … did I just hear this? Is the world going crazy? I challenged him with, "When I get home in the morning from third shift will you come home with me and tell me this right in front of him? You put your car in my garage so he does not see it. When he comes in from work, you tell him this. I want to see his face."

Surprisingly, he showed up early, parked in the garage, and confronted Jose face to face. Jose did not deny it. I told Jose to leave and to not come back. He knew me well enough that adultery, combined with the steroid usage was the end of the marriage. The sad part was that Jose was the only "father figure" Nathan had known since birth. Larry never developed a relationship with Nathan the way he should have. He just deferred to Jose. In every way except genetically, Jose had been a good father to Nathan.

There must have been other girls but I was so busy working I did not have time to find out what he was doing. Jose knew that I was serious and that there was no chance of reconciliation. It was the perfect storm for ending a good but loveless marriage. Nathan was confused and devastated. He was closer to Jose than Little Larry but he knew his mother was not happy. Jose tried to gain visitation rights during the divorce. He spent a lot of money trying to make sure he could keep Nathan in his life. Because he was not Nathan's biological father the court denied his request. Because of his lifestyle in the last year I was adamant that Nathan not be under Jose's influence in any way. Nathan was almost five years old by that time. Jose still tried to periodically stay in contact with Nathan up until high school. When I explained to Nathan what Jose had done, he made the decision and agreed with me.

Later, my friends at Kelly Springfield told me Jose married a girl from the Dominican Republic and had three children. I knew he was probably a good dad but I doubted that he stopped cheating. Twenty years later, Jose still works at Kelly Springfield Tires. The pay and benefits make it hard to give up. My sister saw him throughout the years. She said he no longer looks fit and handsome as he did when we were married. I know firsthand that working in a factory building tires takes a heavy toll. Hard labor in a factory does not build the body up—it tears it down.

An Indian Prayer

O'Great Spirit,
Whose voice I hear in the winds,
And whose breath gives life to all the world,
Hear me! I am small and weak; I need your strength
and wisdom.
Let Me Walk In beauty, and make my eyes
Ever behold the red and purple sunset.
Make My Hands respect the things you have
Made and my ears sharp to hear your voice.
Make Me Wise So that I may understand the
Things you have taught my people.
Let Me Learn the lesson you have hidden
In every leaf and rock.
I Seek Strength, not to be greater than my
Brother, but the fight my greatest
Enemy-myself.
Make Me Always Ready to come to you with
Clean hands and straight eyes.
So When Life Fades, as the fading sunset,
My spirit may come to you
Without shame.
From "Red Cloud Indian School"

Life with Jeff

This Indian Prayer from the Red Cloud Indian School has special meaning to me. I am moved by the words of Indian prayers in general. The music of the Indian people has a mystical effect on me. When I hear the instruments being played at powwows I am overcome by emotion. I have a visceral reaction to the lyrical instruments and beating of the drums. I feel as if I am part of the earth and the heavens at the same time—a feeling of peace and serenity washes over me.

My husband is an intensely private man when it comes to sharing his personal life with others and he will not appreciate my sharing these thoughts openly. I had the same cosmic connection when I met Jeff, when we fell in love, and when we created our children. Love in our relationship is powerful and often unspoken. Our love is communicated through our actions as much as through our words. We are joined as one soul, I think. We have shared the best and the worst of times with equal humility and awe. Finding your soul mate on earth is a precious gift from God.

Jeff's wisdom and support made some of the best things in my life possible. He encouraged me to stop working at Kelly Springfield Tire Factory, and come home to raise our three daughters. This was a luxury I did not have when my sons were born. As soon as our girls were old enough to start school, he encouraged me to return to college and pursue my interests in art and art history. When it was the opportune time to pursue a master's degree and teaching credentials, Jeff vigorously championed me. He put actions behind his words and that has made all the difference in the woman I have become.

Jeff listened and shared my dreams and he took the actions necessary to help me realize them. He didn't just give me lip service! Ironically, I spent the first thirty years of my life fighting my situation and begging my spouses to support my dreams of college. I no longer trusted men to honor their promises. I was jaded and thought men were deceitful and selfish. Oddly, I felt unsuccessful until I had finished college.

After we married and got our daughters all in school, by 2005 I had my master's degree with honors! I was hired at North Myrtle

Beach High School to teach art history, contingent upon obtaining my teaching credentials within one year. Jeff's support and sacrifices and my hard work and self-discipline paid off. I was a college graduate—with honors!

How does that happen to a woman like me who grew up in poverty, domestic violence, and divorces? I had survived two failed marriages, mothered five children, suffered two miscarriages, and brought my mentally ill mother into our home and took care of her. With my family's help we cared for her at home until she died of lung cancer six years later. Without Jeff's encouragement, intellect, and planning, none of the good stuff dreams are made of would be mine! Now here I am wearing a cap and gown dancing down the aisle while the band plays "Pomp and Circumstance"!

For the first time in my life I was absent that feeling of being a "loser." My world was almost perfect! I had a wonderful marriage, five healthy, beautiful children, and the job of my dreams. I was so proud that my mother lived to share that wonderful experience with me. She was so proud of me and I will never forget her smiling face at my graduation.

Sadly, my mother passed away the following October in 2006. She lost her battle against lung cancer after a lifetime of smoking and factory work. I am so grateful that Jeff supported her and was so kind to her during all those years living with us. Despite shortages of money, time, and room—there was no shortage of love in our house. Thankfully, having a new job that I loved helped me keep my mind occupied after her death.

I had a strong respect for my husband long before my stroke and aneurysm. I admired his intellect and character. Jeff was an avid reader—devouring several books a week. Not your stereotypical bookworm, he was fun, witty, and had a commanding presence. During our twenty-two year marriage he has consistently shown his strength of character. He takes pride in being a good husband, father, and son. He is respectful toward our respective families and to people in general.

Reviewing my life while writing this, I marvel that I can finally appreciate that Jeff and my two sons are such fine men. They demonstrated their courage and love in our darkest hour and in all the months that followed. They taught me that there are decent, respectable loving men in the world who have no ulterior motives. These three men love me and my children unconditionally and always try their best to do the right thing. Although I am prejudiced—their character is impeccable, they are bright, handsome, and mine! My daughters will have to search far and wide to find such good men for husbands. I have been richly blessed.

I thought I did have a wonderful life before I met Jeff. I was making good money, raising my boys alone, paying my bills on time, and enjoying myself. I had no idea that Jeff was possible and that God had a plan for me that I never dreamed of. By His grace, I am blessed with a "love story" that would fill another book.

Reflections on My First Two Marriages

Writing this has forced me to revisit and re-evaluate my life. I could have made better decisions, and exercised more wisdom, even after the brain damage. I liked to think that I knew what was best for me and opinions of others were not paramount in making decisions. Even as I aged, I thought I was smarter at figuring things out and stubbornly clung to character traits that no longer served me well. Instead of getting smarter I realized there are things about myself that I do not like. I realize that others suffered as much as I did, that many decisions I made were based on selfishness, and I am embarrassed about many things I did and said. Knowing that I have a traumatic brain injury does not excuse things I've done and said since that fateful day in the spring of 2007.

When my sons were ages 6 and zero I divorced their father. I believe we married for the wrong reasons. In retrospect, it was a business plan rather than a marriage plan. Years later, we did fall in love but our dreams and aspirations were on two separate paths. He never wanted children. I hope he recognizes today that Larry and Nathan are the best part of his life and his true legacy. We both tried to make the marriage work, but it was too little, too late. I know now that God doesn't make mistakes, I just didn't listen to His plans.

When I met and married Jose, I wasn't listening to God then, either. Jose was by far one of the worst decisions of my life. I married him for the wrong reasons and we both suffered the consequences.

My decisions were based on getting revenge against my ex-husband and lust for a body builder, not love. That memory of my attitude and behavior is humiliating to me but I accept my part in it.

Meeting Jeff

When I met Jeff, I was out dancing at a club in Fayetteville. My youngest sister, Carol, loved dancing and going to the clubs. As her oldest sister, I wanted to take her to more upscale clubs where she could socialize and dance. (Soon after this, Carol married a man named Eddie Guyton who worked at the tire factory for many years before I did. They have been together all these years and have a good marriage and beautiful family. They own a beautiful home in Hope Mills. Their daughter has beautiful red hair and stands out in a crowd. Carol works as a teacher and loves working in special education).

Jeff was a non-commissioned officer, a staff sergeant in the Army Special Forces. He had spent years at Fort Lewis, Washington, in an Army Ranger battalion, then changed station to the 82nd Airborne Division, and finally ended up in Special Forces. He was stationed at Fort Bragg and had just returned from field duty when we met that night. He had a buddy who needed to meet a date at the club. Jeff drove him there and sat in a booth reading, according to my sister. It just so happened to be the same night I took Carol there. Carol and I had a good time there dancing and socializing. We were at Syd's, a very popular bar with several bouncers. After I sat down Jeff came over to our table and introduced himself. He was attractive to me and vice versa. I thought he had Native American facial characteristics and asked him about his background. He said his paternal great-great-grandmother was American Indian. He was comfortable with himself and confident.

He loved books and so did I. I was very interested in him but hoped he wouldn't call me after I found out he was eight years younger than I was. I told him that I was divorced and had two young sons. I did not want to become involved with anyone under false pretensions. We danced and talked. I was impressed with his wit and knowledge. He was quite different than other men I met in the nightclub scene. Despite living near a military base all my life, I had never dated anyone from Fort Bragg. I had dated several military men in Valdosta, Georgia, when I was in the Air Force.

We were smitten with each other. My best girlfriend was stationed in Georgia, an Army captain attending the Army's Advanced Course. I was immediately anxious to call her and ask questions about the Army. I knew nothing about his military job and he did not talk much about what he did and changed the subject. We talked throughout the evening. She thought that was so weird that someone would come to a club and read a book! He said he walked behind me after I came back to my table from the ladies' room. I was dressed in black and he later told me he liked my shape and the way I walked. (Of course he was just out of the field so that probably had something to do with it!)

I was the designated driver for Carol that night and only had a few drinks. After Jeff sat down at our table, she danced more than I did after that. Jeff and I were more interested in talking than dancing. I gave him my phone number and wondered if I would hear from him again. I also wondered if I even wanted him to call.

Jeff did begin calling and we dated several times before I introduced him to my sons. The next time he came over he rode a motorcycle and my boys thought Jeff was really cool on a bike! We did not have cell phones 25 years ago so it was easier to avoid phone calls. The last thing I wanted was to get into a serious relationship. He called me several times and I turned him down. I actually had other plans but I was also reluctant to date a man younger than I was. Jeff was serious and mature compared to other men his age. I did try to talk him out of dating because I was working long hours, raising my sons, and had little free time to socialize. Jeff found out that my divorce from Jose was not final and was not happy about that fact. Although Jose was not Nathan's biological father, he had raised Nathan from birth and actually sought weekly visitation rights in our divorce settlement. Our marriage was over and I did not think it was in Nathan's best interest to be influenced by a man I considered to be of poor character.

On our first date, Jeff took me to the Kyoto's Japanese Restaurant. The chefs prepare the food teppanyaki-style at the table. We still go there to celebrate special times together. In the South, dressing for dinner is the norm. Jeff was from the casual California coast. He wore jeans, a sweater, and great snakeskin boots. He was so tall, dark, and handsome. He looked great but apologized after he saw that I wore high heels and semi-dressy attire. Other than his military dress uniform, he was unused to "dressing up". I thoroughly enjoyed the dinner and conversation. He was different from the other men I had known and dated in the past. I think you would call him a "Renaissance Man." He knew something about almost everything due largely to his intellectual curiosity and prolific reading habits. He was not trying to impress me—he knew what he was talking about and seemed to be one of those genuinely nice guys. He had a cool, confident demeanor and level gaze that looked right into you.

After a week or two I invited him to dinner at my house to spend a little time with my sons. I needed to know how he reacted around children and I would be able to observe his style first-hand. He talked a lot and seemed very comfortable with the boys and vice versa. From our first evening together, I experienced a strong physical attraction that did not need to be said. I told him during dinner that I was taking a vacation in a few weeks. I was going to spend several days hanging out with my boys and then going to the beach on the weekend.

After that we saw each other more frequently. Jeff talked and played with the kids with ease. Nathan was five years old and suffered with eczema. His skin was very dry and I had to use oatmeal skin conditioner in his bath. We were not sure what allergy he had so my Collies were not allowed inside the house because of Nathan's allergies. Nathan's skin condition did not seem to bother Jeff. One evening, Jeff took Nathan down to the store to get gas. He knew nothing about kids and treated them like little adults. I thought it would be okay if Nathan just went with Jeff to the store while I stayed home with Larry.

Chagrined, Jeff returned home with Nathan dripping wet and took him straight to the bathtub. When he was gassing up the car, he let Nathan hold on to the hose nozzle while Jeff washed the windows. Although he did not take his eyes off Nathan as he washed the windshield, he saw Nathan suddenly pull the gas nozzle out of the tank and aim it straight up in the air. The gasoline drenched Nathan's tender body and clothing. Jeff grabbed a water hose and washed him off as much as possible. Nathan screamed all the way home and Jeff was mortified by his miscalculation of a child's capability. He had never spent any time with small children. Jeff felt so badly it was the last time they went anywhere alone together for a long time.

The boys thought of Jeff as a MacGyver hero character on television. MacGyver could do anything and everything that hero men do. Now it was the boys' turn and they miscalculated Jeff! Jeff was constantly teaching the boys woodcrafting tricks, bringing them magnets, etc. Jeff thought it would be neat to teach the boys how to start a fire with steel wool and a battery. He picked up some good steel wool at a Home Depot store and decided to test it out with the battery while sitting in his new truck. The steel wool erupted in a ball of flame that Jeff quickly batted into the door, where to his chagrin a burn spot remained for the life of the truck. Jeff came to see us often and when the boys went to bed we watched movies at home and talked into the wee hours.

When it was time to take my vacation the following week, I was thinking seriously about inviting Jeff to go to the beach for a weekend getaway. First, I talked to my girlfriend at work and she encouraged me to go for it! It was short notice, but Jeff jumped at the invitation and volunteered to drive. At that time, there were two places at the beach where I loved to go dancing. I went there frequently throughout the 1980s with Jose. I had not made room reservations but I definitely wanted to go dancing at these clubs.

I was so excited about going to the beach with him. I worked so hard all year just to take a few days at the beach. It doesn't even matter when it rains I just wanted the serenity of being at the beach. We had a wonderful time and ate at several romantic places. That weekend went by so fast. Neither one of us wanted to leave. I do not think we danced, I don't remember that part … I could not even tell you if it rained. We did not leave the room or talk very much on the last day!

The following week I was mad at myself for having feelings for someone in the military who I knew would not be there long. He had told me he was staying in the military again and had asked to go to the 10th Special Forces Group in Germany. He had been working for a long time to get this transfer. I was thinking that it would be nice to enjoy him while he was here. He was a good lover and I was definitely going to miss that.

We became serious about our feelings toward each other. We had many dates and talked about things that were important. I told him I would never marry anyone in the military because I did not want to be a lonely military wife. I also told him I cannot have any more children. He asked me why and I told him my doctor had to remove my cervix to the point I would not hold a pregnancy. I did not question it because I knew I did not want any more children. I think Jeff had about three more months to decide whether he wanted to continue military service. He had to sign to "re-up" or get out. We had a wonderful time during those months and talked about everything. I was honest with him and my boys liked him a lot. He spent a lot of time talking to them. We could not get enough time with each other.

Jeff invited me to go to Washington, D.C., to see all of the museums. We were enjoying our time alone and had a lot of fun. We stayed at the bar in the hotel right near the museums and did not have to worry about driving. We knew we did not want to talk; we wanted to get to the room as soon as possible. We both had worked that week but were not tired. He talked to me about his family and I told him a little about me. He was concerned that I was married to "the bodybuilder" and he had told his sister "I am not sure what she sees in me." I do not remember what she told him but I remember what I told him many times. He also knew I told him exactly what I thought even if it might keep him from seeing me again. I told him I was so glad he was more invested in developing his mind instead of his body. I told him I did not love Jose and I believe I married him because Larry said I couldn't. How silly does that sound? The decisions we make when we are young cause us all to shake our heads when we get older.

We did not mean to drink so much because we could hardly walk out of the bar to our room. We were staying in a hotel that had a fire alarm evacuation in the middle of the night. There was not a fire but we still had to go outside in the downtown area. We did not think that we would have to get dressed and go down in front of everyone. It was so funny. We did find our way back to our room but we never did that again! We were both green the next day and did not enjoy the museums.

Jeff's roommate was an officer on his Special Forces team, a captain named Pete. Jeff told me Pete had two girlfriends from Denmark coming to visit. We were just dating and I said "Don't worry about me, I have plenty to do. I have a housekeeper—but I am still behind in my housework." (Actually, I was so jealous because

I was sure they were probably young and beautiful. Jeff did not have a clue how I felt. Those were feelings I had not experienced for a long time.)

I guess he had a little jealousy, too. One night one of Jeff's friends was leaving Fort Bragg, and they all went out. I went out as well on my own and saw Jeff at Syd's. His roommate Pete told him later, "Jeff, you should not be seeing her all the time. After you met and left the bar, she was there several times dancing and hanging out with other guys. She left with one of them after you started dating." I smiled and said, "Yes, we work together at Kelly Springfield but we are just friends. He knows there is nothing between us, and I appreciate that he drives me there and home because he does not drink." I told him that his friend was wrong about the reason and besides we had just met each other there anyway.

Jeff did not call me the next week. I could not stop thinking about him. I am not sure if that had anything to do with the Danish girls or if he was trying to forget about me. That was a hard week and I was so mad at myself! I did not want to have a serious relationship with someone eight years younger than I. I was sure his parents tried to talk to him about the risks of being with an older woman twice divorced with two small children. I know I would caution my sons if they met someone like me and I would have discouraged them. I called Jeff and asked to meet him and we met at a Pizza Hut and worked things out.

I called my best friend in the military, Linda Farley, many times to ask her questions. I wanted her opinions about Jeff and how I was feeling. Jeff was getting studio photos and offered to get one together while he was in his Ranger's uniform. I was flattered and was glad to take a picture. I told Linda that he was leaving probably in a few months for Germany. I told Linda that it cannot get serious because his parents do not have any grandchildren and I could not have anymore. He said that does not matter but he does not know how much he would miss that opportunity.

I invited Jeff to meet Linda Farley. I did not tell him she was going to test him and tell me what his military background was. Jeff wore a lot of medals on his uniform but I did not know what each one signified and he didn't talk about their meaning. He was quite vague about his job; all I knew was he jumped out of planes and "ran around in the woods." He would tell funny stories about deployments or things that happened but kept all the stories light. We drove to Georgia to visit Linda. I hoped she did not find anything wrong with him because I knew she would have to have a significant reason why I should not pursue this relationship. I was so happy to see her. Everything went well and she assured me he was a keeper! She explained what each of those medals meant. She said he was Ranger qualified, Special Forces, and Halo. I asked him why he never told me about his military work. He still did not talk about it much.

While I was there I saw puppies for sale near her town. The man said they were a German shepherd and wolf mixed breed. I knew exactly what they should look like. Jeff and I both loved large dogs and I had lost my Collie from old age. Larry and Nathan were old enough for a German shepherd. This man had some of the prettiest German shepherd puppies and we decided to get two of them. I was going to take the black one at my house and Jeff had the largest male. He could bring his back to me when he moved to Germany. Those were the smartest large dogs. My boys were so excited to see the puppies. We still had to make sure that Nathan did not have an allergic reaction to them. He seemed fine with them. We did not discuss the approaching departure date to Germany. I would have kept both dogs anyway.

This was the first time I had not fully focused on my job and on getting ahead at work. I dreaded going to work and hurried to get home like a child. I did not work the double shifts and had taken every other weekend off. These were the extra steps needed to take for promotions to management. Larry took the boys a little more than he used to. Jeff and I spent as much time together as possible. It was not easy or convenient between his schedule and mine. The last four years I had been on a mission to become the first female plant manager.

We knew we were in love with each other, but we did not talk about getting married for two major reasons. He was still in the military and going to Germany, which was a deal breaker for me. In addition, I was told I could not have any more children. During the following month I went to the doctor for my annual pap smear and mammogram. I asked the doctor about my ability to become pregnant because a portion of the cervix was removed in 1985. This test was

1989. I asked him if there was a way I could have another baby. Surprisingly, he said that everything looked normal despite partial removal. I was shocked when he said that I could certainly try to get pregnant. I said, "I am glad I asked."

Happily, Jeff decided to refuse the assignment to 10th Special Forces Group that he had worked so hard to get; he was getting out and making arrangements to find another job. We were very seriously contemplating marriage. I still had a concern that someday he would regret not having a child of his own. I told him what the doctor said about the possibility of carrying a baby full term. I also told him that I did not want to get married unless I got pregnant first. He protested that he would be perfectly happy being a dad to Larry and Nathan. I told him Jose delayed my divorce again to try and get visitation with Nathan. Jeff knew I did not want that to happen. We started talking more about marriage.

The day that made my final decision to marry him was the first month he was out of the military and had been looking for a job. He came back to the house one day for lunch and I was in the kitchen. Both the boys were in school. I did not realize how intimidating Jeff could be. Jose came to the door and said he wanted his passport to go to the Dominican Republic. I turned the corner to get the passport and Jeff was standing taller than Jose with that intimidating glare and a .357 Magnum revolver in his hand. I can't remember what Jeff said but Jose never bothered me again! You might say that was scary! Not at all to me! Do you remember my childhood? I wish a man could have had the balls to protect my mom and us we would not have suffered the way that we did. So this was getting even better!

Jeff and I planned our future together. He wanted to get married because he wanted me to have his name. We just wanted to get married privately without any fanfare. I told him about South Carolina and how easy it was to marry there. I repeatedly told him I did not want to get married unless I knew we could have a baby and it was safe. He had said he only wants to get married one time. That was even more of a reason to make sure I could have another baby. We decided we would try that first. I told him the women in my family get pregnant easily. He bought a beautiful engagement ring for me.

Jeff entered the military from high school and within a few years was nominated by his commander and accepted at the West Point

Preparatory Academy. This was a real testament to his intellect and leadership qualities. Jeff was too young, I think, to settle in with an academic role. He much preferred the role of soldier in the field and opted out of West Point. His parents were disappointed that he chose a different career path that would make education more difficult later on but they respected his decision. Jeff's first job in North Carolina after military service was working in the insurance business and he hated it. He began looking for another job right away. We were busy but happy. Jeff tried a few other jobs but could not find his niche. Fayetteville was a military and factory town. Jeff didn't belong in either one. He had enough money left that he had a little time to find something he enjoyed. I made enough money to keep us fine. He also considered going back to college. I told him I wished I had done that.

By January 1990, I was pregnant. When I was in the second trimester and my divorce from Jose was final, we were married in South Carolina in June. Jeff seemed disappointed that we went in one side of the chapel and out the other side. Admittedly, we had a whirlwind-romance and made sudden decisions about our future together. Within a six month timespan, Jeff left the military, I got pregnant, my divorce was final, Jeff was job-hunting, and we were married in South Carolina. My age was still a factor in having a child. But we both knew what we wanted and knew that we were soul mates—so why wait?

I was still determined in my quest to become the first female manager in the plant. I did not allow any of our decisions to slow me down at work. I did have some complications with gestational diabetes in the last trimester. I had to be careful to check my sugar and eat healthy.

I started re-educating myself about pregnancy and newborns. It had been six years since Nathan was born and I wanted to have the latest health trends for newborns. They changed the way you put a baby in the crib to go to sleep. My doctor told me if I breastfeed my baby she most likely would not have the allergies like Nathan did. I started going to women for breastfeeding advice. I thoroughly enjoyed being pregnant and I think it was because Jeff was so excited. Compared to my previous husbands it was a joyful experience to have a supportive and happy expectant father like Jeff. I enjoyed being pregnant with Larry and Nathan by myself. With Jeff it was a true celebration to give birth to a child. I just knew she was a girl.

The most significant problem I had with Christina was the last-minute need for an epidural. I was in extreme pain and didn't know why it was different this time. She ended up being a breech birth because she turned at the last minute. Everything seemed to go fine until the shift change at 7:00 P.M. As soon as that nurse was in the room she called for an emergency "C" section. I was so glad. That child weighed almost 10 lbs.!

Jeff's parents, Dick and Peggy, sent me an entire "baby shower" in one shipment. This was their first grandchild. I did not have a baby shower because I had one with Larry. Peggy must have enjoyed choosing all of the cutest things for girls! We did not have to buy a single item for Christina's layette or nursery. We opened gift boxes for an hour and thoroughly enjoyed their excitement and support.

After Christina was born, I was pushing hard at work to get the managerial promotion I wanted. During this time Jeff worked at Sears and raised Christina, Larry, and Nathan while I worked extra hours. He cooked, looked after the kids, worked, and got them off to school every morning. He enjoyed being a dad and husband. Although he was more accustomed to the role of a military man I knew that he was totally contented when I heard him singing one day nursery rhymes in the shower! When Christina was about three years old she watched Mother Goose and the "Little Mermaid" videos over and over. One day I heard him saying the rhymes and singing in the shower instead of his colorful Army cadences. These are the most special things that I realize today are priceless. I am so happy that I can enjoy the memory. What if I could not remember something this simple? Based on the nature of the brain injury sustained, I should not have been able to recognize my family or say their names. I am so happy I can hear him sing that right now in my mind.

Jeff was always looking for new opportunities for us. We went through a period of time when we were part of Amway. They were wonderful people. Amway distributed good food, vitamins, and other products. Most of the sales force and distributors were very religious. There were several business philosophies touted in books and tapes that were highly motivating. Amway conventions were well attended and promoted confidence in our ability to grow our income. We met people who believed in the things we felt were most important in raising a family, good character and strong family values. Jeff and I were very strong in our beliefs. We believed that the people who worked hard and did the right thing usually ended up as millionaires. We enjoyed the functions and conventions surrounding free enterprise. In some respects it was similar to attending church—the spiritual message was there. Dedication to hard work and family was paramount.

Jeff and I progressed through the ranks and improved our financial standing which helped us launch the next business endeavor. We are no longer part of Amway, but our involvement helped solidify our unity of purpose in life. We wanted to be successful in our business, in marriage, and parenting. We are so glad that our commitment, respect, and love taught us to work through the difficult times and remain close. We worked very hard to compromise, understand, and discuss our disagreements. We were so strong-minded that "compromising and listening" were our biggest challenges. We learned to listen to each other, talk things out and come to a decision. I think it is safe to say that when it came to compromising—I made the most sacrifices early on.

We each had our own bank accounts and I had the hardest time letting him pay the bills. I had always been so dependent in the past, mainly because my first husband ran our marriage like a business. He was very control-oriented. Jeff's life changed dramatically from the freedom of a bachelor in the military to the rigors of marriage, child care, and parenting. The kids were six years apart in age. Jeff had some rough days dealing with the behaviors, demands, and diapers! I worked about twelve hours a day, sometimes six days a week, while he managed to change jobs, cook, and take care of the kids. The company switched from eight- to twelve-hour shifts. The managers had to work fourteen continuous hours daily. Luckily, we had a wonderful lady living across the street who took care of Christina. Her name was Ann Fields. She had one son and her husband was away a lot in the military. She was British and the perfect pre-school baby sitter for Christina. Like Jeff and I, she was firm with Christina and managed her behavior very well. Ann visited us later in Myrtle Beach with her mother from England. We enjoyed seeing her and felt so lucky to have someone like her to help us with Christina. Christina was very smart like Jeff and she would take advantage of anyone that she could. She knew "Miss Ann" would not let that happen.

We also let Christina stay with our friend, Honey Barr. Her son and daughter-in-law (Clark and Consuelo Barr) became our closest friends in the Amway business. Clark and Jeff had a lot in common in the military. Clark was funny and smart and had the same quick wit that Jeff did. Honey lived with the Barrs and practically raised his two daughters, Darcy and Felicia. (I was so proud of Consuela. In 2004 when I received my master's degree in art, she was also awarded her degree in Spanish.) We are about the same age. We were living in Myrtle Beach when Clark's mother died and the marriage ended. The two girls were in middle school and moved in with us until Clark was able to relocate. Consuelo did not speak much English when the girls were younger and she stayed mostly with her sister. Proudly, Darcy and Felicia grew up as lovely young ladies who finished high school and went to college. They are both beautiful and look a lot like their Honduran mother. These were important people in our lives who shared the ups and downs of life together.

Jeff did very well in his business ventures and I was impressed. I was also impressed that he had more patience than I did. At times, we were too strict in our discipline. We played a private game with each other called "Sound of Music." This was our "secret code," without letting the kids know, that we were disagreeing with each other. Like Captain Von Trapp, Jeff loved his children, but tended to treat them like they were in the military! I had been in the military and had to be a tough manager at the plant which turned us both into task masters. But at home, we wanted to maintain some balance. By using the "Sound of Music" phrase, we were reminded that our kids were not in the military and that one of us was being too strong on discipline. It worked beautifully! Children will drive you crazy if you let them.

Larry and Nathan's dad did more things with them as they got older and Jeff never tried to replace their dad. Those boys grew up as good men that any woman would be proud to marry. They watched Jeff's commitment to family and hard work. They protested but he was a firm and fair dad and husband. I have constantly emphasized to all five of my kids that it was not easy to find a man like Jeff— someone with all the traits I dreamed of in life all rolled up in one person. By example, Jeff set the standard for being a perfect dad, husband, and businessman. Simply said, he is a winner. Both of the boys are wonderful men and I am so proud of both of them. They all worked as a team when I needed them most. The boys trusted Jeff and they learned from him. They watched Jeff in crisis, making crucial decisions, keeping the family close, sharing information and responsibilities. Jeff is a naturally inclusive leader who engages every human resource to participate in his "field of operation." They witnessed Jeff's attentiveness to me, my medical crisis, and to their younger sisters more than two hundred miles away. I think Larry and Nathan grew up to full manhood that month. Now, years later, they are very close to Jeff and call him frequently for his advice. They make their own decisions as men, but enjoy the privilege and benefits of Jeff's wisdom. I will always be grateful to God that Jeff was the head of our family when the stroke occurred.

I have family and friends who do not have that commitment or clarity of purpose that is present in my household today. Advice is cheap, but I believe everyone has a true soul mate and that life is too short to settle for less than love. We all make poor decisions in life, but in matters of the heart, I firmly believe in correcting course. My friend says, "No matter how far down the wrong road you have gone—turn around." I am sorry that I made poor decisions in relationships early on, but I am so grateful that I had the courage to make the changes that allowed me to maintain my dignity in life.

Without Jeff in my life, I do not believe Larry and Nathan would be the fine men that they are. Jeff is the reason that I have my daughters Christina, Carmelita, Elena, and my grandson Jaxon. Looking back at my marriages, I am glad I did not settle for less than the moon! I believe in being forthright, discussing problems, and fighting for fair change. But mutual respect is paramount and without it I believe in moving on to a greater good. Today, I know that I must pray about tough decisions, seek counsel from close friends and family, and have the courage of my convictions and to take the next indicated step boldly. Like recovery from a stroke—the first step forward is often the hardest. I have learned to be assertive without being aggressive. I have learned that I deserve to be on this earth and that I am not any better or any less than anyone. I have made some modest peace with the fact that there were some very mean, miserable people who abused me as a child. I no longer assume the role of avenger—that is

God's job. I choose not to associate with people who live and dwell in their problems and never seek solutions. The only drama I tolerate in my life today is the drama of living with teenagers! Enough said!

When Christina was five years old and starting kindergarten, Jeff told me he would love to have another child. I finally became a manager at Kelly Springfield and was proud of my accomplishment. But promotions at work were no longer my top priority. I enjoyed spending more time with him and our family. We knew that I could continue to manage at Kelly Springfield and work until I was within six weeks of delivery. Jeff had a job that he enjoyed with Chase Mortgage and he did very well there, but he still wanted something different and he wanted another child—which made me happy, too.

We knew I would be pregnant right away but we were soon disappointed that we had a miscarriage. We got pregnant again and I was concerned because I was forty years old and older than Jeff. Was this the right thing to do? On my next appointment we were pregnant with twins. I knew my grandmother had three sets of twins that were still-born. About a month later we had another miscarriage and had to spend the day at the hospital for a dilation and curettage. My doctor told me to wait a few months before trying again and to see him as soon as I was pregnant.

The next pregnancy gave us our beautiful Carmelita. She was a special gift to us because she would not have been born if the prior pregnancies came to full term. I cannot imagine our lives without Carmelita. I had started having mild contractions too early in the third trimester and the doctors ordered me off work. Interestingly, I loved art all of my life, but never had time to paint when I was working and raising children. The only time I painted was when I was pregnant or the six weeks of parental leave. It was an added joy to be pregnant and painting at the same time.

Several weeks prior to our due date, I had some significant bleeding one day and the baby's movements felt different. I knew something was wrong and Jeff took me to the hospital. After a few hours of waiting, the doctor wanted to send me home because he said I was not dilated and not ready. I was becoming agitated and fearful. I said "I might not be ready but something is wrong. How do you explain the blood that I saw? You need to check further because I can feel that something is wrong. She is like the perfect child; I got to know her and I feel that something is wrong." The doctor still wanted to send me home until Jeff stepped in and insisted on another ultrasound.

Thankfully, they performed another ultrasound and it revealed a life-threatening condition for me and the baby called "placental abruption." The doctors performed an emergency caesarian which saved us both. We could have had a very tragic outcome if I had not been adamant about my "sensing" that something was very wrong. It is unscientific to say "I can feel something is not right." This complication occurs when the placenta peels away from the uterine wall prior to delivery. It can be caused by sudden trauma, like a car accident or fall. It can also be caused by a leakage of the amniotic fluid surrounding the baby inside the placenta. When abruption occurs the baby is deprived of oxygen and nutrients and the mother suffers heavy bleeding—sometimes intermittently. Regardless of the cause, the condition is fatal if not treated immediately. I do not know the precise cause of my condition, but one of the risk factors is maternal age over forty, and I was at risk and didn't know it. This was another miracle in my life.

Jeff enjoyed the mortgage company so much that he decided to start his own business at the end of the year. After Carmelita was born we started looking for larger house for our growing family. We also wanted to live closer to Kelly Springfield to reduce the commute time and live in a good school district. By that time Larry was out of high school and working for his dad full time. He had been working in several of his dad's businesses part time until he graduated. With full-time employment, Larry rented the house Jeff and I owned where the kids had grown up. Jeff and I found a lovely two-story home with a big yard to accommodate dogs and kids. We decided to rent it then buy if we really liked living there.

Christina had already started school. She was always the princess in our home. Her brothers doted on her as the baby sister and we were thrilled that we had a child together. When Carmelita was born, Christina did not like sharing *her family*. The typical sibling rivalry occurred and it was a big adjustment to her world.

Jeff was doing well and decided to find someone who would be interested in his business as an investor. We knew several people in the Amway business who might be interested and had investment resources. Jeff developed a good business plan and found an investor right away. His first business was called Allstate Mortgage Company. His business grew fast and he hired a lot of employees and profits exceeded his expectations. It was a great year. I continued to work and Jeff started hinting that I should come home to stay. To lure me away from working, Jeff said he would pay me the same salary to stay at home and be a mom. I had never had an opportunity like this! I told Jeff if he continued to do well in his business, I would retire.

With management responsibilities my work was increasingly demanding. I was working up to fourteen hours a day. I hated being away from the kids that long. I had already been working there for sixteen years. I had even gotten used to the heat. The area I managed had no air conditioning and the summer heat and humidity were brutal even though there were fans in some of the employee areas. I managed between forty to sixty people a day. The area was so large I had to move around the plant on a tricycle or go-cart. It was hard to think about leaving because I had worked with these people so long they were like part of my family. I cared about them and how their families were getting along. On the other hand, I did not relish the job of dealing with the unions. Most employees did their job but we had a few who caused problems with the continuous operation. If one person takes too long for a break, stays outside too long to smoke or eat, it affected all of us. The union was a challenge, protecting some of the bad workers over the good ones. I was evaluating the pros and cons of retiring. I enjoyed my job, the money was good, and I had to take a leap of faith. I made a hard decision to retire.

Jeff's business was doing so well that he opened another office in Charlotte, North Carolina, and one in Myrtle Beach, South Carolina. Life had never been better. Jeff had a beautiful new Corvette and a Cadillac Escalade that seated the whole family. We went on cruises and vacations often in Myrtle Beach. We always stayed at Kingston Plantation in Myrtle Beach. Always looking ahead, Jeff and I tried to decide what we would do in the future and where we wanted to live. Carmelita was still in diapers and he wanted one last baby. I told him I did not want to spend so much time away from them if we had another child. We knew this was the last time due to my age and the necessity of two prior caesarians. My body had experienced enough pregnancy complications. We agreed to have another baby.

It was a great arrangement! I was able to retire, Jeff "paid" me the same salary I was earning at the factory, and I would be part-owner of the business. We also decided we might live in Myrtle Beach. I got pregnant within two months, and in the third trimester of a successful pregnancy I turned in my retirement papers. That was scary. I had a lot of faith in Jeff and God but I was used to my own money that I earned myself. I was getting excited about staying home with the kids and painting again.

Everything went well until the end of the pregnancy. Similar to the condition with Carmelita, I was at home and started having premature contractions. I had one large blood clot and knew there was another problem. I did not feel scared as I did with Carmelita, but I was on guard about my condition. Again, Jeff took me to the hospital to deliver early. I was not taking any chances because of the blood clot and my previous experience with Carmelita. The nurses were not at all concerned and directed me to walk the entire floor "to speed things up." I was firm about my situation and said, "Before I start walking, can you please examine me to be sure everything is okay? Where did the blood clot come from?" She said, "I haven't seen any blood." I was getting more anxious and I told her that with my last pregnancy I had a similar problem that resulted in an emergency C-section. I felt like a hypochondriac and slightly embarrassed. Thankfully, Jeff supported me and did not budge. Jeff insisted that I see a doctor immediately.

Another doctor came in to examine me. He said, "No blood, you need to walk the entire floor to speed things up." I just cannot stand the cockiness of a doctor talking about my body which they cannot feel! I asked, "Where does that blood I saw come from? I did not imagine it. The baby is still moving but I want to be checked." Jeff insisted on a sonogram and another doctor came in to join the group forming around my bed. Again, the sonogram revealed another placental abruption! I had another emergency caesarian and it could have been fatal otherwise. Elena was so blue when she was born and she stayed that way for a week. Jeff's parents now had three little Weatherspoon granddaughters. They came out from California right after Elena was born. Elena's safe birth was another miracle in my life.

By 1998, Jeff's business was going exceptionally well. As often happens in partnerships, the principles had disagreements and dissolved the business. Jeff established a new business on his own in South Carolina. We loved Myrtle Beach and I was happy to move there. I resisted at first because of the distance from my Mom. Jeff told me he had no problem if I visited her every week. The first year was a major struggle financially. I was no longer working, all three girls were little, we had relocated, and Jeff was heavily focused on growing his new company.

The house was beautiful and I enjoyed staying home with the children. Next we decided to look for a condominium on the beach at Kingston Plantation and moved there the following year. Jeff made good decisions for us and we discussed everything together about the business, school districts, child-rearing, and our dreams for the future. It was uncomfortable at times because I wanted to maintain my independence to some degree. Again, I had to take a leap of faith and I trust his decisions.

Jeff decided to buy a German shepherd for the family and partly for security reasons and we chose one that was trained for small children. We knew we could keep this Germen shepherd when we moved to the condo. We found a place that trains German shepherds for protection. These dogs were well-trained and responded to commands in three different languages. We chose German and were trained to use the key commands in German. We stayed overnight in a hotel with the dog before we moved. We needed to test his personality toward us and practiced commands. We used a "bucket" with a leash to practice. The dog would only "contact and bite" if given a command. Jeff and I were able to take the dog anywhere and feel confident. The dog was so large and menacing that people felt intimidated. We ended up leaving him at home on most outings except for exercise. The three girls loved him, especially Christina. We wanted personal safety for our family and a good pet for the girls. They do not bark like untrained dogs. I do not remember most of the details of this story. I know that the dog we chose did not like to bite. We saw him in action on command. Whenever we returned home, the dog entered the house first and checked the house for intruders. When he completed his search, he returned to the door and we knew we were safe. His name was Balou and he was a wonderful dog for our family.

I had the hardest time not tripping over him. He followed me wherever I went in the house and laid as close to me as he could possibly get. The little girls were were in diapers when we got Balou and now they were three and four years old. They could fall down on top of him and he would just let them play. Nathan lived with us at that time, too. He had so much fun with the dog, too. Balou was exceptionally well-trained and a valuable watch dog. We could have friends over without any attempts by Balou to attack. German shepherds often develop hip dysplasia as they age. Their hips begin to deteriorate by age ten. Jeff was concerned about buying such an expensive dog that might develop this malady. The trainer guaranteed that Balou would not suffer hip dysplasia and I never understood how he could make this commitment!

Balou was specifically trained to find a lost child. All he needed to search was a sock, shoe, or personal item that belonged to the missing child. He was also trained to attack on command but he did not like it. Balou was featured in a news program about search dogs before we bought him. One day Carmelita and Elena had a lunch nap. I was listening to music and painting. As usual, Balou was right at the back of my heels. In a flash of movement, Balou leaped six feet from the floor and moved aggressively toward the door. All of his teeth were bared and he was growling loudly. Alarmed, I turned and saw a tall stranger closing my front door. We changed the locks when we moved in and I never expected anyone to have a key. I looked out the peep hole and saw that he was still there. Through the door, the man said that he had a key and was looking for someone he knew. I asked him, "Do you know how close you came to being bitten"? I told him to leave immediately. Balou had immediately sensed the threat and reacted exactly as he was trained to do. I had a bad feeling about that incident and was very glad Balou protected us. We changed the locks again but wondered where he got the key to a new lock and what he intended to do. We never saw him again. It was a high security complex and a key was required to get inside the building. Another key was required to access the stairwell. We still wonder how that intruder got in to our home and why.

Several months later, we took Balou for a walk around the grounds of the complex. People were always walking their pets, feeding the ducks, and milling about the grass and grounds. In a flash, Balou was in the attack stance. He was all teeth and not pulling away as if I had put him on guard. There was a man in the bushes who appeared unexpectedly. Balou was on full alert. The man took off running and Balou would not release. I did not command until the man was away. Maintenance men were working on the grounds and I told them what happened. I kept Balou inside house because I felt something was wrong. I never saw him act like that again.

We enjoyed living at the beach. Most of the people who lived in our complex had timeshares and came to Myrtle Beach only for summers and holidays. The rest of the year we enjoyed a great deal of privacy. We usually enjoyed having the sauna, Jacuzzi, and gym all to ourselves. The girls loved the indoor heated pool—they were all water rats and swam every day they possibly could. These are some of the wonderful memories I have recovered by writing. I wonder what important things I can no longer recall.

Like most Americans, the events of September 11, 2001, were life-changing for me. It is still the most catastrophic incident in American history during my lifetime. This is one awful memory that I am grateful I still have, however. I think it brought Americans closer together and we were unified against a common enemy. The unthinkable happened when we were attacked on our own soil. My brother Terry was a platoon sergeant in the 82nd Airborne Division and deployed several times to Iraq and Afghanistan.

All Americans were on high security alert for a long time following the assault on our freedom. People worried about going in public places, like malls, churches, and sporting events where large numbers of people were gathered. Historically, our fight for freedom was conducted on foreign soil. Most Americans were willing to sacrifice everything to preserve our freedom and independence from tyranny. My brother Perry supported his own son's military service knowing he would be deployed to Afghanistan or Iraq. They were willing to die for their country.

We watched the news daily following all the events of 9/11. As many have said, America lost its innocence that day. Jeff sold his small plane because the small airport atmosphere was so difficult. I suddenly appreciated my life more, being home with my girls, and recognizing that time was going by so fast. We had a new awareness of the most precious things in life.

Soon the girls would be old enough to start school. Every Thursday I drove up to Fayetteville, North Carolina, to visit my mother, family, and friends. Mom would make dinner for us and then I drove back to the beach where we lived. Mom's mental status was erratic and I was very mindful of her medications and behavior. I was not well-versed in mental disorders and I knew I had to learn everything I could about her condition. She was finally diagnosed with bipolar disorder and managed by her family physician rather than a psychiatrist. I remember reading that this disorder tends to run in families. It seems that many famous artists also suffered from mental disorders and alcoholism. I learned that people with bipolar disorders often feel "normal" after drinking alcohol because it slows down the "hyper" part of their behavior. That terminology was rarely used to identify suicidal tendencies among artists. I remember reading a particular book about a female doctor who was bipolar. It reminded me so much of my mother's behavior when I was a child. I intuitively assumed the role of her protector knowing that things were not right in her mind at times. Undiagnosed until 1990, our family was in complete denial about the seriousness of her condition. I had always accepted that she was never the same after my sister Helen's death. I thought that was the precipitating cause of her erratic behavior at times. Even in our adulthood we were in total denial that something was wrong with our mother. We witnessed her talking excessively and being overly happy at times. And there were the really bad days that her behavior was maddening. Yet we did not recognize it as mental illness. We were completely in the dark.

Loving My Mother to the End of her Life

One Thursday I visited my mother and she was quiet different. I wanted to ask her some questions about her medications, the appearance of her house, and her behavior. But I was careful not to say anything negative that might give Felton fodder for attacking her when I left. When it was time for me to leave, she clung to me and I could tell she did not want me to go yet. She knew I had to get home before it was too late at night.

Her change in behavior bothered me and made me feel guilty

the rest of the week. I sensed something was changing and she was disturbed by it. The following Thursday she was uncontrollable. She was talking incoherently and could not stay on task while cooking. She was a very good cook and trying to make rice, which she was burning in a pot! She was more agitated than usual and just not herself. I saw her take her medication earlier that day. I left to visit my sisters and said my goodbyes to Mom. I had to get back to Myrtle Beach earlier than usual. I was headed home on I-95 and I had that nagging feeling again that something was just not right. I turned around, knowing I needed to check on her for some reason. Sometimes she was too talkative because she took the maximum amount of lithium. When I walked into her house, Felton was angry and in her face while she was trying to cook. He was mad that she had burned dinner. He was cussing her out and telling her she could not do anything right. Mom was crying and very upset. She hardly acknowledged I was back.

Carmelita and Elena were still in their car seats asleep and I went alone in her house. I knew instantly that she was in trouble and Felton was turning violent. She was definitely manic. I knew what he was capable of doing if I had joined the violence. I knew it was fruitless to try to talk to her logically—she was having an episode and out of control. As calmly as I could, I told Felton, "You probably should let me take her home until she gets her medication stable." She was not even cogent enough to get some clothes together or pack anything else she should have needed overnight. I found her medications and all of the bottles were empty. According to the labels, she should have had another week's supply. I bundled her up along with the essential items I could find and loaded her into my car.

Luckily, my daughters were very sound sleepers. Mom talked non-stop and repeated herself for the two-hour ride back to Myrtle Beach. I was worried about the behavior of my mother in front of the kids. Those two hours were painful for me. She had been doing so well following her diagnosis and medication regimen. I thought it was obvious that the lithium and haloperidol were taken inappropriately for some reason. I was flying blind trying to manage a situation that I had very little experience with. Still unmanageable at home, I called the emergency room to ask questions about intermediate steps I could take until she could be seen by a doctor the next day. She was up moving around without sleep for two days. The girls were afraid and we tried to reassure them. Jeff understood my mother's mental condition but we were both uneasy about what might happen.

Jeff kept the girls occupied as I watched over her during the continuing manic state she was in. She was a heavy smoker so she stayed in a second floor condo on the beach where we live. I told the psychiatrist she did not appear to be suicidal but her behavior was manic. She was rocking back and forth relentlessly and rapidly speaking the same phrases over and over. I did not sleep for two days because I thought she was so agitated that she might jump off the second story balcony, not because she was suicidal but because she thought she could do anything—even fly. Nothing I could say could change her behavior and I was aware of that. Jeff was worried about the gravity of the situation and we knew she needed medical intervention. The next morning I contacted her doctors in Fayetteville and asked to have her medications refilled by telephone at a local pharmacy. In the meantime, we decided to take Mom to the local community hospital at Waccamaw.

I learned a lot about managing her medications there. The lithium was prescribed as a mood stabilizer. It is most effective for individuals with "pure" or euphoric mania (where there is little depression mixed in with the elevated mood). In bipolar disorder, anti-depressants must be used in combination with a mood stabilizing medication. In her case, she was using the anti-depressant without a mood stabilizer which pushed her into a manic state. The blood work showed "O" level of lithium in her system resulting in the sustained manic state. Somehow her medications were altered, dosed incorrectly, or the result of human error. I suspected that Felton intervened with her medication regime as punishment for something she did or did not do.

The anti-psychotic medication that my mother took with lithium was haloperidol (Haldol). With her full manic episode she needed to be hospitalized with around-the-clock care and support. In the severe manic state individuals do not sleep—sometimes for days. I did not want to leave her alone in the hospital and Jeff was supportive of whatever I needed to do. I recorded notes about her behavior in a journal to use when I visited her psychologist. Even though she was in bad shape, she deserved my respect. Her doctor only spoke limited English and Mom could not understand her. I went into all sessions with Mom and served as an interpreter and to keep her calm. One of the books that helped me understand mental illness was entitled *An Unquiet Mind, a Memoir of Moods and Madness* by Redfield Jamison, Ph.D. As caring family members, it is imperative to research, read, and learn as much as possible about mental disorders afflicting our loved ones.

Mom was eventually stabilized and returned to our home for aftercare. I took her to appointments with the psychologist and met with her doctor to learn how to manage her medications effectively. I had not quite decided what was to be done about Felton—but I knew that Mom could not survive if she returned to that environment. We decided to take things one day at a time until she was stable.

With some coaxing, Mom attended a church with us and went to a support group for people with bipolar disorder. I asked her to go at least a few times and then she could stop as soon as she wanted. Thankfully, she went once a month for about six months. She was quiet and listened to the others but did not participate herself. I was glad she continued as long as she did. Most of the group members shared their attempts to commit suicide. She told me she did not want to go back to the group because it was sad and she did not want to think about killing herself. I did not force her to attend after that.

The love Jeff showed to my mother during her illness and her time living with us was amazing. He was generous with his time and patient beyond belief. He had no training or experience with any of these issues, yet he jumped in with both feet and did what needed to be done. It confirmed my belief that I had truly found my soul mate on earth. It took my mother two years living in our home to relax and feel safe. For the first time in decades she could sleep without the fear of having to protect herself from an abusive husband. It was at the end of two years when she said, "Linda, I have never seen Jeff yell or get angry." I smiled and told her that "He gets angry but we never argue in front of the children. We want them to feel safe." She gave me one of her special smiles that was all I needed to know that she understood we were also trying to make her feel safe and enjoy her time. We had so many challenges over the next few years and a lesser man than Jeff could not have steered us through those rocky times. At that moment, everything was turning out all right.

The condo at Kingston Plantation was now home to a 100-pound

German shepherd guard dog, three adults, and three children. We were crowded, to say the least. Without hesitation, Christina gave up her room for her grandma and moved in with the little girls. We had expected to live there the rest of our lives right on the beach. But we needed more room and Jeff suggested that we should rent a house to give us the room we needed. We found an older house on Chesapeake Road that was ideal for our needs. There were separate quarters downstairs for mom, including a dinette, sink, and small refrigerator. She loved the quiet and the privacy. There were five bedrooms and a large unfinished room that Jeff turned into an office. We did not expect that having Balou would become the major problem. Despite the Realtor's assurances that the dog was acceptable, the owner required an exorbitant insurance policy to cover liability. We really needed that house and did not want to have the girls changing schools. It broke our hearts to let Nathan take Balou into "retirement." We knew Balou would get a great countryside home with Nathan outside Fayetteville.

We all enjoyed cats so the girls got kittens from Santa Claus that year. Jeff was not very fond of cats and not at all pleased about a sack full of kittens on Christmas Eve! Christina chose a black cat that she loved, and the little girls got orange tabbies. Kids and animals are always a challenge. The tabbies could not be house trained and wet in the girls' beds! We found them homes in the country where they could be happy outside, so they had to go and the girls were upset again.

When Mom was diagnosed with lung cancer, we were determined to keep her with us and take care of her. We knew she would live longer and be happier. Elena and Carmelita were in high school I decided to go back to college. I thought about going to nursing school again, like I started to do when Larry was a baby. I thought the money was good and with mom's condition it would help me care for her. I also loved science. I decided to look at the curriculum at Coastal Carolina College. When I was there, I saw that Horry County needed art teachers. I had painted as a hobby since I was a child and I was very good. I had never considered art as a possible career. I learned that the Horry County School District was desperate for qualified teachers. Thus, the district paid the tuition and awarded an annual stipend of $5,000 if students agreed to work in the district for five years following graduation. I was very interested and the timing was exactly right.

Jeff and I discussed it at length and I had a few months to make up my mind before the semester began. The more I thought about it, I knew it was something I wanted to do. We both realized that I would be fully focused on my studies and getting through each semester. I am just an average student and feel like I have to work twice as hard as others to succeed in school. As always, Jeff encouraged me and thought it was a great decision. He said he would help with taking care of my mother and he was already a great dad. He was a better cook than I was and the whole family knew it! I do not think he realized at the time just how focused I would be! I wanted to start now and finish yesterday. I was on a mission to get through school as quickly as I could and get into teaching.

I doubled my course load during the summer sessions. Dr. Susan Slavik was my advisor and I was so lucky to have her. She understood how serious I was about getting my degree and her help was invaluable. I wrote and studied everything that she told me to do. We were about the same age but she was brilliant. She was responsible for testing us in the master's level courses. She was tough and demanding. She would not assign a grade until the student met the precise standards established. She expected every student to meet those standards—or fail.

The most difficult course I took was Dr. Slavik's "Principles and Methods of Teaching Content." *The* applied arts were easy, but the research and assessments were hard for me. (Writing this—I wish I could remember the principles and methods without looking at my notes. I repeatedly try reading and learning it again—but I have not managed to retain it. After the stroke, I tried to learn and read the materials again and had to put them away. Every six months I would try again. Some of the words I remembered and others will take more time. I get discouraged because my vision is impaired and comprehension takes a great deal of effort. I have to use the dictionary frequently. On the bright side, I am euphoric when I realize I remembered and retained something from my last study session! It has been five years since the stroke and I have progressed from a second-grade reading and comprehension level to a high school level.)

My "History of Western Art" class by Dr. Morgan required mastery over a mountain of information. She lectured the entire class and I had written an hour of her lectures three times a week. She did not want us to interrupt her during lectures. Her personal art is incredible. The sculptures I had seen were of the female body or shoes. She used her own barbed wire to achieve the texture she desired. Her work has been sold to several celebrities. Her work was feminine and her sculpture "Rose Thorn" was in great demand. I wish I could take all of my classes again and again....

Dr. Treelee McAnn was my professor in the life drawing class. I would say I probably learned most about drawing from her. All of the students were in their twenties and I was twice as old as they were! I finally met a student my age in this class. She would take time to grade every piece of student art completed in pencil, pastel, or charcoal. She would place tracing paper on top of the student's drawing to determine what body part was disproportionate. This was an effective teaching strategy for me. I am a visual learner. I still look at her comments about my work. She would write notes to explain why a drawing was good or why it was bad. I did not take that for granted. If I had not saved my compositions I would be unable to visualize and relearn techniques that are lost somewhere in my brain.

In 2004, two of my art works were accepted in a literary art magazine, Archarios. Those were "Heritage" mixed media and "In the Spirit of..." oil canvas. I have both of these works in my studio. The expectations were high on a huge volume of creative work. Most of my art works related to the American Indian, my mother and patriotism. I had forgotten how much art was created to get a master's degree in art!

Looking at the textbooks and *The Artist Magazine* help me remember, at least for that moment in time. I have so many books, compositions, and notes that I mastered once. I was able to easily identify the artists and their basic medium. Today, I understand when I review the material but I cannot explain or discuss the information without comprehensive notes. I don't think my students would enjoy having a robot for a teacher*!* These are some of the most significant artists' I had studied and appreciated: Harley Brown, Chris Saper, John Singer Sargent, and Robert Carter Clark.

I have enjoyed the support and help of many local artists since my

310

stroke. These artists have been instrumental in helping me to restore my style and relearn techniques. As a visual learner, it helps me to watch their application and style. I am learning every day. I was a member of the Waccamaw Arts and Craft Guild prior to the stroke. The techniques we share have been priceless learning tools for me. I cherish the memories I have with them before and after the stroke. Some have died and some are older and generously share their skill and wisdom with the guild members.

My three sisters are a huge part of the achievements I enjoyed in my art education and career. Since high school they urged me to paint on canvas and create wall murals for them long before I had any professional training. They loved my work and bragged about my skills to others. My biggest fans were my mother and my grade school art teacher, Mrs. Weathers. They led by example. I learned from my mother to never give up no matter what and to love family unconditionally. Mrs. Weathers taught me to focus on the future and my strengths rather than the chaos around me. She taught me everything she knew about art. Recalling their words and their love, they continue to be the wind beneath my wings. I think about one of them every day.

Although I have been a private person all of my life, I am compelled to share my story in writing. I may be living on borrowed time—or I may live to be one hundred—but I want others to know how wonderful married life can be. I wish more than ever that my mother could have experienced the joy of a serene life. With Jeff, I have been able to realize my dreams. I know that my purpose in life is to be a good wife, devoted full-time mom, and child of God. I sound like someone with a 1950s perspective, but I intend to spend the rest of my life with Jeff. I don't think he could accomplish his full potential in three life times. One of his traits that I admire most is his self-confidence. His presence fills a room and there is no doubt about his ability to motivate people and assume a leadership role. He makes it look so easy. He is a true intellectual who keeps a wealth of knowledge to himself unless he is asked. He never brags about what he owns or what he knows. He is the Rock of Gibraltar in our home and always has been.

Jeff is relentless in his pursuit of knowledge about anything and everything. He has been a voracious reader for the 24 years we have been married. He loves to read books on world history, aircraft, artillery, medicine, science, and especially biographies. He has skydived, scuba-dived, learned to fly, and owned his own small plane. When my mother experienced mental illnesses, Jeff researched psychiatry and psychology as much as I did to help us understand her behavior and treatment. Yet, Jeff is also a real caveman! He is a jeans and T-shirt kind of guy. He has handled guns since he was a child and has a huge collection. He is an intense advocate of the Second Amendment. He is a geek when it comes to computers and current technology. In fact, he has been part of an international "video games geek squad" for more than a decade. Luckily, he is not an artist or connoisseur of fine art, this is the only discipline that I know more about than he does.

Jeff goes about life effortlessly. Whatever stressors he has or feels, he shoulders them pretty much alone. He handles stress better than anyone I have ever seen. Eventually, he discusses everything with me, usually after he has figured out the best course of action. He is not a man who takes orders easily and is at his best when he is the leader of the pack. He is entrepreneurial, self-educated, and the "real McCoy." With Jeff, what you see is what you get.

On the homey side, Jeff is a real family man. He loves his children unconditionally. He is a stern disciplinarian when he needs to be and believes in "tough love." He usually treats our kids like young adults and talks to them matter-of-factly about almost everything. We have been fairly consistent over the years about our philosophy of child-rearing. We tried not to fight or disagree in front of the children because we wanted them to feel safe and secure. We have done our best to teach our kids the value of family, hard work, and good character. He did not blink when I needed to bring my mother to live with us or when various family members and close friends needed temporary shelter in our home. He is respectful to others— even when he isn't fond of them! To be perfectly honest, I could probably dedicate equal space and time discussing his defects, but it would serve no purpose and I would have to think a long, long time to fill up the space. Simply put—Jeff is a good man and I am proud to be his wife until death us do part.

The first year teaching at North Myrtle Beach High school was one of the best years of my life. I learned that one teaching position was opening at Myrtle Beach High School in 2004-05. There were other positions in neighboring towns—but the commute would require relocating our home and changing school districts for the girls. I had my eye on that one job and knew that I had to graduate early to compete for the position. I told Jeff that I wanted to finish a year earlier than usual and he readily agreed to help me with the girls, my mother, and the household chores. (What man signs on for that duty without blinking an eye?)

It worked out great and I was granted special permission from the dean to carry 24 semester hours during the summer session. I received excellent grades and was on the Dean's List. I worked as hard as I could and it paid off. I graduated early and was hired into that one desired position before the ink was dry on my diploma! One year later, I was named the Master of Arts Teaching Candidate of the Year in 2004-2005 by Coastal Carolina University within the Spadoni College of Education. My husband, five children, two of my sisters, and my mother were there to celebrate this honor with me. It was an outstanding way to begin my new career as an art educator. Receiving an award for academic excellence from the university was the highlight of my adult life. Finally—I was not less than and I was not a loser. It was unbelievable that the faculty selected me for this honor unanimously. I graduated with a 4.0 GPA.

Two years post-stroke, I started reading my art history texts. I comprehended very little in the beginning. Large chunks of information were missing in my comprehension. The remaining information was distorted because I had no point of reference. It was like picking strips of paper from a shredder and trying to make sense of a series of letters. I was demoralized when I first tried and put the books away for several hours. Then I would try again. Slowly but surely, I am getting better. In my estimation I was performing at a third-grade level. There were books that I wanted to read that were easier, but my vision was distorted and partially blocked. All of my art books were difficult to understand so I kept the easiest one on top of my desk and the hardest were in the bookcase. I finally found that *The Artists Magazine* was the easiest to comprehend. Gradually, I could use a dictionary. Later, I learned to use the Internet. I have a comprehensive list of art terms that is invaluable to me. Typically, I spend two to four hours each day studying and reading. I try to focus only on the information that is currently important to me. I no longer try to learn every detail. It is a slow process and I get discouraged and must remind myself that a few years ago I was partially blind, paralyzed, and aphasic. I have come a long way.

My wonderful son, Nathan, gave me a huge Mother's Day card. On the back of this large card I listed all of the important art terms that I had once recalled with ease. I still keep the list in my studio and refer to it constantly. I am adapting to my limitations—yet trying to break the sound barrier to maximize new capabilities. I will not settle for being less than I can possibly be.

Jeff is so much more resilient than I am. When I face a major problem that requires action, I fight to the death to make it work. When Jeff faces a similar problem, he analyzes, strategizes, and develops a new plan to get where he wants to go. He makes success look easy and I torture it to death! I have learned a great deal watching him and now have the ability to appreciate his talent and his depth of character.

In 2009, I was two years post stroke. Jeff was carrying the load of the entire family, except or the few things I could do to help in our home. My medical bills were devastating, coupled with my loss of income and loss of insurance coverage from my job. Jeff was faced with a huge financial burden. He also had a very sick wife who was uninsured and uninsurable! I know he must have had many sleepless nights but I never saw a chink in his armor.

As always, Jeff was formulating a new plan and looking for a new opportunity to provide for his family. He studied, researched, and analyzed the markets for business development. He found the right opportunity at the right time. He had always worked with his brain—insurance, stocks, and mortgage business. He found a business venture that excited him—working with his back instead of his brain. I had complete confidence in the man I married who had the Midas touch. He decided to start a paving business. He developed a business plan, found an investor, and at the end of his first year turned a very healthy profit. He made it look so easy; the business doubled annually for three consecutive years and thrives to this day.

The first years he worked side by side in the field with his crew. He came home smelling like oil and asphalt and he was hot, dirty, and tired. But he was smiling and happy with every shovel of gravel.

How does he do that? He does back-breaking work with shovels, jackhammers, and backhoes and drives three to four hours a day to different job sites! He gets new business and repeat business. He still comes home grinning like a Cheshire cat, so proud of himself. And at the end of every day, I am proud of him, too.

These reflections in this final chapter may be of little value to anyone except me and my closest family members. It was tremendously therapeutic for me to put the remote past into perspective. It was a cathartic process to review the content of my life from birth until the present day. I am humbled by what I learned about myself. Someone famous once said, "The unexamined life is not worth living." I have relived the "bad old days" and made peace with my past. I am anxiously awaiting knowledge of God's will for me for today and for the future. Every morning when I wake up—that is the first question I ask Him.

The End